Handbook of
Psychiatric
Diagnostic
Procedures

Handbook of Psychiatric Diagnostic Procedures

Vol. II

RICHARD C. W. HALL, M.D.
Medical Director, Psychiatric Programs
Florida Hospital, Orlando
Director of Research, Monarch Health Corp.
Clinical Professor of Psychiatry
University of Florida, Gainesville

THOMAS P. BERESFORD, M.D.
Chief, Psychiatric Service
Veterans Administration Medical Center
Associate Professor of Psychiatry
University of Tennessee Center for the Health Sciences
Memphis, Tennessee

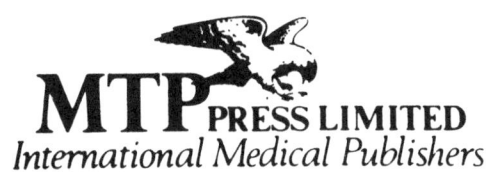
MTP PRESS LIMITED
International Medical Publishers

Published in the UK and Europe by
MTP Press Limited
Falcon House
Lancaster, England

Published in the US by
SPECTRUM PUBLICATIONS, INC.
175–20 Wexford Terrace
Jamaica, NY 11432

ISBN 978-94-011-6730-7   ISBN 978-94-011-6728-4 (eBook)
DOI 10.1007/978-94-011-6728-4

THIS BOOK IS DEDICATED TO:

Anne and Ryan

and

Carol, Eddie, Hal, and Charlie

Contributors

Suha A. Beller, M.D. Assistant Professor and Director of Clinical Services, Section on Geriatric Psychiatry, Department of Psychiatry and Behavioral Sciences, University of Texas Medical School at Houston, Houston, Texas

Thomas P. Beresford, M.D. Chief, Psychiatry Service, Veterans Administration Medical Center; Associate Professor of Psychiatry, University of Tennessee Center for the Health Sciences, Memphis, Tennessee

Fred S. Berlin, M.D., Ph.D. Assistant Professor of Psychiatry, Johns Hopkins University School of Medicine; Co-Director, Biosexual Psychohormonal Clinic, Baltimore, Maryland

Monte S. Buchsbaum, M.D. Professor of Psychiatry, Department of Psychiatry and International Institute on Brain Function and Behavioral Visual Imaging Center, University of California College of Medicine, Irvine, California

Todd W. Estroff, M.D. Assistant Director, Neuropsychiatric Unit, Fair Oaks Hospital, Summit, New Jersey

Michael Feinberg, M.D., Ph.D. Assistant Professor of Psychiatry, Mental Health Research Institute, University of Michigan, Ann Arbor, Michigan

Steven R. Gambert, M.D., F.A.C.P. Professor of Medicine; Director, Division of Gerontology and Geriatric Medicine, Department of Medicine; Director of Center for Aging and Adult Development, New York Medical College; Director of Genetics, Westchester County Medical Center, Valhalla, New York

Mark S. Gold, M.D. Director of Research, Fair Oaks Hospital, Summit, New Jersey

John F. Greden, M.D. Professor of Psychiatry, and Director, Clinical Studies Unit, Mental Health Research Institute, University of Michigan Hospital, Ann Arbor, Michigan

Richard C. W. Hall, M.D. Medical Director, Psychiatric Programs, Florida Hospital, Orlando; Clinical Professor of Psychiatry, University of Florida, Gainesville; Director of Research, Monarch Health Corporation, Marble Head, Massachusetts

Henry H. Holcomb, M.D. Staff Psychiatrist, Laboratory of Psychology and Psychopathology, Section on Clinical Brain Imaging, National Institute of Mental Health, Bethesda, Maryland

Ismet Karacan, M.D., (Med)D.Sc. Professor of Psychiatry and Director of Sleep Disorders and Research Center, Baylor College of Medicine; Associate Chief of Staff for Research and Development, Veterans Administration Medical Center, Houston, Texas

Alvin J. Levenson, M.D. Clinical Professor of Psychiatry, Baylor College of Medicine; Chief, Section on Geriatric Psychiatry, Department of Psychiatry and Behavioral Sciences, University of Texas Medical School at Houston, Houston, Texas

Dennis G. Low, M.D. Associate Chief, Primary Care, Department of Medicine, Santa Clara Valley Medical Center; Clinical Assistant Professor of Medicine, Stanford University School of Medicine, Palo Alto, California

Thomas B. Mackenzie, M.D. Associate Professor of Psychiatry and Medicine, University of Minnesota Medical School, Minneapolis, Minnesota

Michael K. Popkin, M.D. Professor of Psychiatry and Medicine, and Chief, Consultation/Liaison Section, University of Minnesota Medical School, Minneapolis, Minnesota

Maurice Rappaport, M.D., Ph.D. Academic Administrator, Langley-Porter Institute, University of California, San Francisco; Director, University of California Brain Function Study Unit, Research Department, Agnews State Hospital, San Jose, California

Bernard Saltzberg, Ph.D. Head, Information Analysis, Texas Research Institute of Mental Sciences, Texas Medical Center; Professor of Psychiatry, University of Texas Medical School at Houston; Adjunct Professor of Neurology, Baylor College of Medicine; Adjunct Professor, Biomedical Engineering, Rice University, Houston, Texas

Fredrick W. Schaerf, M.D., Ph.D. Department of Psychiatry and Behavioral Sciences, Johns Hopkins University School of Medicine, Baltimore, Maryland

Frederick A. Struve, Ph.D. Professor of Psychiatry and Behavioral Science, Eastern Virginia Medical School, Norfolk, Virginia; Hampton Veterans Administration Medical Center, Hampton, Virginia

William L. Webb, Jr., M.D. Vice-President and Medical Director, The Sheppard and Enoch Pratt Hospital, Baltimore (Towson), Maryland

Daniel R. Weinberger, M.D. Chief, Clinical Neuropsychiatry Section, and Staff Psychiatrist, Adult Psychiatry Branch, Intramural Research Program, National Institute of Mental Health, St. Elizabeth's Hospital, Washington, D.C.

Robert L. Williams, M.D. Chairman and Professor, Department of Psychiatry, Baylor College of Medicine, Houston, Texas

Thomas N. Wise, M.D. Chairman, Department of Psychiatry, Fairfax Hospital; Falls Church, Virginia; Professor of Psychiatry, Georgetown University Medical Center, Washington, D.C.; Professor of Psychiatry, Johns Hopkins University School of Medicine, Baltimore, Maryland

Preface

The first volume of this *Handbook* discussed neuroendocrine diagnostic tests and the diagnostic use of central nervous system amine metabolites. That volume further reviewed the toxicological evaluation of patients and the laboratory evaluation of treatment outcome. It suggested a system for evaluating newly admitted psychiatric patients and defined the scope of diagnostic procedures available in the emergency department. Volume II focuses on the use and interpretation of electrophysiologic and radiologic diagnostic tests in psychiatry and then explores the laboratory evaluation of special groups of patients.

The clinical sections of this volume are designed to assist the physician in instituting a proper workup for specific patients and defining tests which will assist them in the differential diagnosis of various psychiatric disorders. Such workups are critical to exclude possible organic disorders which can present with psychiatric symptoms.

The workup suggested for the various classes of patients will assist the clinician with differential diagnosis, provide base-line information for long-term follow-up, delineate biological perimeters at the beginning of treatment, protect the patient from unrecognized cardiac, renal, hepatic, or endocrine disorders which could be adversely affected by the administration of medications, and provide a rational sequencing of workup for particular disorders to insure the most thorough yet cost-efficient approach to the patient.

The final section of this volume deals with future directions in laboratory diagnosis in psychiatry. It is meant to stimulate the reader's interest and curiosity concerning techniques that will likely be available to him in the near future, if not currently.

It is hoped that these volumes will provide the practicing physician with a state-of-the-art and clinically useful approach to laboratory diagnosis in psychiatry.

RICHARD C. W. HALL, M.D.
THOMAS P. BERESFORD, M.D.

Contents

LABORATORY EVALUATION FOR SPECIAL
GROUPS OF PATIENTS

FUTURE DIRECTIONS

Electrophysiologic Diagnostic Tests

CHAPTER 1

Clinical Electroencephalography as an Assessment Method in Psychiatric Practice

FREDERICK A. STRUVE

In a historic sense, it is appropriate that a chapter on electroencephalography be included in a volume which concerns diagnostic procedures relevant to psychiatry. This is because Hans Berger, the clinician and scientist whose persevering and sharply focused brilliance led to the science of electroencephalography, was himself a psychiatrist. Perhaps because of this and because he had a profound interest in the relationships between physical and biological variables and psychiatric function, he was able to discern what many others had long failed to see. In their brief but informative history of the origins of electroencephalography [1] the Gibbs' note that despite the existence of continuing published animal studies of relevance, the possibility that shifting electrical potentials could originate from and be recorded from the human brain went unrecognized for more than 40 years. As early as 1875, Caton [2] was able to document the existence of electrical potentials derived from the cortical regions of rabbit and monkey brains and this was later followed by related reports by Beck [3,4] and von Marxow [5]. Numerous other animal studies of brain-derived potentials, which need not receive documentation here, continued to appear until Berger, following a series of his own animal experi-

Handbook of Psychiatric Diagnostic Procedures, vol. 2, edited by R. C. W. Hall. and T. P. Beresford. Copyright © 1985 by Spectrum Publications, Inc.

iments, began to publish his classic series of papers [6] on the human electroencephalogram (EEG) in 1929.

Of necessity early investigations by Berger and others focused on establishing the descriptive parameters of the recorded EEG. The range of observed EEG frequencies as well as wave form and morphological features and scalp distributions of various EEG findings had to be classified. Furthermore, the wide variety of subtle as well as dramatic normal alterations of the EEG related to diverse factors such as alertness, somnolence, external stimuli, changes in physiological substrate, chronological age differences and the like had to be documented if the procedure was to have relevance to health and disease. The fundamental aspects of normal EEG activity are now both well known and well summarized in standard electroencephalography texts [1,7-18] and need not be elaborated here.

It was not long before EEG became a tool for study and diagnoses of clinical dysfunction. However, the thrust of the new technique was not in psychiatry, the home of its founder, but rather in the fields of epilepsy and classical neurology. In 1935, soon after Fisher had established [19] that in animals drug-induced convulsions were associated with high voltage EEG changes, the human EEG was successfully used [20] in the study of clinical epilepsy in man. Not much later it was shown by Walter [21] that one could "localize" intracranial tumors by observing alterations of electrical activity recorded noninvasively from electrodes on the scalp. Other early clinical expansions of electroencephalographic application involved development of nasopharyngeal [22] and tympanic [23] electrodes for recording closer to inferior mesial and basal areas, direct exposed cortex recording as well as depth electrode study [24,25] for adjunctive use in neurosurgical procedures, and the emergence of photic and pharmacological techniques to "activate" latent dysrhythmic EEG changes.

Today we recognize clinical electroencephalography as a discipline widely accepted as a valid and useful method of assessing brain function in states of central nervous system (CNS) disease and in those organic impairments secondarily affecting the brain. Its importance in the study of epilepsy [13,14,26-27] and its value with structural brain lesions, tumors, vascular disorders of the brain, and head trauma is, of course widely appreciated [11-15,18,28]. Its usefulness in coma and determination of cerebral death receives continued publicity [29]. Perhaps less well recognized outside of electroencephalography is the method's contributory value in assessing degenerative disorders, infective and noninfective encephalopathies, toxic syndromes, and metabolic, endocrinological, and electrolytic imbalances as well as other areas [13-15,18,28,30-33]. The primary EEG discipline has also helped spawn closely related sister fields of considerable importance. Chief among these is its use in sleep research [34], a field which is producing results of relevance to psychiatry [35-38]. The field of computer-assisted quantitative analyses of EEG spectra [39-41] steadily assumes greater importance in psychopharmacology and the rational use of psychotropic agents. Certainly more esoteric is the recent parallel development of the magnetoencephalogram [42-44] which in many ways closely mimics EEG wave form but which may eventually be superior in specifying the intracranial three-dimensional localization of dysrhythmic events [45].

In order to appreciate the degree of diagnostic relevance of EEG to psychiatry —or for that matter to any category of clinical dysfunction—it is first essential to acquire a fundamental understanding of the limitations of EEG and its reliability as a measure as well as some genuine awareness of what is implied by the terms "normal" and "abnormal." Nothing can be more basic but yet so commonly neglected. For this reason these concerns are introduced at this juncture.

LIMITATIONS OF CLINICAL SCALP ELECTROENCEPHALOGRAPHY

Accessibility of Brain Area—The Constraint of Limited Coverage

Nature's undisputed wisdom in providing the human (and animal) brain with special protection against external traumatic insult has also rendered vast areas of brain tissue inaccessible to measurement by external scalp electroencephalography. Because of its confinement to external scalp electrode placement, EEG methodology is allowed a "reasonable" degree of recording from only approximately one-third of the outer convexity of the cerebral cortex—the so called "electroencephalographically accessible cortex" referred to by Gibbs [28] or the "outer cortical mantle" described by Glaser [46]. Sizable areas of cortical surface—especially mesial, inferior, and deep buried cortical tissue—as well as subcortical and cerebellar structures lie outside of the reach of nonsurgical clinical scalp EEG study. Clearly dysfunction in these inaccessible areas may be invisible and undetectable by current methods. Even over accessible cortical areas, the amplitude of recorded potentials will decrease with increasing distance from the exploring scalp electrode and minimal (that is, low amplitude) electrical dysregulation originating in areas between exploring scalp electrodes possibly could remain undetected. Use of special electrodes (that is, nasopharyngeal) and the observation that during sleep recording [28] some influences from subcortical structures may be visible at scalp tracings do little to lessen this constraint.

Electrical Impedance of Biological Structure—The Constraint of Sensitivity

When graphically recording potentials measured in microvolt units (one-millionth of a volt), substantial amplification is necessary. There are many biological structures that impose varying degrees of impedance between the source of electrical signals and detecting scalp electrodes and, although these are not completely understood in terms of all of the specifics of their effects [13], the attenuation of signals reaching the scalp is real. Not only do the skin, skull, and dura pose obstacles to recording EEG signals (potentials derived from the exposed cortex are considerably stronger than those taken from the scalp) but brain tissue itself has electrical impedance. As a consequence and depending upon the specific circumstance, scalp recorded activity is variable in the extent to which it reflects underlying electrical potential changes. It has been known for a considerable time that cortically and subcortically (depth electrode) recorded events–both pathological and normal wave forms–may at times be either absent from scalp EEG tracings or may appear on the scalp recording in a way that precludes specific identification of their locus of origin [47-55].

In many ways, clinical electroencephalography is similar to the exposed tip of the proverbial iceberg. Certainly an absence of pathological electrical activity at the scalp can never provide assurance that abnormal discharges are not occurring at a depth sufficient to preclude detection.

Frequency Response of the Electroencephalogram— The Constraint of Mechanical Limitation

In a clinical and pragmatic sense, various physical-mechanical limitations of the direct writing electroencephalograph preclude accurate registration of frequencies over 100 Hz. In actual clinical practice involving visual EEG analyses, the effective upper limit of useful frequency response is around 50 cycles per second. Virtually all of what we know of visually analyzed clinical diagnostic EEG concerns electrical activity within the narrow frequency range below that upper limit.

Various specialized recording techniques (that is, ink spray electroencephalography to avoid friction of capillary feed writing units, electrostatic recording with specially treated paper, cathode ray oscilloscope photographic techniques, transformation through variable speed tape recorders, and so forth) have suggested the existence of brain wave activity in frequency bands over 1,000 cycles per second [56-60]. Such high frequency potentials may contain within them patterned activity such as does the traditional clinical EEG spectra, however, the extreme chart paper speeds necessary for visual resolution of such activity, as well as other technical problems, have precluded determinations of standards of normality and criteria for abnormality. It is possible that with a normal standard EEG, pathological disturbances of high frequency spectra may exist in response to cerebral dysfunction yet remain undetected with standard clinical recording apparatus.

Infrequent Episodic Discharges—The Constraint of Time Sampling I

Some of the most important findings during the EEG examination occur only episodically or sporadically during the tracing [13,14,18,26,28]. That is, we have a situation in which the tracing is normal for a period of time and then this background activity is unexpectedly and suddenly interrupted by a relatively brief discharge of abnormal electrical activity following which the tracing returns to its previous background pattern. Abnormalities occurring in this fashion are generally referred to as "paroxysmal dysrhythmias." Depending upon the type encountered, they may be of serious clinical importance or they may be of relatively little clinical diagnostic value. Paroxysmal dysrhythmias may occur only once in a very long tracing or they may occur frequently—even as often as every few seconds.

The EEG recording must be sufficiently long in duration to provide a "fair chance" for paroxysmal activity to become manifest. However, the question of how long is long enough to avoid false negative recordings is always problematical and difficult to answer. Certainly very short EEGs of less than 30 minutes duration are undesirable and are to be avoided. Experience suggests that a minimum recording length of about one hour (which contains sleep) provides a "reasonable" assurance that pathological paroxysmal activity will be recorded. Longer recording times are often desirable. However, the salient point is that it remains possible that if extremely wide spaced and infrequent paroxysmal discharges exist they may be missed in even a very prolonged clinical recording. A long normal EEG can only suggest "presumptive evidence" that a scalp recordable paroxysmal dysrhythmia does not exist; it cannot be construed as positive evidence of absence of such activity.

Fluctuations in Substrate Physiology—The Constraint of Time Sampling II

To a considerable extent the stability of the EEG tracing is dependent upon the stability and homeostasis of cerebral physiology. Brain waves are particularly influenced by alterations in acid-base equilibrium, cerebral carbon dioxide tension, blood sugar level as well as a host of other physiological variables [13,14,28]. While I will not delineate them specifically at this point, there are a very large number of endocrinological disorders, metabolic dysfunctions, vitamin deficiencies, infectious states, and toxic conditions from either pharmacological or industrial substances which are capable of producing nonspecific abnormalities in the clinical EEG [13,14,28,30,32,33]. Even tobacco use—especially its onset or cessation—may produce slight yet visible alterations of EEG frequencies [61,62]. Most often the many variables mentioned above produce abnormalities in the frequency spectrum of the clinical EEG, however, paroxysmal activity and spike discharges are possible and have been reported.

When any of these factors produce clinical signs of cerebral dysfunction, the EEG is often abnormal. However, even with subclinical dysfunction in the absence of an obvious organic syndrome, EEG changes can occur—although not as frequently. To the extent that any disease process, dietary deficiency, or metabolic error produces a changing, irregular, or cyclic fluctuation in the cerebral physiological substrate—to that extent the EEG may be abnormal at one time and normal at another time with the result that a single EEG examination may fail to detect potential dysfunction.

Failure to Denote Etiology—The Constraint of Nonspecificity of Results

When a discrete EEG abnormality is recorded, it is, with only limited special exception, a "nonspecific" finding in that it does not denote specific underlying etiology [14,28,63]. Furthermore, an EEG abnormality is also "nonspecific" in that it is generally unable to delineate with precision expected discrete correlative symptoms. These limitations on clinical inference apply to those EEG irregularities which are grossly abnormal as well as those electrical dysregulations of more minor importance. We have a situation where a wide variety of pathophysiological disturbances of brain neuronal function are reflected in a much more limited or constricted repertoire of specifically expressed electrical aberrations detected at the scalp. For example, moderate generalized slowing in the EEG (that is, wake EEG frequencies considerably below the range of normal variation) may be caused by factors such as hypothyroidism, lithium toxicity, Wernicke's encephalopathy, hypopituitarism, recent head trauma or encephalitis, porphyria, and cortical atrophy and may occur concurrent with ECT or following idiopathic or iatrogenic seizures. Similarly a CVA, neoplasm, subdural hematoma, brain abscess, aneurysm, or head trauma as well as other dysfunctions can all yield similar types of focal slowing.

The fact that quite similar EEG changes can result from very dissimilar underlying pathophysiologies may be naggingly disconcerting to the psychiatrist. It should not be. Rather electroencephalography represents a methodology that is quite sensitive to cerebral electrical dysregulation and frequently this sensitivity provides clues to dysfunctions that can be clarified by continued careful clinical appraisal of the presenting symptomatology viewed against a comprehensive history and the results of additional tests which may be indicated.

In my judgment, clinical EEG can be of considerable value to psychiatry and it is probably underutilized in institutional and private psychiatric practice. However, the limitations of nonsurgical clinical scalp EEG are important and they are not set forth for mere academic interest. Because of these limitations, the normal EEG must at all times be regarded as a potential false negative and it should never be allowed to override good clinical examinational data suggesting physical dysfunction. It is clear that lesions can be missed by the technique and as Solomon has suggested [64], this is especially likely if the "lesion is deep, small, or old." It is also of value in this context to appreciate the extent to which various types of serious brain pathology may at times yield normal EEG tracings and for illustrative purposes a small selection is shown in Table 1. A normal EEG tracing awake and asleep and with activation procedures can never be construed as positive evidence of "no brain dysfunction" although it may make certain types of pathology (that is, cortical tumor) unlikely.

Table 1.　Incidence of Normal Electroencephalograms in Selected
Pathological Conditions Involving the Brain[a]

Condition	% Normal EEG	References
Intracranial neoplasm		
1.　Cortical	3–13	28, 65–67
2.　Deep	14–62	
Parkinson's disease	32.7	68
Progressive multifocal leukoencephalopathy	16.7	69
Hydrocephalus	7–38	28, 70
Seizure disorders (excluding petit-mal)	30–50[b]	64
Cerebrovascular occlusive disorders	41.3	71
Cerebral palsy	18–50[c]	28
Multiple sclerosis	57	28

[a]A nonexhaustive and limited listing for illustration purposes only. The point being made does not require a survey of additional relevant conditions nor an attempt to survey the work of large numbers of investigators.
[b]Interictal EEGs only. Percentages may vary widely between laboratories depending on factors such as recording length and use of sleep or other activating procedures.
[c]Depending upon the age of the subjects.

INTERPRETER RELIABILITY

It would seem evident that the reliability of clinical interpretation of the EEG constitutes an area of vital and fundamental importance to the diagnostic usefulness of this test. Therefore, it is most perplexing to find that although this notion may be universally accepted, interpreter reliability is almost never subject to formal study and assessment. With only one exception [14] major EEG reference works omit discussion of this topic. Interpretive reliability can be assessed by either contrasting the *independent* interpretations of the same EEGs by two or more electroencephalographers (inter-judge reliability) or by having one electroencephalographer reinterpret a number of EEGs after an elapsed time and without knowledge of his earlier impressions (intra-judge reliability). Both methods are suitable and should be encouraged as self-monitoring assessments in all laboratories. Clearly, if two readers disagree sharply on the interpretations of EEG tracings or if one interpreter is frequently inconsistent with himself over time, then the test can have no ultimate validity.

Formal studies of the reliability of clinical interpretation of the EEG are remarkably few in number [72–82]. Regrettably, some of them fail to demonstrate significant levels of reliability using either the inter-judge [72,77,78] or intra-judge [76] format. A close reading of some of these studies suggests that lack of

Table 2. Summary of Studies Reporting Statistically Significant Levels of Inter-Judge or Intra-Judge Reliability of Clinical EEG Interpretation

Study	Study type	Number of interpreters	Number of EEGs	Percent agreement in interpretation	Statistical significance
Houfex & Ellingson [73]	Inter-Judge	2	140	(1) 85.7% Overall (2) 91.5% Omitting clinically minor disagreement	$\chi^2 = 71.5$, dif. = 1 p < .001
Walker & Jablon [74]	Inter-Judge	2	140	74.3%	$\chi 2 = 22.85$, dif. = 1 p < .001
Little & Raffel [75]	Intra-Judge	1	100	(Not stated)	rho = 0.73, t = 1 p < .001
Wayne et al. [83]	Inter-Judge	2	51	(Not stated)	r = 0.87
Rose et al. [80]	Inter-Judge	2	200	88%	$\chi^2 = 52.73$, dif. = 1 p < .001
Struve et al. [81] Sample 1	Inter-Judge	2	118	(1) 92% Overall (2) 98.3% Omitting clinically minor disagreement	kappa = 0.86 ± 0.08 z = 10.47, p < .001

			Total EEGs	Agreement	Statistical tests
Sample 2	Inter-Judge	2	458	(1) 94.5% Overall (2) 96.6% Omitting clinically minor disagreement	Statistical tests were not done[a]
Sample 3	Inter-Judge	2	225	92%	kappa = 0.854 ± 0.06, z = 14.14, p < .001
Sample 4	Inter-Judge	2	286	88.1%	kappa = 0.7798, z = 14.29, p < .001
Small et al. [82] (1)	Intra-Judge	1	>147	96%	Statistical tests were not done[a]
(2)	Inter-Judge	2	Majority of sample (1) above	80%	Statistical tests were not done[a]
All inter-judge samples combined [73,74,80,81]			Total EEGs 1,567	Agreement—91% (weighted average) Omitting minor disagreements	

[a]Although statistical tests were not reported, the magnitude of agreement shown would suggest that appropriate contingency analyses would have yielded significant results. The findings are included for this reason.

interpretive skill may in part contribute to the negative results—as, for example, when inability to reclassify tracings the same way regarding the presence or absence of sleep and other variables are reported [76]. However, several other investigations [73-75,80-82] using large sample sizes have shown statistically that highly significant levels of interpreter reliability can be achieved in assessing clinical material. Table 2 summarizes these latter studies (which combined involve ten discrete reliability assessment samples) and shows inter-interpreter agreements ranging from 74.3% to 98.3% with an overall 91% weighted average for interpreter agreement calculated for the combined sample of 1,567 cointerpreted EEGs (author's calculations). Table 2 also shows that minor or irrelevant disagreements (that is, such as borderline slow versus normal [81]) occur which reduce agreement. Such small discrepancies, which are estimated from the Table to occur in 2% to 6% of the tracings, have no real clinical import or relevance and do not impair diagnostic value.

One source of unreliable EEG evaluations suggested above was simple lack of interpreter skill. The prevalence of this problem has not been ascertained although it must play at least a small part in the dissatisfaction some psychiatrists and others may have for the value of EEG findings. Recently, Hooshmand [84] reviewed a sample of 96 electroencephalograms and their reports (secured from 41 different electroencephalographers) for patients referred to a seizure control clinic. He concluded that 17.7% of the EEGs were overinterpreted and that 7.2% were so poorly taken that an interpretation could not be made. Sources of interpretive error in the original reports involved a variety of gross recording artifacts (that is, pulse artifact, loose electrode, eye movements, and so forth) being interpreted as abnormal potentials of brain origin. In instances such as these the clinical validity of reported results is absent. A second source of inter-interpreter disagreement may occur among highly skilled and experienced electroencephalographers who clearly are able to "see the same phenomena" in the electroencephalogram but who may place different clinical emphasis on various discrete findings or who use differing qualitative "cut off points" in classifying subtle variations as significant or not. Such disagreements are not over the contents of the tracing but instead on the meanings attributed to the observed patterns. It is important to stress that differences among skilled interpreters will rarely involve classification of major electroencephalographic abnormality but instead will be confined to findings considered controversial or of minor importance. The nonelectroencephalographer should also appreciate that the demarcation between normal and abnormal—especially regarding frequency and asymmetry judgments—is not always crisp and sharp but involves a transitional grey area within which interpretive differences may exist without significant clinical consequence.

A subsidiary reliability issue is the degree of test-retest reliability of EEG findings from each patient across occasions. Small and associates were the first to suggest the importance of determining the "consistency" of EEG findings over time and they report measures of this variable for several minor EEG dysrhythmias which frequently occur among psychiatric patient samples [85-87]. Although others [88] have also reported significant test-retest EEG associations for EEG findings obtained from psychiatric patients, the issue has not continued to receive attention in the literature.

NORMAL VERSUS ABNORMAL: THE MISLEADING DICHOTOMY

There are two closely related areas of conceptual confusion, which still continue to impede optimal acceptance of clinical electroencephalography as diagnostically useful in psychiatry. One of these is the simplistic but erroneous notion that a dichtomous normal-abnormal classification of EEG findings in an of itself contains clinical relevance. The second involves serious conceptual errors that emerge when such a dichotomization is uncritically applied to findings derived from normal populations.

Psychiatric practitioners not infrequently ask if their patient's EEG is "abnormal" and, if the answer is yes, they may be enthusiastic or less so depending upon their "a priori" expectations. Should they wish to conduct a study of a defined clinical population they may ask what proportion the EEG consultant thinks may have "abnormal" tracings. Certainly, questions of what percentage of schizoaffective disorders, character disorders, dysthymic conditions, hyperactive children, alcoholics and so forth display "abnormal EEGs" seem truly ubiquitous in professional dialogue and in print. The apparent permanence of such questions notwithstanding, the term abnormal EEG is, by itself, clinically quite ambiguous. It is essential to realize that there are a great many different ways in which an EEG can be abnormal and this fact frequently is totally obscured by our tendency to think and reason in dichotomous terms. A few EEG patterns are considered abnormal by some investigators but normal by others simply because the body of empirical research is conflicting and the findings subject to still unresolved controversy. Other EEG findings may be statistically unusual and even accepted as abnormal but their clinical correlates are slight and they may occur in the EEG's of some persons free of major complaint. Should a psychiatrist receive "abnormal EEG" reports—without explanatory clarification—involving findings with limited clinical expressivity or treatment relevance, he or she may well question how meaningful an "abnormal EEG" really is. However, the majority of discrete EEG abnormalities are confined to clinical populations and many of them are associated with diagnostic possibilities of grave seriousness. Depending on how one views classification, there are probably more than 30 or 40 discrete and separate EEG abnormalities that stand in contrast to the normal tracing and their meanings may differ considerably in terms of clinical expressivity and potential diagnostic or pathophysiological correlates. For purpose of heuristic illustration I have arbitrarily abstracted only 11 of the many separate and distinct EEG patterns

Table 3. Prevalence of Selected EEG Patterns Among Normal Control Subjects.[a]

EEG pattern	Comments	Normal control subjects (see text)		
		Age	Sample size	Prevalence
14 and 6/sec. positive spikes	Mild abnormality. Controversial. Many consider a normal variant	15–19	1,361	17.3%
Generalized slightly slow (S-1) awake	Mild abnormality. What some call "slight excess of theta activity"	Adults	1,000	7.6%
Slightly abnormal fast (F-1)	Mild abnormality	Adults	1,000	6.2%
Small sharp spikes	Mild abnormality. Controversial. Some consider a normal variant	25–29	360	5.5%
Generalized very slow (S-2) awake	Moderately abnormal. Continuous 5-7/sec. activity mixed with 3-4/sec waves	Adults	1,000	0.7%
Generalized exceedingly slow (S-3) awake	Very abnormal. Essentially diffuse delta activity	10–60	1,288	0.0%
Hypsarhythmia	Very abnormal	0–9	2,188	0.0%
Petit-mal discharges	Diffuse 3-4/sec. Spike and wave	0–60	3,476	0.0%
Anterior temporal spike focus	Negative or biphasic spike or spike-wave. "Sharp wave discharges" not included	10–60	1,288	0.0%
Hemisphere spikes	Negative or biphasic spike or spike-wave over one hemisphere	0–60	3,476	0.0%
Focal moderate slow (S-2 focus) to focal very slow (delta focus)	Moderate to severe abnormality	10–60	1,288	0.0%

[a]Data abstracted from Gibbs and Gibbs [1,28]. Sample sizes vary because author selected age ranges where peak prevalence (if any) occurred.

listed in Volumes 1 and 3 of the Gibbs' atlas series [1,28] and in Table 3 the prevalence of each finding among their normal control subjects is shown. For controversial findings and more minor clinical abnormalities prevalence rates range from 5% to 17% among normal subjects. However, as more serious abnormalities are listed, confinement to clinical populations becomes complete and the search for etiologically relevant pathophysiological dysfunction more urgent.

When a report of EEG abnormality is received, the cavalier statement that 10%, 15%, or 20% of the normal population have "abnormal EEGs" is often invoked in an effort to diminish whatever value the EEG observations in question may have had. This high prevalence—usually 10% to 15%—of abnormal EEGs among normal subjects has been commented on frequently [64,89-94] in works related to the use of EEG in psychiatry and as a result has now become a common, albeit misunderstood, mainstay of the clinical folklore. Again, however, EEG findings are not dichotomous and one must specify which distinct EEG abnormality one is talking about when the question of normal population prevalence is raised.

In Table 4 (adults) and Table 5 (children) the prevalence of EEG abnormality "in general" among normal control populations as reported by various investigators is displayed. Within each table, studies are combined to yield a weighted average prevalence figure of 17.8% for adults and 12.9% for children and both estimates are in accord with the common notion that abnormal EEGs occur in about 15% of the normal population. Using these same tables, whenever possible I remove all controversial abnormalities (that is, 14 and 6 positive spikes, 6/sec. spike and wave, small sharp spikes and so forth) as well as minor or borderline abnormalities (that is, sporadic theta, minimal generalized slow or fast activity and so forth) in order to generate a grouping of abnormalities that would consensually be considered of moderate to serious importance. These tables clearly indicate that the prevalence of at least moderate EEG abnormality among normal controls is vastly lower than figures for overall abnormality and in many sutdies the decrease in prevalence rates caused by omitting controversial or minor findings is striking. As the combined study weighted average estimates in Tables 4 and 5 suggest—and contrary to common opinion—EEG abnormalities of at least moderate importance occur in less than 4% of normal subjects. Among psychiatrists, interest in paroxysmal EEG dysrhythmias has often been high, apparently because of the potential association between such abnormalities and seizure manifestations or so called behavioral "seizure equivalents." In Table 6, several studies that focus on the prevalence of accepted paroxysmal abnormalities within normal control subjects are summarized. Prevalence rates ranging from zero to 5.6% are reported and the weighted average prevalence rate for all studies combined is only 1.14% for a combined total sample of 11,560 child and adult normal controls. In constructing Table 6, all controversial paroxysmal EEG findings (that is, 14 and 6 positive spikes, small sharp spikes, 6/sec. spike and wave and so forth) as well as photically

Table 4. Prevalence of (I) All EEG Abnormality (including borderline) and
(II) Moderate to Serious EEG Abnormality only Among Adult Normal
Control Subjects[a]

Study	Reference	Sample size	I. All EEG abnormalities	II. Moderate to serious abnormality only[b]
Williams	95	221	7.7%	Cannot determine[c]
Finley & Campbell	96	250	29%	7%
Silverman	97	60	15%	5%
Rossen & Gordon	98	200	16%	6%
Cohn	7	251	14.4%	6.7%
Gibbs & Gibbs	1	1,000	15.8%	2%
Hill	99	147	20%	4.8%
Buchthal & Lennox	100	682	15.1%	5.2%
Moore et al.	101	120	12.5%	Cannot determine[c]
Chamberlain & Russell	130	43	11.5%	0%
Rodin	131	40	57.5%	2.5%
Kitamura & Asakura	103	229	4.3%	Cannot determine[c]
Blanc et al.	102	2,000	20.5%	2.5%
O'Connor	104	500	10%	3.6%
Romain	105	9	11%	0%
Pacheco e Silva	106	1,000	23.4%	1.7%
Total N (all studies) = 6752, Abnormal = 17.8% (weighted average)				Total N = 6182, Abnormal = 3.2% (weighted average)

[a]Calculations of weighted averages for combined studies made by author.
[b]See text for explanation.
[c]Cannot determine from primary source.

induced paroxysmal changes were omitted. Stevens [132] has commented on
the high prevalence of a positive photoconvulsive EEG response to stroboscopic
flash in nonepileptic subjects—especially adolescent females—and she lists several
documentary references to this important observation.

Normal Control Group Definition

In Tables 3-6, I tried to illustrate that the oft quoted high prevalence of abnormal EEGs among normal people undergoes striking shrinkage when minor,
borderline, or controversial "abnormalities" are omitted from consideration.

Table 5.   Prevalence of (I) all EEG Abnormality (including borderline) and
(II) Moderate to Serious EEG Abnormality Among Normal Children
Control Subjects[a]

Study	Reference	Sample size	I. All EEG abnormalities	II. Moderate to serious abnormality only[b]
Secunda & Finley	107	76	15%	Cannot determine[c]
Henry	108	583	11.9%	5%
Gottlieb et al.	109	270	15%	Cannot determine[c]
Kennard & Willner	110	102	7%	Cannot determine[c]
Miller & Lennox	111	373	10.4%	1.7%
Herrlin	124	70	28.6%	0%
Brandt & Brandt	112	135	3%	3%
White et al.	114	13	0%	0%
Hutt et al.	115	60	0%	0%
Whitehouse et al.	116	28	50%	7.1%
Small	117	25	0%	0%
Stevens et al.	118	57	Approx. 29%[e]	9%
Capute et al.	119	33	15%	3%
Gubbay et al.	120	23	21.7%	0%
Small	121	34	14.7%	5.8%
Small et al.	122	16	43.8%	12.5%
Total N (all studies) = 1898, Abnormal = 12.9% (weighted average)				Total N = 1450, Abnormal = 3.5% (weighted average)

[a]See text for explanation.
[b]Cannot determine from primary source.
[c]Primary source not obtained, cannot determine from secondary source.
[e]Two control groups reported paper. Figure for all EEG abnormality (29%) is given for "control groups" and it is not clear what the percentage would be for their more stringent control sample. The 9% listing for moderate EEG abnormality is based on their stringent control group.

In fact, with several serious EEG abnormalities the incidence in normals will drop to zero. Unstated above is the important fact that normal control groups vary quite markedly in the rigor with which they were selected and as a result several such groups probably contain unknown proportions of subjects with either current symptomatic behavior or historical record of relevant cerebral insult. Over thirty years ago, Williams [95] observed that the amount of EEG abnormality among normal controls decreased very substantially as control subjects were required to pass increasingly stringent screening procedures to rule out current and past

Table 6. Prevalence of Accepted Paroxysmal Patterns Among Normal Control Subjects[a]

Study	Reference	Sample size	Age	Paroxysmal patterns[b]
Thorner	123	1,000	Adult	0.3%
Rossen & Gordon	98	200	Adult	0%
Gibbs & Gibbs	1	1,000	Adult	0.9%
Hill	99	147	Adult	4.1%
Buchthal & Lennox	100	682	Adult	2.6%
Miller & Lennox	111	373	Children	0.3%
Herrlin	124	70	Children	0%
Corbin & Bickford	125	71	Children	5.6%
Brandt & Brandt	112	135	Children	0.7%
Blanc et al.	102	2,000	Adult	1%
O'Connor	104	500	Adult	3.6%
Gibbs & Gibbs	28	2,572[c]	Children	1%
Hutt et al.	115	60	Children	0%
Maulsby et al.	126	200	Adult	0%
Bennett	127	1,332	Adult	0.4%
Doose et al.	128	118	Children	0.8%
Stevens et al.	118	57	Children	≈2%[d]
Eeg-Olofsson et al.	129	743	Children	2.6%[e]
O'Connor	133	300	Adult	0.3%

Total sample size (all studies) = 11,560
Prevalence (weighted average) Paroxysmal Patterns = 1.14%

[a]Weighted average for all studies combined calculated by author.
[b]See text for explanation.
[c]Children are defined by present author as ages 0 to 14.
[d]This figure is estimated from printed histogram data.
[e]The original authors list far higher figures for paroxysmal findings. The present author has omitted findings possibly controversial, those of unclear clinical expressivity (that is, diffuse bilateral synchronous paroxysmal activity during drowsiness and light-sleep—referred to as "pseudo petit mal" in the Gibbs' Atlas [28], and photically induced changes. These authors present a landmark series of important papers and the informed reader will want to review their primary work in detail.

psychiatric, medical, and cerebral dysfunction. Later Stevens and associates [118] reported that moving from less stringent to more stringent criteria for screening behavior problems out of their control group resulted in a decrease in the prevalence of moderate to severe EEG abnormality of from 19% to 9%.

On the infrequent occasions in which seemingly normal control populations have been examined more closely, meaningful amounts of relevant medical, neurological, convulsive, or neuropsychiatric history or current symptoms have been found. Prevalence figures for such findings among normal controls have ranged from 3.4% of 174 "active and nonhospitalized" adults studied by Kooi [134] through 5% [106] and 9.8% [100] of large samples of airmen to 22.8% of a sample of 259 naval controls in good physical health at the time of the EEG [95]. Thus, one sees that it is always possible that some moderate EEG abnormalities among "normal subjects" may occur in patients who under closer scrutiny may be symptomatic or have a prior relevant medical condition or event. In his excellent review of paroxysmal EEG patterns in "normal" subjects, Chatrian [136] takes a forceful stance on this issue and writes that ". . . even control populations selected on the basis of stringent criteria of normality may include a small proportion of concealed and/or clinically inapparent disturbances of brain function capable of giving rise to deviant EEG findings of a paroxysmal nature."

In light of such findings, how well selected are the normal control groups used in assessing EEG findings? In a few studies, "control groups" are not normal at all and instead should be viewed as comparison groups of one sort or another. This is especially true when experimental patients are severely disturbed children inpatients and "control subjects" are outpatients with more minor problems [113] or when, in a Metrazol activation study [135] "control subjects" consist of those patients referred for EEG study who were nonepileptic. Some studies list their control group as "volunteers," either paid [131] or unpaid [97] or simply refer to them as "unscreened controls." [109,111] A common practice is to accept subjects as normal control individuals if they are in apparent good health at the time of testing [98,104,107,130] or as the Gibbs' state [28] ". . . without significant diseases, constituting a representative sample of the general normal population." This may seem inherently sensible but in my judgment a weakly screened representative normal population containing an unknown proportion of undetected disease cannot provide a critical test of the control incidence of EEG signals presumed or suspected to be of pathologic significance. Related to the above and suffering from the same drawbacks are "normal" control groups selected from patients hospitalized for conditions (that is, tonsillectomy, orthopedic surgery, and so forth) judged to be unrelated to brain function [114,116,124]. Air Force pilots, due to the nature of their training and duty, are often reasonably well screened medically [95,104,105] as are some civilian samples [125]. In their classic series of studies, Peterson and Eeg-Olofsson and associates [129,137-139] have given careful attention to the selection of normal subjects and one wishes that all control studies had embraced their philosophy.

Additional Considerations

Space does not permit critique of methodological and technical parameters of all control group studies. However, there are factors operating in many studies which could lead to false negative EEGs with the consequence that prevalence figures for some EEG findings might best be viewed as lower limit estimates. Small and associates [82,122] as well as Stevens [118] have commented on the importance of "blind" EEG interpretation in normal control studies if bias toward underinterpretation is to be reduced. Small and associates [82,121,122] also stress the importance of including drowsy and sleep activation (to be discussed later) as well as serial EEG study [121] in order to maximize the chance of detecting positive EEG findings. Unfortunately, many studies of EEG findings among normal control populations do not address these concerns.

PRAGMATIC USE OF CLINICAL ENCEPHALOGRAPHY IN PSYCHIATRY

Historically, clinical EEG took two main paths or roads into the realm of psychiatry. One of these involved an energetic search for discrete EEG patterns that could be tied closely to various psychiatric syndromes and hopefully used to strengthen diagnostic precision. Unfortunately, this strategy eventually ended in a blind cul-de-sac and the resulting frustration contributed to the disenchantment with EEG as a useful tool in psychiatry. Although considerably elevated prevalences of EEG abnormality do occur in most psychiatric nosological groupings (as opposed to normal groups), the EEG abnormalities are widely heterogeneous and as Ellingson noted more than 25 years ago [94] discrete EEG findings that are pathonomonic for specific psychiatric disorders have not been found [11,13,64,140-143]. Clinical EEG's second path into psychiatry—and the one still traveled today—involved its value as a laboratory procedure in assessing those functional psychiatric patients suspected of potential organic brain disorder. All too frequently this has been narrowly construed as evaluating brain tumor or seizure disorder suspects when in actuality the sensitivity of the test allows a far wider range of usefulness.

Clinical EEG can be valuable to the psychiatric practitioner either as a routine screening assessment or it can be used selectively for those patients where a high index of suspicion of cerebral dysfunction exists. The following discussion will consider those EEG applications more familiar to the psychiatrist as well as those uses of EEG that are less traditional and less well recognized.

Brain Neoplasm and Brain Abscess

Brain neoplasm and abscess are usually not discussed together. However, although infectious and inflammatory, an abscess is localized and exhibits some EEG characteristics of an expanding lesion. Early classic studies [144-146] have shown that psychiatric symptoms are not uncommon with brain tumor and in the early series of cases described by Soniat [147] over half of the tumor patients had seemingly functional symptomatology which, when present, operated to obscure correct diagnosis. That it is possible that an initial diagnosis of functional psychiatric disorder has been maintained until later progressive developments have revealed the presence of a temporal lobe lesion or cortical neoplasm has been stressed by numerous investigators [148-152]. My laboratory has provided [153,154] EEG evidence for the initial detection of brain tumors with clinical-psychiatric presentations as diverse as rapid onset (that is, not insidious) juvenile delinquency, seemingly functional anorexia, toxic psychosis, schizophrenia and the like although cerebral tumors were very uncommon in our population.

The brain tumor itself is electrically silent and the electrical dysregulation seen in the EEG stems from the tumor's impact on surrounding neural tissue. The characteristic EEG finding in cases of brain tumor is focal slowing [7-9,11-15,18,28] although this may take a variety of forms and certainly is not always present. EEG is most often contributory in supratentorial lesions where estimates of correct lateralization and localization of hemispheric tumors may reach 90% [13,18,28,155]. Often the focal slowing will contain delta (0.5-3 Hz) or delta-theta activity which is more or less continuous but which varies considerably or is mixed in wave form (that is, polymorphic delta activity) and is poorly reactive to stimuli. Less frequently paroxysmal focal spike activity may appear as well [156] even without seizure onset being part of the clinical presentation. Delta activity can also occur episodically (not continuous in the tracing) in more even rhythmic bursts, which are usually high voltage (intermittent rhythmic delta activity) maximal over either anterior or posterior areas. When laterally accentuated, it may suggest the hemisphere of lesion and when bilaterally equal and synchronous may suggest infratentorial involvement. Localized voltage reductions and distortions of expected normal wave forms (that is, sleep spindles) are less common but may be seen.

Infratentorial lesions and deep tumors of the basal ganglia are less well detected by the EEG although a variety of nonspecific electrical dysregulations may occur. By one estimate [155] about one-third of the EEGs are normal in cases of infratentorial tumors as opposed to less than 5% incidence of normal tracings with hemispheric neoplasms. Gibbs [28] has reported a 14% to 57% incidence of normal EEGs with subcortical tumors depending upon location, which contrasts with only a 4% normal EEG incidence for cortical tumors. He also suggests that a variety of disordered sleep EEG patterns may occur in deep tumors but such changes are not specifically diagnostic.

Lateralized focal delta activity or episodic bilateral high voltage Delta with or without other electrical aberration represent serious pathological findings although diagnosis of tumor is not made with the EEG alone. Indeed, Kooi [13] has cautioned that "... there are no electrographic signs by which the diagnosis of brain tumor can be made with certainty."

Subdural and Epidural Hematoma

Ever since the early reports by Walter [157] and Jasper [158] of electroencephalographic "silent areas" overlying extradural or subdural hematoma, EEG has been
used in assessing this pathology. It is unlikely that the psychiatric practitioner will
ever be directly involved in the immediate medical issues raised by a suspected
acute hematoma developing after injury. However, he may encounter a patient
who, following a posttraumatic "silent period" of days or weeks begins to develop
symptoms (which may be psychiatric or behavioral in nature) suggesting further
evaluation for a possible subdural collection. The original trauma may not even be
recalled and focal signs may not always occur but unexplained hyperirritability,
dysphoria, memory difficulty, confusion, which may fluctuate widely in severity,
possibly developing headaches, and so forth may emerge. Patients at most risk are
those prone to head injury such as the senile elderly, the alcoholic, or those in risk
sports or activities.

In a large review, Friedlander [159] concluded that EEG findings usually consisting of lateralized or focal slow activity with or without amplitude asymmetries
(localized voltage reductions) aided localization efforts in 85% of hematoma cases.
My own review suggests that positive findings may occur more often in acute than
chronic cases. Again, EEG findings alone are not specifically diagnostic and as with
neoplasms patients with a high index of suspicion are nowadays often referred directly to the newer computerized scanning procedures if they are readily available.

Other Vascular Disorders

Vascular lesions of the cerebral hemispheres produce lateralized or focal delta
activity when significant cerebral infarction occurs [13,14,28,64] and these EEG
changes may partially resolve or even normalize with time and recovery. However,
of more relevance to the psychiatrist are those behavioral alterations produced by
minor transient ischemic attacks which may mimic functional disturbance. A wide
variety of cognitive (that is, memory, concentration, confusion, and so forth),
mood (dysphoria, excitement, hyperirritability), thought content (suspiciousness,
delusional ideation) and other behavioral symptoms may occur which vary in
abundance and degree with the severity and locational distribution of the underlying pathophysiological changes occurring. Symptom onset may be abrupt and
seemingly inexplicable or insidiously deteriorating. Kolb and Brodie [93] strongly
state that cerebral arteriosclerosis with multiinfarct dementia should be considered
when characterological changes occur in any person beyond age 50. When major
cerebral infarcts are omitted, less pronounced ischemic changes produce only relatively slight changes in the EEG and not infrequently the EEG may be normal.
With pronounced mental status changes (that is, confusion and so forth), positive
EEG tracings are more likely. EEG alterations which may occur include generalized

slowing or slowing seen sporadically in temporal regions with the frequencies usually in the theta (4–7 Hz) range. When present, EEG changes will confirm cerebral organic involvement but will not in and of themselves denote the vascular (or other) basis underlying the EEG change. It must be cautioned that some slowing of alpha activity and increase in theta activity—especially in temporal regions—is an expected concomitant of the normal aging process.

Dementia and Atrophic Changes

The incipient onset of dementia may involve symptomatology which coincides with that of nonorganic psychiatric disturbance. While the distinction is clarified by longitudinal clinical course, early diagnosis may be problematic. In some types of dementia, EEG study may be of initial help in suggesting organic involvement whereas with others its usefulness is more limited. Early signs of progressive dementia [63,93,160] may involve a variety of personality changes along with a decreasing range of interests, increased apathy, and a blunting of emotional nuance eventually leading to flat, nonspontaneous affect. Irritability and even overt angry outbursts may occur as well as depression. Progressive cognitive loss involves functions of memory, concentration, alertness, and attention span and subsequently confusion and impairments of orientation occur. Serial neuropsychological assessments may help to document the early insidious intellectual deterioration.

The EEG findings [13,14,18,28] will vary depending upon the type of dementia under consideration. With Alzheimer's dementia, the EEG is almost always abnormal and in the early stages of the disease a reduction in the amount of alpha activity present along with a slowing of alpha frequency is seen. Later changes include generalized theta activity, which may shift in lateral emphasis along with periods of delta activity superimposed on the background patterns. If advanced disease patients are tested, interhemispheric synchronization of brain-wave activity may begin to break down. Huntington's chorea is another progressive dementia that has a high incidence of abnormal EEGs. In this disease, the EEG alpha activity may be absent and the tracing may be characterized by extremely low voltage activity with some beta frequencies and occasionally random slow waves dispersed throughout the record. Early unexplained personality and cognitive changes combined with a positive genetic history and this type of EEG suggest that a diagnosis of Huntington's chorea may be upheld. Jacob-Creutzfeldt disease, caused by a slow virus, is a third condition with characteristic EEG features. As this disease progresses, generalized slow-wave activity appears and later distinctive generalized polyphasic sharp waves, usually high voltage, which are repetitive at a frequency of about 1 to 2 Hz, appear. We recorded the EEG of a psychiatric admission and obtained only diffuse high-voltage theta activity mixed with some delta waves. However, mental deterioration (along with our EEG report) prompted admission to medical services where another EEG secured two weeks later contained the high voltage 1 to 2/sec. repeating sharp waves typical of this condition. In distinction to the above types of dementia, Pick's disease often yields a normal EEG and when abnormal changes are seen they are nondescript involving less alpha activity with an increase in theta activity. This is also true of simple senile dementias of unknown classification. In our experience patients with CAT scan evidence of significant cortical atrophy usually have EEGs containing abnormal generalized slowing.

Seizure Disorders

There is little doubt that assessment of the suspected seizure patient remains as one of the major recognized uses of clinical EEG in general. It also may represent the primary reason psychiatrists refer patients to the clinical EEG laboratory.

It is not possible to include an extensive discussion of the wide variety of clinical seizure manifestations along with their expected ictal and interictal electroencephalographic correlates; fortunately such material is well covered elsewhere [13,14,18,26-28]. Furthermore, given the purpose of this volume it would serve no purpose to do so. The psychiatrist is not the primary treating practitioner involved in known cases of petit mal, myoclonic, grand mal, akinetic, Jacksonian, and focal seizures and the like, although he or she may manage psychiatric aspects of seizure cases. Rather EEG is useful psychiatrically in establishing a suspected seizure diagnosis at the onset or during the course of psychiatric treatment, in helping to separate out "hysterical" seizures, in identifying behavioral phenomena, which may be based on seizure activity or constitute interictal behavioral aberrations, and in identifying those acute prolonged confusional episodes representing certain types of seizure status.

The EEG in suspected grand mal, myoclonic, and akinetic seizures is not always abnormal but if sleep recordings as well as other activation techniques are included, high incidences of the relevant spike, spike-wave complexes, or other paroxysmal findings of diagnostic importance may be seen. When the first EEG is normal, serial recordings may be useful as well as recordings following 24 hours of sleep deprivation. We have found unequivocal seizure confirmation (EEG changes linked with clinical manifestations) only after as many as five normal tracings and this was fortunate because a diagnosis of hysterical seizures was strongly considered by treating staff. When petit mal absence attacks are suspected when treating the child (or less often the adult), the EEG is a very reliable (about 90% to 95%) confirmatory test and, if this disorder is present, the classic diagnostic diffuse 3/sec. spike-wave pattern is invariably recorded if the tracing is long and is sure to contain vigorous hyperventilation [26]. Patients with hysterical seizures will have normal EEGs, however, EEG normality does not confirm this because up to 50% of grand mal epileptics may also display normal EEG tracings in the interictal period. Often, If EEG's are secured with comments about the recordings normality made within ear shot of the patient, the subject may simply provide a "seizure" during the test and the EEG may reveal it as not genuine.

Infrequently, patients may enter an emergency psychiatric service in various states of mild to moderate confusion, bizarre behavior, disorientation, and being minimally responsive often speaking in monosyllables. An EEG at that time may reveal continuous 2 to 3/sec. spike-wave activity of petit mal status [161-163] or even psychomotor variant status [164], which would rule out functional disturbance or transient toxic disorder. Such "status behaviors" have been viewed as psychotic at times [165-166].

For the psychiatrist the concepts of complex partial seizures, temporal lobe or psychomotor seizures, temporolimbic seizures, and similar nosological coinages are of considerable importance. Seizure discharges originating in portions of the temporal lobe, orbital frontal cortex, and limbic structures may involve—in addition to the more obvious automatisms—a broad variety of psychic, autonomic, and behavioral features that could be mistaken for functional symptomatology. Such wide and diverse symptom manifestations are too numerous to detail here but they have been superbly summarized by Jovanovic [167] as well as many others. Less well appreciated are the variety of interictal behaviors in such seizure patients which may not be recognized as part of the ongoing clinical syndrome. In part these involve hyper- or hyposexuality, excessive religious preoccupation which may border on the delusional, excessive and compulsive writing (hypergraphia) or drawing, as well as personality trait disturbances [168,169]. Interictal florrid psychotic episodes also occur. The quite serious possibility of psychiatric misdiagnosis of such phenomena as functional behavioral syndromes has been commented on [18,143,148,168-170]. The EEG in focal seizures and especially in psychomotor seizure disorders is positive in a majority of cases with focal negative or biphasic spike or spike-wave discharges classically being found. However, other paroxysmal features may also be seen as well. The number of positive confirmations will depend upon several recording variables, one of the most important of which is the inclusion of a drowsy and sleep tracing. Gibbs reported [26] positive EEG confirmation in 87% of 678 patients with a clinical diagnosis of psychomotor epilepsy, whereas Currie and associates [171] reported on 666 patients with temporal lobe seizures of which 92% were found to have focal abnormal EEG changes in the temporal leads.

Iatrogenic Seizure Risk and Side Effect Prediction

Most neuroleptic medications lower seizure thresholds. Furthermore, in some patients neuroleptic exposure can produce paroxysmal EEG changes when premedication EEG tracings are normal [143,172,173]. Infrequently patients treated with neuroleptic medications will develop grand mal seizures—usually with very high doses or during periods of major dose change. We report [174] as does Itil

[143,175] that patients with a variety of paroxysmal EEG patterns in the pre-treatment EEG—even relatively minor dysrhythmias—are at significant risk for iatrogenic medication-induced seizures. EEG findings can thus alert the psychiatrist to this risk so that prophylactic measures can be considered such as using the lowest effective dose or selecting, as Itil suggests [143], neuroleptics with the least epileptogenic potential. In addition to identifying seizure risk, paroxysmal EEG dysrhythmias may relate to a variety of pharmacological side effects including extrapyramidal symptoms [174,176]. One pattern, the B-Mitten dysrhythmia, shows promise as a potential risk variable for dyskinetic movements and clinical tardive dyskinesia in some patients [177].

Endocrine, Metabolic, or Nutritional Disorder and Substance Toxicity

When the psychiatrist treats a patient suspected of having an endocrinological-metabolic disorder or toxic response to environmental or industrial substance, the referral will be directed to the appropriate endocrinological or other medical specialty and not to electroencephalography. Nonetheless, it is important for the psychiatrist to realize that the EEG is sensitive to a wide variety of such disorders and that in the process of either routine EEG testing or securing EEGs for more traditional referral issues, cryptic or unrecognized disease possibilities may be suggested. Almost all of the disorders of endocrine or metabolic dysfunction, certain vitamin deficiency states, and many toxic reactions to substances will produce alterations in the frequency spectrum of the EEG. Most often they will produce generalized slowing, the degree of which may sometimes parallel the severity of the condition and presence of mental or behavioral changes. Frank seizure potentials are rarely found within this general category of disorders but they have been reported in some cases. Some conditions, such as hyperthyroidism and exposure to manganese or carbon disulfide, may produce increased fast activity either alone or in addition to slowing activity, while others (that is, hypoglycemia, Addison's disease) may produce a marked response to hyperventilation activation with rapid onset and prolonged duration of the hyperventilation-induced slowing activity. Normal EEGs are possible and with some (that is, hepatolenticular degeneration) this is more likely than with others.

Table 7 summarizes the salient EEG findings typically seen with these types of disorders. Such EEG abnormalities are always "nonspecific" but they should prompt the practitioner to rethink and review history and all symptoms and make referral for appropriate additional tests or specialist consultation if correlation with such biological dysfunctions seems at all possible. We have frequently found generalized and/or paroxysmal slowing in the routine EEG from patients with functional psychiatric disorder associated on follow-up with unsuspected endocrine disease, cerebral cyst, medication toxicity, cortical atrophy, grand mal seizures, lead toxicity, Jacob–Creutzfeldt disease, head trauma residual, Alzheimer's disease, intermittent petit mal status, demyelinating disease, and the like. This has even been true [178] when the initial preliminary consulting opinion of internal medicine and neurology discounted the EEG results claiming that the patient was euthyroid and neurologically asymptomatic!

Medication Toxicity and Toxic Psychosis

Unauthorized use of prescription drugs is sometimes apparent by characteristic frequency changes in the EEG. Barbiturate abuse invariably produces characteristic beta activity. Benzodiazepines produce a characteristic diffuse 20 to 25 Hz activity maximal over frontal-central areas, which in the case of diazepam is especially marked and of moderate voltage. When on the basis of these EEG changes we suggested covert use of these drugs, follow-up nearly always indicated that we were correct. With toxicity from these agents, psychotropic medications [33] and certain anticonvulsants [180], the usual EEG finding is mild, moderate, or marked generalized slowing with or without superimposed paroxysmal bursts of diffuse delta and with imipramine spike and sharp waves can also be seen. We find that the most frequent cases of medication toxicity involve lithium—even at blood levels within [179] or below the therapeutic range—and secondly, haloperidol.

Toxic psychoses may occur secondary to the biological variables mentioned in the above sections and frequently the EEG is of considerable value in establishing this organic involvement. With suspected toxic behavioral disturbance secondary to hallucinogenic drug use or other illicit drug abuse the EEG is often normal and uninformative. However, when a confusional mental state is part of the suspected toxic syndrome the EEG may be abnormal. Itil has made the valuable observation [143] that serial EEG tracings may be informative in that drug-induced EEG changes will subside with time whereas, if the EEG and behavioral disturbance stem from organic disease or lesion, EEG improvement over the short term will not occur.

Episodic Behavioral Dyscontrol and Episodic (Atypical) Psychosis

Not infrequently diffuse or focal spike discharges or other paroxysmal EEG events will be recorded from psychiatric patients who do not display motor seizures or easily recognized behavioral manifestations of complex partial seizure phenomena. It is unfortunate that these cases are often dismissed without any further thought or study. It is unfortunate because a legitimate argument for a relationship between a variety of episodic symptoms of emotional dyscontrol and either spontaneous or activated paroxysmal EEG features has been made [181-191,198] and continues to influence clinical thought. Patients who seem to display episodic reoccurring periods of psychopathological disturbances of mood, affect, or behavior

Table 7. Typical EEG Abnormalities in Selected Endocrine, Metabolic, Toxic, and Nutritional Disorders [13,14,18,30,33,93]

Condition or substance	Psychiatric component	Basic EEG findings	Hyperventilation response	Epileptogenic findings
Hypothyroidism	Yes	Generalized slowing in theta to delta range with or without paroxysmal bursts of slowing		
Hyperthyroidism	Yes	Either low voltage fast with increase in beta activity or generalized slowing		Rare
Hypoglycemia	Yes	Reduction of alpha frequency initially followed by generalized slowing	Marked response	Rare. May accentuate pre-existing dysrhythmias
Panhypopituitarism	Yes	Mixed alpha and theta in less severe cases. Generalized slowing as condition worsens	Questionable increased response	
Addison's disease	Yes	EEG normal in up to half of the cases. Otherwise bilateral theta-delta either nonparoxysmal or in bursts	Marked response	Rare
Cushing's syndrome	Yes	Most EEGs are normal. Some may show low voltage fast or mild generalized slowing		
Hypocalcemia	?	Generalized slow (theta)	Increased response	Epileptic discharges possible
Hyperparathyroidism	?	Insufficient information		
Pheochromocytoma	Yes	Generalized slowing in theta-delta Range. Some EEGs are normal		

Condition		EEG findings	Additional findings
Acute intermittent porphyria	Yes	Generalized slowing in theta-delta range	Increased response; Paroxysmal slow bursts and spike-wave discharges possible
Hepatolenticular degeneration	Yes	EEG may be normal in up to half of the cases. Otherwise mild, inconsistent slowing. Grossly abnormal EEGs are rare	
Lead exposure	Yes	Generalized slowing mild to moderate depending upon severity of exposure	Paroxysmal activity possible
Manganese exposure	Yes	Most often EEG contains generalized slowing. Some records contain excessive beta (fast) activity	
Carbon monoxide	Yes	Generalized slowing	Paroxysmal activity possible
Carbon disulfide	Yes	Initially there is increased beta activity. With more severe cases generalized slowing occurs	
Pernicious anemia (B_{12} deficiency)	Yes	Generalized slowing with mixed theta-delta frequencies. Some records contain diffuse paroxysmal bursts of slow	Temporal region spike discharges possible
Wernicke's syndrome	Yes	Generalized slowing the severity of which correlated with the severity of the illness	
Nicotinic acid deficiency	Yes	Generalized slowing in the theta-delta range	

either of brief duration (that is, acts) or prolonged episodes of weeks or more which are ego dystonic and disruptive of the patient's background life pattern should be referred for EEG study. We often think of dyscontrol as consisting of violent behavior, probably because as Elliott [192] and others [184] have shown, sudden and unpredictable violence can be associated with a high incidence of neurologic and electroencephalographic abnormality. However, as Monroe has remarked [191], episodic behavioral dysfunction associated with ictal activity in the limbic region can involve a variety of disruptive behavioral symptomatologies which are not necessarily violent. While EEG referral may be valuable and EEG abnormalities may be recorded, limbic system dysregulation is not always reflected at the scalp and a normal EEG cannot rule out an organically based episodic psychiatric syndrome.

In a study of EEG abnormalities in patients receiving phenothiazines, Davies and associates [172] found significant relationships between EEG dysrhythmias and variables such as irritability, destructiveness, depersonalization, emotional lability, and mental status symptoms of confusion, clouded consciousness, and disorientation. However, the most significant statistical relationships occurred between EEG dysrhythmias and the episodic nature of the patient's symptoms. In a subsequent investigation [173] these workers again substantiated these observations with additional data. Several authors listed above in this section [172,173, 187,189,190,192] as well as electroencephalographers [143,170] have noted that patients with paroxysmal EEG dysrhythmia or clinically established episodic syndromes might not respond well to traditional medication approaches and that other psychopharmacological adjustments may be of greater value.

Minor (Controversial) Paroxysmal Patterns

The topic of certain "minor" electroencephalographic dysrhythmias (that is, 14 and 6 positive spikes, small sharp spikes, psychomotor variant, and mitten patterns) occurs often in discussions of EEG-psychiatry relationships because these patterns have their highest incidence in psychiatric populations. None of these patterns are associated with seizure disorders in the traditional sense and they also are found in small proportions of normal subjects (14 and 6 positive spikes an exception and can occur with much higher control incidence among adolescents). Unfortunately, they have been either summarily dismissed as irrelevant or normal [15] or subject to critique [18] appealing more to simplistic emotion than reasoned methodological analyses. These patterns are controversial and in need of considerable empirical clarification. Early positive studies often have, in fact, been seriously flawed as critics note. However, many negative studies contain equally grave methodological flaws which are seldom systematically explored in critical reviews.

A meaningful review of these patterns is not possible within the confines of a general chapter both because of the voluminous amount of literature which would have to be discussed as well as the complexity of the issues involved. For whatever it may be worth, my own personal judgment based on an intensive in depth review of all the literature is that these EEG dysrhythmias do constitute minor yet definite abnormalities, albeit with a low level of clinical expressivity, associated with a variety of behavioral, autonomic, and affective symptoms which cut across diagnostic categories. The interested reader is referred to well conducted studies of autonomic pain [183], controlled study of behavior disturbance [194], and trauma correlates and predictive studies [195,196] of 14 and 6 positive spikes; general correlates [197] and dysphoria [86,199] associated with small sharp spikes; ictal manifestation [200] and confusional "status" [164] associated with the psychomotor variant pattern; and diagnostic and affective dysregulation correlates of the B-mitten dysrhythmia [201,202].

ROUTINE SCREENING VERSUS SELECTIVE REFERRAL

In the majority of psychiatric hospitals and with most private psychiatric practitioners, only selected patients are referred for EEG study and the majority of patients do not receive this test. However, with a minority of hospitals routine EEG screening is provided for all psychiatric patients and it has been suggested [143,154,170] that this practice may be of considerable value. Is there a viable rationale for routine EEG screening? If there is, can we empirically assess the "yield" of positive EEG findings and also determine if routine testing significantly improves upon results obtained using the more traditional selective referral approach.

Covert Physical Disease

Concern with undetected physical disease-producing psychiatric dysfunction is not new and reports from 40 years ago can be found. This is not surprising because almost all psychiatric symptoms are, after all, "nonspecific" and can stem from multiple etiologies—both organic and functional. Depending upon the study and investigative methods used, prevalence rates for unrecognized physical disease among patients with diagnoses of functional psychiatric disorder range from 15% to 50%. The collected literature is now voluminous and clearly cannot be documented in this space, however, the classic studies of Slater [203], Koranyi [204], and Hall [205,206] should be mentioned. When unrecognized physical disease is present it may (1) be the etiologic cause of the psychiatric presentation, (2) be noncausal but aggravating to the psychiatric disorder or (3) occur as incidental but nonetheless worth knowing about and treating if necessary. As has been shown earlier in this chapter, clinical EEG may be sensitive to a wide variety of variables which either directly or indirectly impinge on brain function and in this sense unsuspected EEG irregularities can suggest patients who may benefit from further detailed medical scrutiny.

Electroencephalographic Yield

Reports [85,172,207,208] from psychiatric facilities using routine EEG screening suggest that prevalence figures for abnormal EEGs range from 20% to 50% among psychiatric inpatients. Figures for outpatients are not available. Based on a total sample of wake and sleep EEG evaluations of over 15,000 consecutively admitted psychiatric inpatients collected over twelve years, I reported [154] that after *omitting* controversial EEG patterns (as discussed in the preceding section) the yearly incidence of EEG abnormality ranged from 16.2% to 30.8%. The unweighted simple average over the twelve year period was 24%. It would seem that expected yeild of positive EEG results among unselected psychiatric inpatients is sufficient to support a routine screening operation in most centers.

Contrast with Selective Referral

Since 1976, I have published four separate studies [153,154,209,210] each using essentially the same methodology that contrasts routine screening with selective physician referral in detecting EEG abnormality. All studies combined involve a composite sample of 508 consecutive cases of EEG abnormality obtained from our routine EEG screening program. In all studies, controversial EEG findings were omitted and methods were devised to determine for each patient whether or not the treating physician had any prior suspicion, however mild, that organic dysfunction existed. All patients were dichotomized into those cases where prior suspicion of brain dysfunction or physical illness indicated that selective referral for EEG probably would have been made versus those cases where such referral would not have been made by treating personnel. The results summarized in Table 8 indicate that an overall average of 66.3% (range 56% to 71%) of psychiatric inpatients with abnormal EEGs would not have been referred and hence would not have been recognized without a screening program in operation. Depending on the time period sampled, it was calculated that one out of every six or seven admissions (15%) to one out of every eleven or twelve admissions (8.8%) have EEG suggestions of unsuspected covert presumptive organic involvement which is only detected by way of routine EEG screening. Furthermore, analysis confined to patients displaying the most serious EEG abnormalities revealed that 54.6% of the cases would have been missed with reliance on a selective referral philosophy.

The empirical results suggest strongly that routine screening effectively detects substantial amounts of EEG dysrhythmia which would be otherwise missed if only a selective referral policy is followed.

Table 8. Presence and Absence of Pre-existing Clinical Suspicion of Organicity in Four Series
of Consecutive Patients with EEG Abnormality

Prior suspicion of brain dysfunction	First sample [153]		Second sample [209]		Third sample [210]		Current sample		Combined	
	N	%	N	%	N	%	N	%	N	%
No (would not be referred)	64	71.1	79	70.5	161	64.9	33	56.9	337	66.3
Yes (most would be referred)	26	28.9	33	29.5	87	35.1	25	43.1	171	33.7
Totals	90		112		248		58		508	

ACTIVATION PROCEDURES AND SPECIAL RECORDINGS

A basic EEG recording should be long in order to provide opportunity for pathological events to occur in the tracing. In addition to the basic recording—often called the "resting record"—various activating procedures may be employed which have been shown to increase the yield of positive EEG findings.

Natural or sedated sleep is probably the most effective and useful activating procedure for the clinical examination and this is especially true for the elicitation of a variety of paroxysmal dysrhythmias. The activating value of sleep has been known for more than 35 years following the pioneering work by Gibbs and others and the American EEG Society guidelines [211] now recommended that sleep be routinely included in the EEG examination. It is not only of demonstrable value in evaluating the seizure patient but it is extremely important—and probably should be mandatory—to include drowsy and sleep recordings in the EEG examinations of psychiatric patients. We have attempted [212] to address this latter point as well as to provide pertinent literature references for the effectiveness of sleep studies through 1973. Since then the importance of this activating technique has not lessened. Figures 1a, 1b, and 1c contain combined material from our work [212] and that of the Gibbs [213] and illustrate for a wide variety of discrete EEG patterns the degree to which each pattern depends upon drowsy and sleep recording for its detection.

Hyperventilation is perhaps the next most widely used activating procedure and it is probably used routinely in most laboratories. During the procedure, strenuous overbreathing for about three minutes is encouraged while the tracing and the patient are observed. Activation is based on vasoconstriction with anoxia secondary to reduced carbon dioxide levels in the arterial blood. Although the procedure is generally safe and well accepted by the patient, it may be contraindicated in patients with cardiac or respiratory problems. Done properly, the technique is very effective in eliciting petit mal discharges and the EEG response (generalized slowing) may be marked with hypoglycemia. The procedure may also accentuate dysrhythmias which were poorly visualized in the resting record and it may also elicit a variety of other paroxysmal features. An increasing voltage of generalized slow (termed a "build up") is a normal EEG response especially in children and at times this has been misinterpreted as "abnormal."

Photic stimulation is a commonly used activation technique and consists of intense but brief strobic flashes at various frequencies of from 1 to 30 Hz produced by a lamp positioned about twelve inches from the patient's face. The test can sample independent flash frequencies separately and randomly or a "zoom" technique can be employed in which a continual flash moving from low to high frequency is gradually introduced. Variations can include patterned (that is, geometric) stimulus and periods of eye opening during stimulation. With many sub-

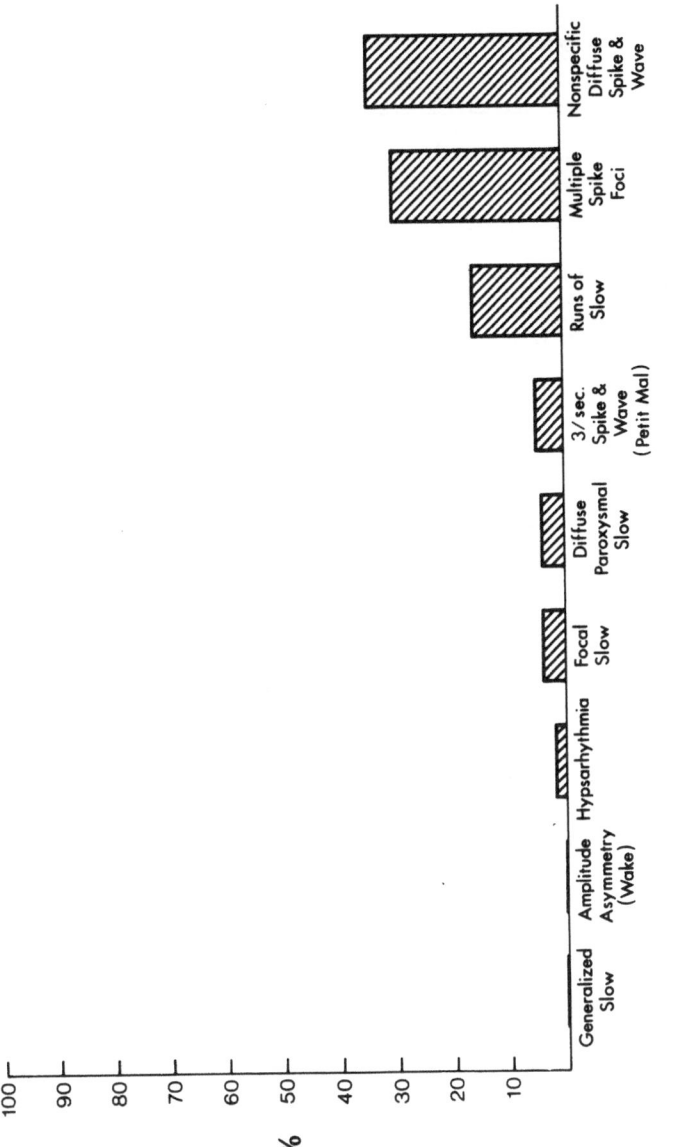

Figure 1a. Percent of discrete EEG dysrhythmias detected only during drowsiness and/or sleep. Of all cases of "generalized slow," sleep was unnecessary for detection. Of all cases of "focal slow," 4% were seen *only* during drowsiness and sleep and 96% were seen during wake. Of all cases of "multiple spike foci," 30% were seen *only during* drowsiness and sleep and 70% were seen during wake, and so forth. Data abridged from Gibbs and Gibbs [213] and Struve and Pike [212].

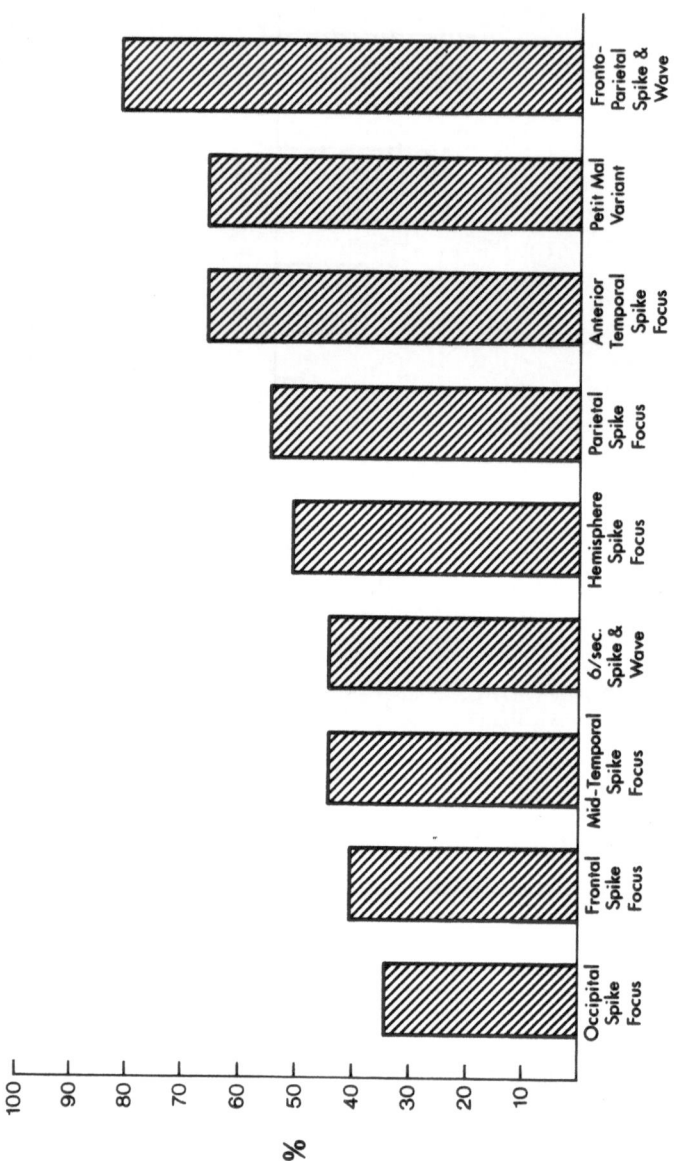

Figure 1b. Continuation of Figure 1a.

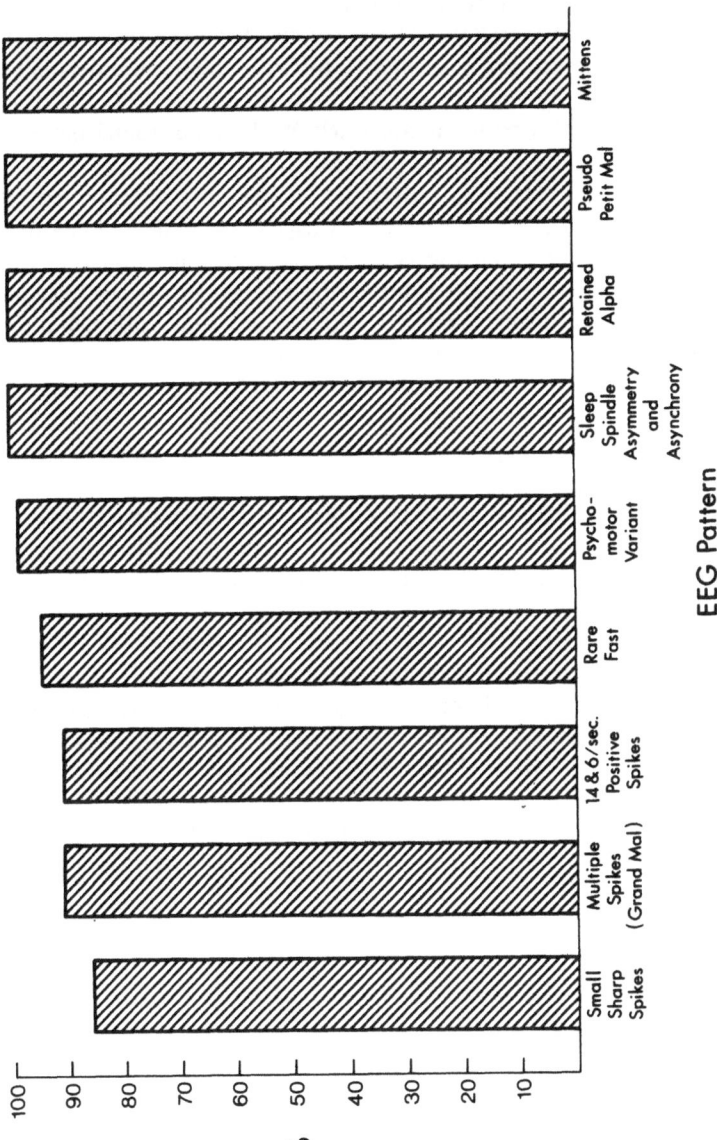

Figure 1c. Continuation of Figure 1a.

jects, photic driving will occur and posterior brain waves will "follow" flash frequencies close to the subject's alpha rate and at higher flash frequencies the alpha rate may drop to a harmonic of half the photic rate. Photomyoclonic or facial and eye muscular responses may occur and some subjects complain of a variety of unpleasant subjective sensations. The procedure has exceptional value in suspected photogenic seizures and may be helpful with seizure disorders in general. However, seizure discharges can be elicited from healthy subjects [132] and the potential for false positive results is not small. We have not found the technique particularly useful with our psychiatric patients.

Sleep deprivation [214] is an activation technique insufficiently used in general EEG work and in the EEG evaluation of psychiatric patients in particular. A period of 24 hours of continual wakefulness has activating properties over and above the simple induction of sleep during the tracing. In private EEG referrals there is always a problem of compliance with the procedure although a properly motivated patient should cooperate in a conscientious manner.

Pharmacological activation including metrazol [215] with suspected seizure patients and alpha-chloralose for psychiatric patients [182] are not widely used in the EEG evaluation of psychiatric referrals although the latter procedure has more relevance to psychiatry and should receive more widespread application. Esoteric activation techniques, such as elicitation of paroxysmal EEG changes by emotionally charged verbal stimuli [216] or alcohol activation in patients with alcohol associated violence [217], have theoretical and potential pragmatic relevance but have not been adopted within the field.

Attention is sometimes given to use of special electrodes capable of recording mesiobasal areas not reached by scalp lead placements [218,219]. From the standpoint of cleaner recordings with fewer artifacts, sphenoidal electrodes may have an advantage, however, since they can only be inserted by a specially trained physician they are seldom used in most laboratories. Nasopharyngeal electrodes are insertable by trained technicians and, whereas the procedure is by no means comfortable, it can be tolerated by most patients. These lead placements may be useful in suspected temporal lobe dysfunctions when the standard wake and sleep tracings are normal. In our experience [220] nasopharyngeal recordings have not been very useful with psychiatric referrals and frequently psychiatric behavioral complications (that is, severe confusion, agitation) or flat refusal prevented their use.

ADVICE FOR THE REFERRING PSYCHIATRIST

Despite published guidelines [211] electroencephalographic laboratories vary widely in their operational procedures, specific areas of expertise, and characteristics of referral population served. What are some of the characteristics that the referring psychiatrist should look for?

First, one can obtain considerable information about an EEG laboratory by talking to one's patients after they have been tested. It is absolutely essential to select a laboratory which routinely employs drowsy and sleep recording with every record. Avoid laboratories that use sleep "only when indicated" and the like because there is no way in which one can know what the sleep recording will contain until it is obtained. Much of the EEG abnormality in psychiatric patients is paroxysmal and enhanced by sleep activation. Furthermore, EEGs should be of long duration—at least 45 minutes to an hour if not longer. The laboratory should have the capability of using photic stimulation and nasopharyngeal lead recordings and be willing to do sleep-deprived EEGs when needed. A laboratory receiving large numbers of psychiatric referrals is most desirable as is an electroencephalographer with some interest in psychiatric dysfunctions and—if possible—some degree of committment to research in EEG-psychiatry areas. A laboratory involved in teaching students or residents is a good indication that current developments and thinking are used in the service. Both the American Electroencephalographic Society and the American Medical Electroencephalographic Association provide special qualifying examinations for electroencephalographers as well as technologists and these could be investigated as well. An essential consideration is the electroencephalographers' availability to provide clarifying consultation on the EEG reports whenever requested.

Finally, patients should leave the EEG laboratory in exactly the same physical appearance as when they entered. All electrode paste, collodian, cotton or gauze (if used) should be completely removed from the skin and hair by EEG staff following the examinational procedure and the patient allowed to regroom before leaving. No sedated patient should be tested and allowed to leave without an escort.

ACKNOWLEDGEMENTS

Appreciation is extended to Susan Feigenbaum, R.N., who has supervised the author's laboratory in all of its clinical and research activity for more than 13 years. She has proven that clinical patient care and scientific imperatives can coexist. Recognition is also given to technologists Carlton Farnum, Joan Trotman, Lata Shah, and Mary Patrick, as well as to Lillian Pike, who have provided dedicated assistance over many years. The author recognizes the kind support from grants MH 13217, MH 20662, and MH 32369, National Institute of Mental Health, United

States Public Health Service. Finally, the author wishes to thank Beverly Smith for
her competent assistance in final manuscript preparation.

REFERENCES

1. Gibbs FA, Gibbs EL: Atlas of Electroencephalography, Vol. 1. Methodology and Controls. Cambridge, MA., Addison-Wesley Press, 1950.
2. Caton R: The electric currents of the brain. Br Med J 2:278, 1875
3. Beck A: Die Bestimmung der Localisation der Gehirn—und Fückenmarks-functionen vermittelst der elektrischen Erscheinungen. Zentralbl F Physiol 4:473-476, 1890
4. Beck A: Die Ströme der Nervencentren. Zentralbl F Physiol 4:572, 1890
5. Fleischl von Marxow, E: Mittheilung betreffend die Physiologie der Hirnrinde. Zentrabl Physiol 4:437-540, 1890
6. Berger H: Uber das Elektrenkephalogramm des Menschen: I Mitteilung. Arch F Psychiat 87:527-570, 1929
7. Cohn R: Clinical Electroencephalography. New York, McGraw-Hill, 1949
8. Schwab RS: Electroencephalography in Clinical Practice. Philadelphia, W B Saunders, 1951
9. Strauss H, Ostow M, Greenstein L: Diagnostic Electroencephalography. New York, Gruen & Stratton, 1952
10. Fois A, Low NL: The Electroencephalogram of the Normal Child. Springfield, IL, Charles C Thomas, 1961
11. Hill D, Parr G (eds): Electroencephalography. New York, Macmillan Publishing Co, 1963
12. Hess R: EEG Handbook, Sandoz Monographs. Sandoz Ltd, 1969
13. Kooi KA: Fundamentals of Electroencephalography. New York, Harper & Row, 1971
14. Kiloh LG, McComas AJ, Osselton JW: Clinical Electroencephalography, 3rd ed. London, Butterworths, 1972
15. Craib AR, Perry M: The EEG Handbook, 2nd ed. Beckman Instruments Inc, 1975
16. Rémond A, Lairy TC, Chatrian GE: Handbook of Electroencephalography and Clinical Neurophysiology, Vol. 6. The Normal EEG Throughout Life. Amsterdam, Elsevier, 1975
17. Kellaway P, Petersen I (eds): Clinical Electroencephalography of Children. Stockholm, Almquist and Wiksell, 1980
18. Klass DW, Daly DD: Current Practice of Clinical Electroencephalography. New York, Raven Press, 1979
19. Fischer MH: Elektrobiologische Auswirkungen von Krampfgiften an Zentralnerven System. Med Klin 29:15-19, 1933
20. Gibbs FA, Davis H, Lennox WG: The electroencephalogram in epilepsy and in conditions of impaired consciousness. Arch Neurol Psychiat 34:1133-1148, 1935
21. Walter WG: The location of cerebral tumours by electroencephalography. Lancet 2:305-308, 1936

22. MacLean PD: A new nasopharyngeal lead. Electroenceph Clin Neurophysiol 1:110-112, 1949
23. Arellano AP: A tympanic lead. Electroenceph Clin Neurophysiol 1:112-113, 1949
24. Lennox M, Ruch TC: Ventricular electroencephalography—description of technique. J Neurosurg 3:219-222, 1946
25. Walter WG, Dovey VJ: Electroencephalography in cases of sub-cortical tumor. Neurosurg Psych 7:57-65, 1944
26. Gibbs FA, Gibbs EL: Atlas of Electroencephalography, Vol. 2. Epilepsy. Reading, MA, Addison-Wesley, 1952
27. Ajmone Marsan C, Abraham K: A seizure atlas. Electroenceph Clin Neurophysiol (suppl 15), 1960
28. Gibbs FA, Gibbs EL: Atlas of Electroencephalography, Vol. 3. Neurological and Psychiatric Disorders. Reading, MA, Addison-Wesley 1964
29. Rémond A, Harner R, Naquet R: Handbook of Electroencephalography and Clinical Neurophysiology, Vol. 12. Altered States of Consciousness, Coma, Cerebral Death. Amsterdam, Elsevier, 1975
30. Wilson WP: The electroencephalogram in endocrine disorders. In Wilson WP (ed): Applications of Electroencephalography in Psychiatry. Durham, NC, Duke Universtiy Press, 1965
31. Green RL: The electroencephalogram in alcoholism, toxic psychoses, and infection. In WP Wilson: Applications of Electroencephalography in Psychiatry. Durham, NC, Duke University Press, 1965
32. Rémond A, Radermecker FJ: Handbook of Electroencephalography and Clinical Neurophysiology, Vol. 15A. Infections and Inflammatory Reactions, Allergy and Allergic Reactions. Degenerative Diseases. Amsterdam, Elsevier 1977
33. Rémond A, Glaser GH: Handbook of Electroencephalography and Clinical Neurophysiology, Vol. 15C. Metabolic, Endocrine and Toxic Diseases. Amsterdam, Elsevier, 1977
34. Williams RL, Karacan I, Hursch CJ: Electroencephalography (EEG) of Human Sleep: Clinical Applications. New York, John Wiley & Sons, 1974
35. Fink M, Foster FG, Kupfer DJ, et al: EEG sleep diagnosis of medical disease in depression. Neuropsychobiology 3:167-178, 1977
36. Neil JF, Merikangas JR, Foster FG, et al: Waking and all-night sleep EEG's in anorexia nervosa. Clin Electroenceph 11:9-15, 1980
37. Akiskal HS, Rosenthal TL, Haykal RF, et al: Characterological depressions: Clinical and sleep EEG findings separating "subaffective dysrhythmias" from "character spectrum disorders." Arch Gen Psych 37:777-783, 1980
38. Feinberg M, Gillin JC, Carroll BJ, et al: EEG studies of sleep in the diagnosis of depression. Biol Psych 17:305-315, 1982
39. Itil TM: Electroencephalography in psychiatry. In HCB Denber (ed): Psychopharmacological Treatment—Theory and Practice. New York, Marcel Dekker, 1975
40. Itil TM: Computer-analyzed electroencephalogram to predict the therapeutic outcome in schizophrenia. In CF Baxter, T Melnechuk (eds): Perspectives in Schizophrenia Research. New York, Raven Press, 1980
41. Itil TM: The use of electroencephalography in the practice of psychiatry. Psychosomatics 23:799-813, 1982

42. Cohen D: Magnetoencephalography: Evidence of magnetic fields produced by alpha-rhythm currents. Science 161:784-786, 1968
43. Reite M, Zimmerman JE, Edrich J, et al: The human magnetoencephalogram: Some EEG and related correlations. Electroenceph Clin Neurophysiol 40: 59-66, 1976
44. Hughes JR, Hendrix DE, Cohen J: Relationship of the magnetoencephalogram to the electroencephalogram: Normal wake and sleep activity. Electroenceph Clin Neurophysiol 40:261-278, 1976
45. Barth DS, Sutherling W, Engel J, et al: Neuromagnetic localization of epileptiform spike activity in the human brain. Science 218:891-894, 1982
46. Glaser GH: The normal electroencephalogram and its reactivity. In GH Glaser (ed): EEG and Behavior. New York, Basic Books, 1963
47. Abraham A, Ajmone Marsaw C: Patterns of cortical discharges and their relation to routine scalp electroencephalography. Electroenceph Clin Neurophysiol 10:447-461, 1958.
48. Heath RG, Mickle WA: Evaluation of 7 years experience with depth electrode studies in human patients. IN ER Hamey, DS O'Doherty (eds): Electrical Studies on the Unanesthetized Brain. New York, Paul B Hoeber, 1960
49. Walter WG, Crow HJ: Depth recording from the human brain. Electroenceph Clin Neurophysiol 16:68-72, 1964
50. Cooper R, Winter AL, Crow JH, et al: Comparison of subcortical, cortical and scalp activity using chronically indwelling electrodes in man. Electroenceph Clin Neurophysiol 18:217-228, 1975
51. Heath RG: Depth recording and stimulation studies in patients. In A Winter (ed): The Surgical Control of Behavior: A Symposium. Springfield, IL, Charles C Thomas, 1971
52. Heath RG: Brain function and behavior. J Nerv Ment Dis 160:159-175, 1975
53. Gloor P: Contributions of electroencephalography to the neurosurgical treatment of the epilepsies. In DP Purpura, JK Penry, RD Walter (eds): Neurosurgical Management of the Epilepsies. Adv Neurol 8:59-105, 1975
54. Olivier A, Gloor P, Andermann F, et al: Occipitotemporal epilepsy studied with stereotaxically implanted depth electrodes and successfully treated by temporal resection. Ann Neurol 11:428-432, 1982
55. Spencer SS, Spencer DD, Williamson PD, et al: The localizing value of depth electroencephalography in 32 patients with refractory epilsepy. Ann Neurol 12:248-253, 1982
56. Lion KS, Winter DF, Levin E: Electrical activity of the brain measured in the frequency range above 200 cycles per second. Electroenceph Clin Neurophysiol 2:205-208, 1950
57. Farina M, Veten L: Oscillographic recording of high frequency waves (50-500 cps) over the human scalp Electroenceph Clin Neurophysiol 7:455, 1955
58. Rodin E, Wasson S, Porzak J, et al: High frequency cerebral electrical activity during various behavioral states. Electroenceph Clin Neurophysiol 14: 453-464, 1962
59. Hall RA, Yeager C, Yarbrough RB: Observations on high frequency electroencephalograms. Electroenceph Clin Neurophysiol 22:262-265, 1967
60. Dawson WW, Stewart HL, Perry NW, et al: Pooling of visual evoked signals from humans: A demonstration of components above 100 Hz. Nature 220: 980-984, 1968
61. Itil TM, Ulett, GA, Hsu W, et al: The effects of smoking withdrawal on quantitatively analyzed EEG. Clin Electroenceph 2:44-51, 1971

62. Conrin J: The EEG effects of tobacco smoking—a review. Clin Electroenceph 11:180-187, 1980
63. Ellingson RJ: The limitations of electroencephalography. In JW Prescott, MS Read, DB Coursin (eds): Brain Function and Malnutrition: Neuropsychological Methods of Assessment. New York, John Wiley & Sons, 1975
64. Solomon S: Neurological evaluation. In HI Kaplan, AM Freedman, BM Sadock (eds): Comprehensive Textbook of Psychiatri, Vol. 1, 3rd ed. Baltimore, Williams & Wilkins, 1980
65. Martinius J, Matthes A, Lombrosco CT: Electroencephalographic features in posterior fossa tumors in children. Electroenceph Clin Neurophysiol 25: 128-139, 1968
66. Velsaco M, Zenteno-Alaniz G: Significance of EEG signs in the diagnosis of 136 intracranial neoplasma verified histologically. Clin Electroenceph 2:65-77, 1971
67. Decker DA, Knott JR: The EEG in intrinsic supratentorial brain tumors: A comparative evaluation. Electroenceph Clin Neurophysiol 33:303-310, 1972
68. Tucker RP, Kooi KA, Newkink TA, et al: A comparative study of the EEG in patients with Parkinson's disease with and without dementia. Clin Electroenceph 3:152-159, 1972
69. Farrell DF: The EEG in progressive multifocal leukoencephalopathy. Electroenceph Clin Neurophysiol 26:200-205, 1969
70. Graebner RW, Celsia GG: EEG findings in hydrocephalus and their relation to shunting procedures. Electroenceph Clin Neurophysiol 35:517-521, 1973
71. Elwan O, Taber Y, Barradah O: Electroencephalographic changes in chronic cerebrovascular occlusive disorders. Clin Electroenceph 5:92-102, 1974
72. Blum RH: A note on the reliability of electroencephalographi judgments. Neurol 4:143-146, 1954
73. Houfek EE, Ellingson RJ: On the reliability of clinical EEG interpretation. J Nerv Ment Dis 128:425-437, 1959
74. Walker AE, Jablon S: A follow-up study of head wounds in World War II. VA Medical Monograph, Washington DC, US Government Printing Office 1961
75. Little SC, Raffel SC: Intra-rater reliability of EEG interpretations. J Nerv Ment Dis 135:77-81, 1962
76. Woody RH: Intra-judge reliability in clinical electroencephalography. J Clin Psychol 22:150-154, 1966
77. Woody RH: Inter-judge reliability in clinical electroencephalography. J Clin Psychol 24:251-256, 1968
78. Volavka J, Matousek M, Roubicek J, et al: The reliability of visual EEG assessment. Electroenceph Clin Neurophysiol 31:294, 1970
79. Majkowski J, et al: Reliability of electroencephalography. Polish Med J 10: 1223-1229, 1971
80. Rose SW, Penry JK, White BG, et al: Reliability and validity of visual EEG assessment on third grade children. Clin Electroenceph 4:197-205, 1973
81. Struve FA, Becka DR, Green MA, et al: Reliability of clinical interpretation of the electroencephalogram. Clin Electroenceph 6:54-60, 1975
82. Small JG, Milstein V, DeMyer MK, et al: Electroencephalographic (EEG) and clinical studies of early infantile autism. Clin Electroenceph 8:27-35, 1977
83. Wayne HL, Shapiro AK, Shapiro E: Gilles de la Tourette's syndrome: Electroencephalographic investigation and clinical correlation. Clin Electroenceph 3: 160-168, 1972

84. Hooshmand H: A look at the EEG report. Clin Electroenceph 9:118-123, 1978
85. Small JG: The six per second spike and wave—a psychiatric population study. Electroenceph Clin Neurophysiol 24:561-568, 1968
86. Small JG: Small sharp spikes in a psychiatric population. Arch Gen Psych 22:227-284, 1970
87. Small JG, Sharpley P, Small IF: Positive spikes, spike-wave phantoms, and psychomotor variants: A survey of these EEG patterns in psychiatric patients. Arch Gen Psych 18:232-238, 1968
88. Struve FA, Pike LE, Ross DC: Consistency of EEG abnormality over time: A test-retest reliability approach with psychiatric patients. Clin Electroenceph 10:96-104, 1979
89. Bergman PS, Green MA: The use of electroencephalography in differentiating psychogenic disorders and organic brain diseases. Am J Psych 113:27-31, 1956
90. Hanretta AG: Psychiatric utilization of electroencephalography. Dis Nerv Syst 26:409-417, 1965
91. Wender PH: Minimal Brain Dysfunction in Children. New York, John Wiley & Sons, 1971
92. Satterfield JH: EEG issues in children with minimal brain dysfunction. Semin Psych 5:35-46, 1973
93. Kolb LC, Brodie HKH: Modern Clinical Psychiatry, Philadelphia, WB Saunders, 1982
94. Ellingson RJ: The incidence of EEG abnormality among patients with mental disorders of apparently nonorganic origin: A critical review. Am J Psych 111: 263-275, 1954
95. Williams D: The significance of an abnormal electroencephalogram. J Neurol Psych 4:257-267, 1941
96. Finley KH, Cambell CM: Electroencephalography in schizophrenia. Am J Psych 98:374-381, 1941
97. Silverman D: The electroencephalogram of criminals: Analyses of four hundred and eleven cases. Arch Neurol Psych 52:38-42, 1944
98. Rossen R, Gordon M: Electroencephalographic findings in a naval "control" group of 200 men. Dis Nerv Syst 8:373-378, 1947
99. Hill D: EEG in episodic psychotic and psychopathic behavior: A classification of data. Electroenceph Clin Neurophysiol 4:419-442, 1952
100. Buchthal F, Lennox M: The EEG of metrazol and photic stimulation of 682 normal subjects. Electroenceph Clin Neurophysiol 5:545-558, 1953
101. Moore FJ, Kellaway P, Kagawa N: Metrazol activation as a diagnostic adjunct in electroencephalography—a reevaluation. Neurol 4:325-338, 1954
102. Blanc C, LaFontaine E, Laplane R: Meaning and value of EEG in aeronautical medicine. Aerospace Med 35:249-256, 1964
103. Kitamura K, Asakura T: Clinical significance of spike and sharp wave in EEG (abstract). Electroenceph Clin Neurophysiol (suppl 12):16, 1958
104. O'Connor P: Analysis of 500 routine EEG's of R.A.F. aircrew cadets (abstract). Electroenceph Clin Neurophysiol 17:341, 1964
105. Romain LF: An electroencephalographic study of flying personnel utiliaing nasopharyngeal electrodes. Aerospace Med 40:1385-1387, 1969
106. Pacheco e Silva A: Value of the electroencephalogram in the selection of 1,000 aviators. Clin Electroenceph 8:150-154, 1977

107. Secunda L, Finley HK: Electroencephalographic studies in children presenting behavior disorders. N Engl J Med 226:850-854, 1942
108. Henry CE: Electroencephalograms of normal children. Monographs of the Society for Research in Child Development, Vol IX, Serial No. 39, No. 3. Washington, DC, National Research Council, 1944
109. Gottlieb JS, Knott JR, Ashby MC: Electroencephalographic evaluation of primary behavior disorders in children. Arch Neurol Psych 53:138-143, 1945
110. Kennard MA, Willner MD: Significance of paroxysmal patterns in electroencephalograms of children without clinical epilepsy. Res Publ Assoc Res Nerv Ment Dis 26:308-327, 1947
111. Miller CA, Lennox MA: Electroencephalography in behavior problem children. J Pediatr 33:753-760, 1948
112. Brandt S, Brandt H: The electroencephalographic patterns in young healthy children from 0 to five years of age. Acta Psychiatr Neurol Scand 30:77-89, 1955
113. Taterka JH, Katz J: Study of correlations between electroencephalographic and psychological patterns in emotionally disturbed children. Psychosom Med 17:62-72, 1955
114. White PT, DeMyer W, DeMyer M: EEG abnormalities in early childhood schozophrenia: A double-blind study of psychiatrically disturbed and normal children during promazine sedation. Am J Psych 120:950-958, 1964
115. Hutt SJ, Hutt C, Lee D, et al: A behavioral and electroencephalographic study of autistic children. J Psychiatr Res 3:181-197, 1965
116. Whitehouse D, Pappas JA, Escala PH, et al: Electroencephalographic changes in children with migraine. N Engl J Med 276:23-27, 1967
117. Small JG: Epileptiform electroencephalographic abnormalities in mentally ill children. J Nerv Ment Dis 147:341-348, 1968
118. Stevens JR, Sachdev K, Milstein V: Behavior disorders of childhood and the electroencephalogram. Arch Neurol 18:160-177, 1968
119. Capute AJ, Niedermeyer E, Richardson F: The electroencephalogram in children with minimal cerebral dysfunction. Pediatr 41:1104-1114, 1968
120. Gubbay SS, Lobascher M, Kingerlee P: A neurological appraisal of autistic children: Results of a western Australian survey. Dev Med Child Neurol 12:422-429, 1970
121. Small JG: EEG and neurophysiological studies of early infantile autism. Biol Psych 10:385-397, 1975
122. Small JG, Milstein V, Jay S: Clinical EEG studies of short and long term stimulant drug therapy of hyperkinetic children. Clin Electroenceph 9:186-194, 1978
123. Thorner MW: Procurement of Electroencephalographic Tracings in 100 Flying Cadets for Evaluating the Gibbs Technique in Relation to Flying Ability. USAF School of Aviation Research Report No. 7-1, 1942
124. Herrlin KN: EEG with photic stimulation: A study of children with manifest or suspected epilepsy. Electroenceph Clin Neurophysiol 6:573-589, 1954
125. Corbin HPF, Bickford RG: Studies of the electroencephalogram of normal children: Comparison of visual and automatic frequency analyses. Electroenceph Clin Neurophysiol 7:15-28, 1955
126. Maulsby RL, Kellaway P, Graham M, et al: The Normative Electroencephalographic Data Reference Library. Final Report, Contract NAS 9-1200. Washington, DC, NASA, 1968

127. Bennett DR: Spike-wave complexes in "normal" flying personnel. Aerospace Med 38:1276-1282, 1967
128. Doose H, Gerken H, Völzke E: Genetics of centrencephalic epilepsy in childhood. Epilepsia 9:107, 1968
129. Eeg-Olofsson O, Petersén I, Sellden U: The development of the electroencephalogram in normal children from the age of 1 through 15 years: Paroxysmal activity. Neuropädiatrie 2:375-404, 1971
130. Chamberlain GHA, Russell JG: The EEGs of the relatives of schizophrenics. J Ment Sci 98:654-659, 1952
131. Rodin E: Metrazol tolerance in a "normal" volunteer population: An investigation of the potential significance of abnormal findings. Electroenceph Clin Neurophysiol 10:433-446, 1958
132. Stevens JR: All that spikes is not fits. In C Shagass, S Gershon, AJ Friedhoff (eds): Psychopathology and Brain Dysfunction. New York, Raven Press, 1977
133. O'Connor PJ: The value of routine electroencephalography. Practitioner 211:178-181, 1973
134. Kooi KA, Güvener AM, Tupper CJ, et al: Electroencephalographic patterns of the temporal region in normal adults. Neurol 14:1029-1035, 1964
135. Cure C, Rasmussen T, Jasper H: Activation of seizures and electroencephalographic disturbances in epileptic and in control subjects with "metrazol." Arch Neurol Psych 59:691-717, 1948
136. Chatrian GE: Paroxysmal patterns in "normal" subjects. IN A Rémond, GC Lairy (eds): Handbook of Electroencephalography and Clinical Neurophysiology, Vol. 6. The Normal EEG Throughout Life. Amsterdam, Elsevier, 1976
137. Petersén I, Eeg-Olofsson O, Selldén U: Paroxysmal activity in EEG of normal children. IN P Kellaway, I Petersén (eds): Clinical Electroencephalography of Children. Stockholm, Almquist & Wiksell, 1968
138. Petersén I, Eeg-Olofsson O: The development of the EEG in normal children from the age of 1 through 15 years: Non-paroxysmal activity. Neuropädiatrie 3:277-304, 1971
139. Eeg-Olofsson O: The development of the EEG in normal young persons from the age of 16 to 21 years. Neuropädiatrie 3:11-45, 1971
140. Small JG, Sharpley P, Small IF; EEG abnormalities in functional mental disorders. Electroenceph Clin Neurophysiol 23:77-97, 1967
141. Low MD: Evaluation of psychiatric disorders and the effects of psychotherapeutic and psychotomimetic agents. In DW Klass, DD Daly (eds): Current Practice of Clinical Electroencephalography. New York, Raven Press, 1979
142. Keitner G, Grof P: The routine EEG—How is it used in clinical practice? Psychiatr J Univ Ottawa 6:144-148, 1981
143. Itil TM: The use of electroencephalography in the practice of psychiatry. Psychosom 23:799-813, 1982
144. Keschner M, Bender MB, Strauss I: Mental symptoms in cases of tumor of the temporal lobe. Arch Neurol Psych 35:572-596, 1936
145. Strauss I, Keschner M: Mental symptoms in cases of tumor of the frontal lobes. Arch Neurol Psych 33:986-1005, 1935
146. Keschner M, Bender MB, Strauss I: Mental symptoms in cases of subtentorial tumor. Arch Neurol Psych 37:1-15, 1937
147. Soniat TLL: Psychiatric symptoms associated with intracranial neoplasms. Am J Psych 108:19-22, 1951
148. Mulder DW, Daly D: Psychiatric symptoms associated with lesions of the temporal lobe. JAMA 150:173-176, 1952

149. Waggoner RW, Bagchi BK: Initial masking of organic brain changes by psychic symptoms: Clinical and electroencephalographic studies. Am J Psych 110:904-910, 1954

150. Strauss H: Intracranial neoplasms masked as depression and diagnosed with the aid of electroencephalography. J Nerv Ment Dis 112:185-189, 1955

151. Remington FB, Rubert SL: Why patients with brain tumors come to a psychiatric hospital. Am J Psych 119:256-257, 1962

152. Malamud N: Psychiatric disorder with intracranial tumors of the limbic system. Arch Neurol 17:113-123, 1967

153. Struve FA: The necessity and value of securing routine electroencephalograms in psychiatric patients: A preliminary report on the issue of referrals. Clin Electroenceph 7:115-130, 1976

154. Struve FA: Clinical EEG assessment of hospitalized psychiatric patients: An empirical contrast of selective referral versus routine screening in detection of covert disease. Psychiatric Medicine (in press)

155. Hess R (ed): Brain tumors and other space occupying processes. In: Handbook of Electroencephalography and Clinical Neurology, Vol. 14. Amsterdam, Elsevier, 1975

156. Kirstein L: The occurrence of sharp waves, spikes and fast activity in supratentorial tumours. Electroenceph Clin Neurophysiol 5:33-40, 1953

157. Walter WG: Traumatic extradural haemorrhage: Clinical application of electroencephalography. Bristol Med Chir J 57:86-90, 1940

158. Jasper HH, Kershman J, Elvidge A: Electroencephalographic studies of injury to the head. Arch Neurol Psych 4:328-350, 1940

159. Friedlander WJ: Clinical evaluation of focal depression of voltage in electroencephalography. Neurol 4:752-761, 1954

160. Whittier JR: Hereditary Chorea (Huntington's Chorea): A paradigm of brain dysfunction with psychopahtology. In C Shagass, S Gershon, AJ Friedhoff (eds): Psychopathology and Brain Dysfunction. New York, Raven Press, 1977

161. Anderman F, Robb JP: Absence status: A reappraisal following review of thirty eight patients. Epilepsia 13:177-189, 1972

162. Niedermeyer E, Khalifeh R: Petit mal status ("spike-wave stupor"). Epilepsia 6:250-262, 1965

163. Goldman JW, Glatstein G, Adams AH: Adult onset absence status: A report of six cases. Clin Electroenceph 12:199-204, 1981

164. Anderson RL, Vanderspek HG: Psychomotor variant status epilepticus. Clin Electroenceph 5:129-132, 1974

165. Wells CE: Transient ictal psychosis. Arch Gen Psych 32:1201-1203, 1975

166. Weissberg MP: A case of petit mal status: A diagnostic dilemma. Am J Psych 132:1200-1201, 1975

167. Jovanovic UJ: Psychomotor Epilepsy: A Polydimensional Study. Springfield, IL, Charles C Thomas, 1974

168. Waxman SG, Geschwind N: The interictal behavior syndrome of temporal lobe epilepsy. Arch Gen Psych 32:1580-1586, 1975

169. Geschwind N, Shader, RI, Bear D, et al: Behavioral changes with temporal lobe epilepsy: Assessment and treatment. J Clin Psych 41:89-95, 1980

170. Lutz EG: Electroencephalography in psychiatry. Front Psych 12:13-14, 1982

171. Currie S, Heathfield JWG, Henson RA, et al: Clinical course and prognosis of temporal lobe epilepsy. A survey of 666 patients. Brain 94:173-190, 1971

172. Davies RK, Neil JF, Himmelhoch JM: Cerebral dysrhythmias in schizophrenics receiving phenothiazines: Clinical correlates. Clin Electroenceph 6:103-
115, 1975
173. Neil JF, Merikangas JR, Davies RK, et al: Validity and clinical utility of
neuroleptic-facilitated electroencephalography in psychotic patients. Clin
Electroenceph 9:38-48, 1978
174. Struve FA: Paroxysmal EEG dysrhythmias in psychiatric patients—do they
indicate vulnerability to side effects? Presented at the Third World Congress
of Biological Psychiatry, Stockholm, June 28-July 3, 1981
175. Itil TM, Soldatos C: Epileptogenic side effects of psychotropic drugs. JAMA
344:1460-1463, 1980
176. Rifkin A, Quitkin F, Kane J, et al: Are prophylactic antiparkinson drugs
necessary? A controlled study of procyclidine withdrawal. Arch Gen Psych
35:483-489, 1978
177. Struve FA, Ramsey PP, Willner AE, et al: Neuropsychological and electroencephalographic correlates of neuroleptic induced involuntary movements:
Implications for tardive dyskinesia. In RN Malatesha, LC Hartlage (eds):
Neuropsychology and Cognition, Vol. 2. The Hague, Martinus Nijhoff, 1982
178. Fader BW, Struve FA: The possible value of the electroencephalogram in
detecting subclinical hypothyroidism associated with agitated depression:
A case study. Clin Electroenceph 3:94-101, 1972
179. Muniz C, Forman AJ, Wilder BJ, et al: Lithium toxicity with low serum
levels: Report of a case. Clin Electroenceph 7:31-34, 1976
180. Wilder BJ: Drug action and correlation with blood levels in the EEG. Clin
Electroenceph 5:160-171, 1974
181. Monore RR: Episodic behavioral disorders—schizophrenia or epilepsy. Arch
Gen Psych 1:205-214, 1959
182. Monroe RR, Mickel W: Alpha chloralose—activated electroencephalograms
in psychiatric patients. J Nerv Ment Dis 144:59-68, 1967
183. Monroe R: Episodic Behavior Disorders: A Psychodynamic and Neurophysiologic Analysis. Cambridge, Harvard Universtiy Press, 1970
184. Mark V, Ervin F: Violence and The Brain. New York, Harper & Row, 1970
185. Maletzky BM: The episodic dyscontrol syndrome. Dis Nerv Syst 34:178-185,
1973
186. Stevens J, Milstein V: Severe psychiatric disorders of childhood: Electroencephalogram and clinical correlates. Am J Dis Child 120:182-192, 1970
187. Bach-y-Rita G, Lion JR, et al: Episodic dyscontrol: A study of 130 violent
patients. Am J Psych 127:1473-1478, 1971
188. Struve FA, Saraf KR, Arkos RS, et al: Relationship between paroxysmal
electroencephalographic dysrhythmia and suicide ideation and attempts in
psychiatric patients. In C Shagass, S Gershon, AJ Friedhoff (eds): Psychopathology and Brain Dysfunction, New York, Raven Press, 1977
189. Andrulonis PA, Donnelly J, Glueck BC, et al: Preliminary data on ethosuxi-
mide and the episodic dyscontrol syndrome. Am J Psych 247:1455-1456,
1980
190. Monroe RR: Neurophysiologic evidence for a "third" psychosis. In C Perris,
G Struve, B Jansson (eds): Developments in Psychiatry, Vol. 5. Biological
Psychiatry 1981. Amsterdam, Elsevier, 1981
191. Monroe RR: Episodic dyscontrol. In C Perris, G Struve, B Jansson (eds):
Developments in Psychiatry, Vol. 5. Biological Psychiatry 1981. Amsterdam,
Elsevier, 1981

192. Elliott FA: Episodic dyscontrol: Neurological findings. IN C Perris, G Struwe, B Jansson (eds): Developments in Psychiatry, Vol. 5. Biological Psychiatry 1981. Amsterdam, Elsevier, 1981

193. Kellaway P, Crawley JW, Kagawa N: Paroxysmal pain and autonomic disturbances of cerebral origin: A specific electro-clinical syndrome. Epilepsia 1:466-483, 1960

194. Hughes JR, Means ED, Stell BS: A controlled study on the behavior disorders associated with the positive spike phenomenon. Electroenceph Clin Neurophysiol 18:349-353, 1965

195. Struve FA, Feigenbaum ZS, Farnum CD: Prediction of 14 & 6/sec. positive spikes in EEGs of psychiatric patients. Clin Electroenceph 3:60-64, 1972

196. Struve FA, Ramsey PP: Concerning the 14 & 6 per second positive spike cases in post traumatic medical-legal EEGs reported by Gibbs and Gibbs: A stastical commentary. Clin Electroenceph 8:203-205, 1977

197. Koshino Y, Niedermeyer E: The clinical significance of small sharp spikes in the electroencephalogram. Clin Electroenceph 6:131-140, 1975

198. Fois A, Lippi A: Nonictal symptoms associated with severe electroencephalographic epileptiform abnormalities. Clin Electroenceph 1:22-31, 1970

199. Small JG, Small IF, Milstein V: Familial associations with EEG variants in manic-depressive disease. Arch Gen Psych 32:43-48, 1975

200. Hughes JR, Cayaffa JJ: Is the "psychomotor variant—rhythmic mid temporal discharge" an ictal pattern? Clin Electroenceph 4:42-52, 1973

201. Struve FA, Becka DR, Klein DF: The relationship of the B-Mitten pattern to process and reactive schizophrenia: A replication. Arch Gen Psych 26:189-192, 1972

202. Struve FA, Klein DF: Diagnostic implications of the B-Mitten EEG pattern: Relationship to primary and secondary affective dysregulation. Biol Psych 11:599-611, 1976

203. Slater E: Diagnosis of "hysteria." Brit Med J 1:1395-1399, 1965

204. Koranyi EK: Morbidity and rate of undiagnosed physical illness in a psychiatric clinic population. Arch Gen Psych 36:414-419, 1979

205. Hall RCW, Popkin MK, Devaul RA, et al: Physical illness presenting as psychiatric disease. Arch Gen Psych 35:1315-1320, 1978

206. Hall RCW, Gardner ER, Stickney SK, et al: Physical illness manifesting as psychiatric disease II. Analysis of a state hospital inpatient population. Arch Gen Psych 37:989-995, 1980

207. Tucker GJ, Detre T, Harrow M, et al: Behavior and symptoms of psychiatric patients and the electroencephalogram. Arch Gen Psych 12:278-286, 1965

208. Gibbs FA, Novick RG: Electroencephalographic findings among adult patients in a private psychiatric hospital. Clin Electroenceph 8:79-88, 1977

209. Struve FA: EEG findings detected in routine screening of psychiatric patients —relationship to prior expectation of positive results. Clin Electroenceph 8:47-50, 1977

210. Struve FA: Utilization of clinical electroencephalographic assessment in the psychiatric hospital: Considerations concerning the issue of routine screening versus selective physician referral. J Psychiatr Treat Eval 2:55-62, 1980

211. American Electroencephalographic Society Guidelines, in EEG—1976. American Electroencephalographic Society, 1976

212. Struve FA, Pike LE: Routine admission electroencephalograms of adolescent and adult psychiatric patients awake and asleep. Clin Electroenceph 5:67-72, 1974

213. Gibbs FA, Gibbs EL: How much do sleep recordings contribute to the detection of seizure activity. Clin Electroenceph 2:169-172, 1971

214. Mattson RH, Pratt KL, Calverley JR: Electroencephalograms of epileptics following sleep deprivation. Arch Neurol 13:310-315, 1965

215. Bancaud J: EEG activation by metrazol and magimide in the diagnosis of epilepsy. In A Rémond (ed): Handbook of Electroencephalography and Clinical Neurophysiology, Vol. 3D. Amsterdam, Elsevier, 1976

216. Small JG, Stevens JR, Milstein V: Electro-clinical correlates of emotional activation of the electroencephalogram. J Nerv Ment Dis 138:146-155, 1964

217. Simon R, DiVito H: Alcohol activation of electroencephalographic abnormalities in persons with a history of violence precipitated by drinking alcoholic beverages. Clin Electroenceph 7:145-148, 1976

218. Dejesus PV, Masland WS: The role of nasopharyngeal electrodes in clinical electroencephalography. Neurol 20:869-878, 1970

219. Binnie CD, MacGillivray BB, Osselton JW: Electrodes and their use. In A Rémond (ed): Handbook of Electroencephalography and Clinical Neurophysiology, Vol. 3C. Amsterdam, Elsevier, 1976

220. Struve FA, Feigenbaum ZS: Experience with nasopharyngeal electrode recording with psychiatric patients: A clinical note. Clin Electroenceph 12: 84-88, 1981

CHAPTER 2

Sleep Electroencencephalography

ISMET KARACAN and ROBERT L. WILLIAMS

INTRODUCTION

In the past fifty years, sleep electroencephalography has emerged as a promising method for diagnosis in psychiatry, for permitting the diagnostician to distinguish between insomnias of anxiety and insomnias of drug abuse, between the excessive sleepiness of depression and that of separate clinical entities like sleep apnea, or, more generally, between sleep complaints of physiological and psychological origins. Beyond these distinctions, sleep electroencephalography has contributed to our conception of sleep; through EEG research we have abandoned the notion of sleep as a period of mental and physical inactivity and replaced it with a picture of sleep as a vital component of our circadian and ultradian rhythms.

Handbook of Psychiatric Diagnostic Procedures, vol. 2, edited by R. C. W. Hall and T. P. Beresford. Copyright © 1985 by Spectrum Publications, Inc.

HISTORY

The development of electroencephalography as a clinical aid began with certain neurological discoveries regarding sleep. Gayet in France [1] and Mauthner in Austria [2] were the first to suggest an association between "lethargic syndrome" (hypersomnia) and lesions in the mesencephalon. Evidence of the brain's role in sleep was provided by von Economo [3] who, during a world-wide encephalitis epidemic, associated hypersomnia and insomnia with separate sites of encephalitic brain degeneration.

A parallel series of discoveries yielded the means for exploring the neurological aspect of sleep. In studies that were dismissed by contemporaries as mere curiosities, Caton [4] found currents in electrodes that had been placed on the heads of monkeys; Ladd [5] attained similar results with human subjects. But it was a psychiatrist, Hans Berger [6], who realized the potential of these discoveries in his 1924 experiments, which demonstrated that the brain's electrical activities originate in the neurons, that those currents respond to sensory stimulation, and that epileptic seizures produce abnormal brain activity.

With the gradual acceptance of Berger's work, EEG analysis gathered momentum. Loomis et al [7], citing their results from full-night EEG monitoring sessions, stated that sleep consists of five stages (which they labelled A-E), distinguishable by amplitude and frequency of the electrical activity involved. Their descriptions have remained valid with only minor modifications. In 1935 Gibbs et al [8] showed the clinical applicability of electroencephalography by providing the first EEG descriptions of narcoleptic patients. Through these studies researchers began to develop ideas of normative and deviant EEG patterns.

The new method was soon applied to psychiatric patients. Diaz-Guerrero et al [9] conducted sleep experiments on manic-depressives and depressed patients, and their findings inaugurated the long historical association between sleep electroencephalography and psychiatry.

The discovery of the rapid eye movement (REM) stage of sleep by Aserinsky and Kleitman [10] was the next major breakthrough in sleep research. REM, it was demonstrated, is linked to tachycardia and variability of heart rate, increased respiration, nocturnal penile tumescence, and the dream process. Dement [11] augmented their discoveries by experiments which suggested the human "need" for REM sleep: following nights of REM sleep deprivation, subjects exhibited higher percentages of the REM stage. Additional research [12-14] has since shown REM to be a period of heightened brain activity, almost a third mode of consciousness (separate from both waking and non-REM sleep), an essential component in the sleep of all mammals and a possible factor in the memory processes.

In 1965 Oswald and Priest [15] expanded the clinical potential of electro-encephalography by conducting sleep evaluations of the effects of sleeping pills. And in the late 1960s and 1970s, further efforts were made to utilize sleep electro-encephalography as a diagnostic tool. We conducted a study at the University of Florida College of Medicine (1959–1972) to establish normative values for sleep EEG-EOG variables in individuals aged 3–79 years and published our results in 1974 [16]. The *Manual of Standardized Terminology, Technique, and Scoring System for Sleep Stages of Human Subjects* [17] was another attempt to establish guidelines for the scoring of sleep recordings in adults.

Thus, since the early 1900s, electroencephalographic research and the revision of our paradigm of the sleep process have been fast-growing and related entities. With continued EEG study we move closer to a comprehensive theory of sleep, and as data on both normal and abnormal sleep increase, the relevance of sleep EEG research becomes more apparent.

METHOD

Evaluation of Sleep Complaints Outside the Sleep Clinic

The function of both non-EEG and EEG evaluations in sleep complaints is to obtain an accurate picture of the complaint, to document physiologic and psychologic concomitants, and to isolate individual components. The diagnostician initiates this process by obtaining as much information as possible regarding the patient's sleep complaints and sleep history by clinical interviews and sleep questionnaires. Topics to be covered include:

1. The primary sleep complaint, its onset, and the events surrounding its onset.
2. History of the patient's method of dealing with the complaint, including past medications, therapies, etc.
3. Scrutiny of the patient's daily work and social habits, including use of alcohol, drugs and caffeine.
4. History of the patient's sleep habits and sleep hygiene.
5. Detailed description of any related sleep complaints, such as allergies, respiratory difficulties, postsleep headaches, and muscular paralysis at sleep/wake transitions.

Sleep diaries which record (over a period of two weeks to one month) the details of each night's sleep, as well as pertinent circumstances of the previous day, may be illuminating; often a diary provides more objective assessment of existing sleep patterns than do the patient's own highly generalized accounts of an "average night's sleep." Similarly, interviews with the patient's bed partner often yield significant information regarding sleep-induced phenomena like snoring, leg-movement, and sleep walking, of which the patient is usually unaware.

General psychological instruments, such as the Minnesota Multiphasic Personality Inventory [18], the Profile of Mood States [19] or the State-Trait Anxiety Inventory [20], should be applied, particularly if the examining psychiatrist detects possible signs of psychopathology as the source of sleep difficulties. Depressives, for example, especially depressed children and young adults, tend to use napping as a form of avoidance; accordingly, recognition of depressive tendencies in a case of excessive sleepiness would be a major diagnostic step.

A meticulous physical examination is also mandatory. Neurologic, endocrine, or allergic disorders may be at fault, while conditions such as respiratory difficulties, high blood pressure, obesity, or generally poor physical condition may be part of the etiology or a symptom of the sleep disorder.

Through these measures the psychiatrist may be able to arrive at a satisfactory diagnosis. If, for example, questionnaires reveal that excessive caffeine intake may be related to insomnia, then moderation or abstinence may be prescribed and regular follow-up examinations performed. However, if the sleep disorder is chronic and serious insofar as it interferes with normal activity, if it is clearly not secondary to or symptomatic of a physical disorder, use of medication, an identifiable psychiatric disorder, gross pathologies such as disease, drugs, psychosis, or jet-lag; and if rigorous efforts to control the problem by drugs, improved sleep hygiene, or relaxation therapy have failed, then we advise the diagnostician to refer the patient for sleep laboratory studies. In the event of this step, the preliminary work of the psychiatrist will be helpful in establishing how the sleep tests are conducted and which variables will be monitored.

The Sleep Electroencephalography Examination

The sleep EEG is conducted in a laboratory room controlled for sound, illumination, temperature, and humidity, and equipped with a comfortable bed and lavoratory for the patient's convenience. The sleep clinic provides optimum sleeping conditions for the patient.

Patients must be prepared for the evaluation. If daily naps are uncommon for the patient, the clinician should request that naps (particularly afternoon naps) be avoided, because they may delay sleep onset or affect the architecture of nighttime sleep. Alcohol, drugs (especially psychoactive drugs) and excessive caffeine are similarly to be avoided if they are not a regular habit. However, if usage of these substances is routine, it should be maintained so that its effect on sleep habits can be monitored; the clinician may desire subsequent sleep EEGs, without the drugs, for purposes of comparison. Finally, the patient must be thoroughly briefed regarding the laboratory procedure, in order that the tests may be run as smoothly as possible.

Electroencephalography is only one part of the broader evaluation method of polysomnography, in which a number of physiologic variables of sleep are recorded simultaneously on a continuous single sheet of polygraphic paper. In all cases it is necessary to monitor the electroencephalogram, the electro-oculogram and the chin electromyogram [21]. Electroencephalography records the brain's electrical activity. The electro-oculogram (EOG) detects the presence of rapid eye movements. The electromyogram (EMG), which is recorded from three electrodes placed on the patient's chin, evaluates muscle tone, which differs in REM and non-REM (NREM) sleep.

The problem may further require that the sleep clinician also measure respiration and limb movements. These variables may be monitored on a single channel each on the first night to see if disturbances of either are concomitant with disturbed sleep: if not, then both channels may be disregarded on later nights. If this relationship is seen, the clinician may observe them more closely on the second and third night. Respiratory effort is measured by a strain gauge placed around the patient's chest, while airflow is monitored by thermistors placed next to the mouth and nostrils [22]. Two electrodes placed on the anterior tibialis muscle record limb movement [23].

Although male erectile dysfunction is not a sleep complaint, it may be evaluated by means of polysomnography that includes monitoring nocturnal penile tumescence (NPT) [24-27]. This procedure distinguishes between psychogenic and organic impotence by isolating individual factors in the dysfunction.

Prior to sleep evaluation, erectile dysfunction patients are subjected to the same physical and psychological examinations as dyssomnia patients; in addition, they receive special vascular, neural, and neuromuscular tests to check for physiologic dysfunctions. NPT is then measured on three successive nights. Mercury-filled, high accuracy strain gauges connected by lead wires to a polygraph amplifier are placed just beneath the corona of the penis and at the base. Measurements of the flaccid penile circumference are taken and then used as baselines for sleep-induced erections. At the moment of maximum estimated NPT, the patient is awakened; his penis is photographed and then measured for rigidity. The patient is asked to evaluate the erection according to his own subjective estimate of his erection potential (thus, some measure of the patient's reliability as a judge is obtained). As a final measure, all NPT evaluations include EEG and EOG measures to determine whether erectile dysfunctions are a result of sleep disorder.

Scoring of the polysomnographic records involves an arbitrarily designated unit of time called an "epoch" [28]. One page of polygraph recording paper (300 mm) forms a convenient unit, and recommended paper speeds of 10 and 15 mm/

second result in epochs of 30 and 20 seconds, respectively. In addition to consistent units of scoring time, EEG scorers must have artifact-free calibration records with which to compare patient records. Trained scorers must have better than 95% agreement in compiling these calibration records. To expedite interpretation, all channels are recorded on a continuous single sheet of polygraphic paper.

The core of variables which sleep clinicians may examine can be divided into four categories:

1. Overall Sleep Quantity
   a. Time in Bed (TIB)—measured from the time the subject is settled in bed until the polygraph is turned off in the morning.
   b. Sleep Period Time (SPT)—TIB minus the time it took to fall asleep and the time the subject lay awake in the morning.
   c. Total Sleep Time (TST)—SPT minus any time spent awake after initial sleep onset.
2. Sleep Initiation—chiefly, sleep onset latency, measured from the time the lights are out to the time of initial sleep onset.
3. Sleep Maintenance
   a. Number of awakenings, amount of awake time.
   b. Number of stage shifts.
   c. Sleep efficiency index—calculated by dividing TST by the TIB.
4. Sleep Architecture
   a. Percentage of each sleep stage—can be calculated from TST, but, more frequently calculated from SPT so that waking periods can be assigned a percentage value.
   b. Number of REM periods, length of REM periods, REM cycle (time from beginning of one REM to the beginning of the next), REM interval (time from the end of one REM to the beginning of the next), and REM density (number of actual eye movements within a brief segment of REM.)

Following each night of polygraphic recording the patient is asked to evaluate the quality of his sleep. If subjective reports of refreshing sleep do not conform to normative data (as is sometime the case), they will at least give the diagnostician some idea of what the patient *does* find adequate (and after all, the ultimate measure of sleep is whether or not it satisfies and refreshes the individual); if the patient reports troubled sleep, the diagnostician will have specific complaints to correlate to the EEG findings.

Furthermore, patients should be followed during the course of any treatment (e.g. drugs, recommended improvements of sleep hygiene) to determine whether these treatments have had any effect. Results at the treatment stage can confirm or refute previous diagnoses.

NORMATIVE DATA

Sleep variable norms for males and females of all ages must be available, because sleep patterns undergo drastic alterations within an 80 year lifespan. In the following sections a summary analysis of an average night's sleep is presented and the patterns of sleep, read by age and sex, are described. For a fuller picture of available norms we suggest that the clinician examine the results of the University of Florida study, in *Electroencephalography of Human Sleep: Clinical Applications* [16].

Sleep Stages and Their Characteristics

As noted earlier, the five-stage descriptions of Loomis et al have, with only slight modification, continued to be used in sleep medicine. These stages, along with their most characteristic EEG wave form, may be summarized as follows:

Stage 0 (Wakefulness)—EEG contains alpha and/or low-voltage mixed-frequency activity.
Stage 1—Relatively low-voltage, mixed-frequency EEG without REMs; slow eye movements are often present; vertex sharp waves may be seen; EMG activity is not suppressed.
Stage 2—12-14 cycles per second (cps) sleep spindles and K-complexes on a background of relatively low-voltage, mixed-frequency EEG activity.
Stage 3—Moderate amounts (20-50%) of high-amplitude (75 μV or greater) slow-wave (delta) activity.
Stage 4—Predominance (above 50%) of high-amplitude delta activity.
REM—Stage 1 EEG features with bursts of REM.

The cycle of these stages seems well-established within the eight-hour sleep period, just as the sleep period itself seems consistently rooted in the 24 hour circadian rhythm. On each night the average adult has 4-6 cycles; the first sequence is: waking, stage 1, stage 2, stage 3, stage 4, stage 3, stage 2, REM. Each cycle that follows differs only slightly: REM, stage 1, stage 2, stage 3, stage 4, stage 3, stage 2. Measuring each cycle from the beginning of one REM to the beginning of the next (the REM cycle), we find an average cycle length of 90 minutes, although the contents of those cycles do tend to change slightly during the course of a night's sleep. Early in the sleep period, slow-wave sleep constitutes the largest portion of the cycle, but in the later cycles it may be greatly diminished or even absent. Furthermore, the duration of REM periods tends to lengthen in later cycles; young adults go from initial REM periods of 15 minutes to periods of 45-minute REMs in their third and fourth cycles.

The chief physiologic distinctions between NREM and REM sleep are in brain activity, body motility, and autonomic activation. When a healthy person passes from waking to NREM (at the moment of "disengagement"), that moment can usually be pinpointed within a few seconds of accuracy on the polygraphic chart by the appearance of NREM's slower frequency brain waves. Progression from stage 1 to stage 4 is characterized by a synchronization and slowing of EEG wave activity. Stages 1 and 2 exhibit a fair degree of body movement and muscle tone, but stage 4 is considered to have the lowest level of physiological, neurological and psychological activity, as well as the highest threshold for arousal, of any stage. In sum, stage 4 bears the closest resemblance to the archaic concept of sleep as a period of "shutdown" (although some endocrine changes such as the increased secretion of growth hormones occur predominantly in this stage).

In contrast, REM sleep can be described as an intensely active brain in a paralyzed body. Its physiologic characteristics include autonomic activation, enhanced dream recall, decreased body motility, and episodes of nocturnal penile tumescence.

The phasic activity which gives the REM period its name is not the only form of autonomic activity present. Muscle twitches may occur, as well as sporadic changes in cardiac and respiratory rates. Concurrently, the brain becomes intensely if irregularly aroused. For these reasons, REM is sometimes referred to as "desynchronized" sleep.

Secondly, dream recall is greatest when test subjects are awakened during REM sleep. The exact reason for this is unknown, but researchers have long suspected some elusive connection between REM, dreaming, and the memory process.

Loss of muscle tone occurs in REM. Because loss of muscle tone begins immediately following REM onset, EMG readings are a reliable guide to REM onset (although not as reliable as observation of eye movements). Tendon and respiratory reflexes as well as voluntary actions appear blocked in this period.

In physiologically healthy males, episodes of nocturnal penile tumescence (NPT) regularly coincide with REM sleep (females undergo a corresponding genital tumescence, but its measurement is exceedingly difficult) [26]. Recurring in cycles of approximately 90 minutes (from the beginning of one NPT episode to the beginning of the next), the NPT episodes last more than 30 minutes each. Penile circumference and rigidity tend to increase in each successive cycle. Since NPT seems to be altered only by physiologic factors such as vascular insufficiency, NPT monitoring provides a reliable method for distinguishing organic from psychogenic impotence, and for subsequently selecting a treatment course (surgical, psychological, behavioral, etc.) for the impotent patient.

Sleep and Age

Normative sleep data, when analyzed according to age and sex, reveal that in the aging process there is a progressive change in sleep patterns. This relationship can be illustrated by an age-by-age tracing of the percentage of sleep stages for both males and females (Table 1).

Stages 3 and 4 diminish more than the other sleep stages as age advances; in men aged 70-79, stage 4 is totally absent. REM sleep also diminishes somewhat with age.

Other variables in the sleep patterns change with age, as shown in Table 2. Total Sleep Time and the Sleep Efficiency Index both decrease throughout the 79 year lifespan. Concurrently, the number of awakenings slowly increases.

SLEEP PATHOLOGIES

From the variety of sleep complaints and their etiologies, four fundamental categories have been described: disorders of initiating and maintaining sleep (DIMS, or insomnia), disorders of excessive sleep (DOES, or hypersomnia), disorders of the sleep/wake schedule, and dysfunctions associated with sleep, sleep stages, or partial arousals (parasomnias). For a more comprehensive nosology, the reader may refer

Table 1. Percentage of Sleep Stages by Age and Sex

Age and sex group	Percent of sleep stage					
	Awake	1	2	3	4	REM
40–49						
M	6.29	7.56	54.75	5.37	3.18	22.85
F	1.63	5.64	54.01	7.51	4.54	26.67
50–59						
M	4.33	7.56	61.71	3.23	1.69	21.48
F	4.96	4.85	57.80	6.49	4.14	21.77
60–69						
M	7.73	9.73	56.79	2.06	0.60	23.09
F	8.93	7.69	54.78	4.50	2.67	21.43
70–79						
M	16.00	9.47	55.49	1.36	0.00	17.68
F	11.69	6.59	52.22	6.30	3.74	19.46

Table 2. Sleep Variables by Age and Sex

Age and sex group	Time in bed (minutes)	Variable			
		Total sleep time	Sleep efficiency index	Number of stages	Number of awakenings
3-5					
M	633.40	610.55	0.96	32.10	1.25
F	604.00	576.45	0.96	35.91	1.68
6-9					
M	589.75	572.88	0.97	30.96	0.67
F	609.65	588.75	0.97	32.10	0.90
10-12					
M	585.00	557.50	0.95	38.23	1.58
F	589.50	562.23	0.95	31.00	1.18
13-15					
M	510.60	488.80	0.96	46.35	3.20
F	502.10	480.40	0.96	39.80	1.90
16-19					
M	475.23	448.62	0.94	36.38	2.81
F	479.60	454.80	0.95	34.40	1.70
20-29					
M	442.23	419.27	0.95	40.91	3.05
F	445.65	429.95	0.96	33.60	1.10
30-39					
M	434.55	421.45	0.97	38.65	2.50
F	443.65	425.70	0.96	32.25	1.40
40-49					
M	429.10	389.10	0.91	40.30	4.65
F	441.45	425.18	0.96	41.00	3.09
50-59					
M	442.58	389.79	0.92	34.88	5.67
F	466.73	430.77	0.93	40.50	4.64
60-69					
M	451.55	407.30	0.90	42.00	7.55
F	465.68	404.95	0.87	40.50	4.36
70-79					
M	493.09	372.86	0.77	40.82	7.09
F	507.05	413.55	0.82	56.10	8.35

to the Association of Sleep Disorders Centers' "Diagnostic Classification of Sleep and Arousal Disorders [29].

Disorders of Initiating and Maintaining Sleep

Until recently, insomnia was rather loosely defined as any inability to obtain normal sleep. Experience has shown that it is preferable to distinguish between primary or idiopathic insomnias, which may be defined as a chronic or subacute inability to obtain adequate sleep, without accompanying gross physical or psychological pathologies, and secondary or symptomatic insomnias, in which sleep complaints can be linked to separate physical or psychological pathologies. Secondary insomnia is by far the more prevalent of the two.

The first type of secondary DIMS, that of psychophysiologic origin, may be divided into transient and persistent types. A transient disorder is characterized by a brief period (less than three weeks) of sleep disturbance, usually provoked by distress of conflict caused by loss or perceived threat. Possible causes of transient insomnia include death of a loved one, divorce, crisis at work, or sleeping in an unfamiliar sleeping environment. DIMS are apt to follow these traumas or dislocations, and for this reason are relatively simple to diagnose.

Should DIMS persist beyond three weeks without the accompaniment of drug usage or gross pathologies, then the condition might be diagnosed as persistent psychophysiologic insomnia. The syndrome may develop as a result of chronic tension, anxiety and/or negative conditioning to sleep. Muscle activity in such patients tends to be high and pulse rates rapid; in EEG recordings, alpha waves are frequent. The patient may have repeated awakenings and anxious dreams. People with persistent idiopathic insomnia often sleep well on vacation or in sleep laboratories, or, in general, whenever the conditioned factors of poor sleep or the pressures of work are absent. They may occasionally demonstrate atypical EEG readings (such as the appearance of stage 2 sleep spindles in REM sleep), but anomalies of this type disappear with the advent of improved sleep. When negative sleep conditioning (e.g., learning to associate one's bedroom, bedclothes, or sleep preparations with the anguish of coming insomnia) is a relatively more important factor than actual stress situations, slow-wave and REM sleep maintain normal proportions.

The diagnostician must be cautious when labelling psychological conditions of stress, anxiety, and depression as causes and sleeplessness as their consequence, for the very opposite is also possible: a few nights without rest may be stress-inducing.

Persistent psychophysiologic insomnia may be treated by a combination of the following:

1. Prescription of hypnotics for brief periods [30].

2. Improved sleep hygiene. This includes maintaining regular arising time (which tends to enforce regular sleep onset time), daily exercise, a quiet, comfortable sleeping environment, avoidance of excessive caffeine or alcohol, allowing proper "unwinding" time before sleep, and cultivating the habit of a light bedtime snack.

3. Relaxation training for relief of tension.

Psychiatric disorders such as psychoses, affective and personality disorders are a second common etiology of secondary insomnia.

Neurotic disorders usually have anxiety at their root; eccentric or compulsive behavior may develop to control anxiety, so that loss of consciousness through sleep may be perceived as the loss of conscious control. For these patients, the clinician should establish at least a three-week correlation between sleep complaints and personality characteristics before venturing the diagnosis. Electroencephalography is likely to reveal sleep fragmentation coupled with reduced slow-wave and REM sleep.

When an affective disorder is obvious, it should be immediately suspected as the source of the sleep disorder. Depressed patients experience restless and unsatisfying sleep, probably as a consequence of awakenings every 60-90 minutes, compounded by shortened REM latency. The most frequent complaint among depressed patients is that of "terminal insomnia," i.e., of premature morning awakenings after which return to sleep is difficult. Bipolar depressives show the same EEG characteristics but are more prone to excessive daytime sleepiness. Manic patients often do not complain about their sleep; rather, their families complain that the manic patient sleeps very little. These patients, although refreshed with rare daytime naps, may sleep no more than 2-4 hours per night. Severely psychotic patients like schizophrenics frequently show progressively delayed sleep onset; sleep may not come until the patient actually collapses from exhaustion. They too may have reduced amounts of slow-wave and REM sleep.

Third, DIMS can also be linked to use of drugs such as hypnotics, sedatives, tranquilizers, alcohol (both chronic and bedtime usage), stimulants, analeptic agents, amphetamines, and excessive caffeine. For diagnosis in any of these cases, the drug must have been used for at least 30 days.

When tranquilizers are involved, DIMS appear because of tolerance or withdrawal [31,32]. While taking the drug, patients have decreased amounts of stages 3/4 and REM, and increased percentage of stage 1/2; stage demarcation may become blurred; stages may change frequently; and spindles, K-complexes, delta waves and REM density may all be reduced. Both 14-18 μHz "pseudo-spindles" and alpha and beta frequencies may increase. Frequent awakenings and progressive delay of sleep onset are also common. During a gradual and supervised withdrawal, both subjective sleep and sleep EEG readings will improve, but in abrupt withdrawal, complete sleep disruption is likely; what little sleep the patient has is mostly concentrated REM, a sleep stage that the tranquilizer has hitherto suppressed.

Stimulants are likely to delay sleep onset, decrease Total Sleep Time, reduce slow-wave and REM sleep, and cause frequent awakenings [33,34]. The classic symptom of an amphetamine-based dyssomnia is the sudden lethargy caused when stimulant effects wear off.

Chronic alcoholics inevitably have complaints of unsatisfying and unrefreshing sleep [35,36]. While drinking persists, stages 3 and 4 are almost completely absent, while REM is disrupted and shortened. Patients undergoing alcohol withdrawal typically demonstrate dramatically prolonged sleep latency and reduced amounts of stages 3/4. However, sleep patterns may return to normal 10-14 days after drinking stops.

Sleep-induced respiratory impairment, or sleep apnea, is more commonly a cause of hypersomnia than insomnia. Nevertheless, the sleep-induced 10+ second cessations of breathing called apneas can result in continuous brief arousals that effectively impair sleep [37].

Nocturnal myoclonus and "restless legs" syndrome are both DIMS in which sleep-initiated muscular (myclonic) contractions in the hip, leg, ankle, and foot are followed by partial arousal or awakenings [38,39]. In nocturnal myoclonus the anterior tibialis EMG shows repeated myoclonic contractions lasting 0.5-10 seconds, with intervals between contractions lasting 20-40 seconds. Episodes are always initiated *in sleep*; the patient is usually not aware of them (although he is aware of unrefreshing sleep); therefore, interviews with bed partners and monitoring of limb movements are essential. Myoclonus occurs primarily among middle-aged and elderly individuals. The "restless legs" syndrome involves, in addition to sleep-initiated leg spasms, the daytime symptom of unpleasant and deep creeping sensations within the calf muscles whenever sitting or lying down, resulting in irresistable urges to move the legs [40,41]. The syndrome is exacerbated by aging and sleep deprivation. Both of these syndromes may also result in excessive daytime sleepiness.

In the absence of accompanying gross physical or psychological pathology, the diagnostician may consider idiopathic or primary insomnia. We conducted a study of idiopathic insomniacs and found their chief sleep characteristics to be longer sleep latency, lower sleep efficiency index, and delayed stage 3 latency [42]. There was some evidence to suggest higher absolute amounts of REM in idiopathic insomniacs than in control groups, but the insomniacs did not exhibit more frequent awakenings or more reduced stage 4 than did control groups. Idiopathic insomniacs must not be confused with individuals who simply require less-than-average sleep time. The latter may have a total sleep time equal to that of the insomniacs but differ insofar as they subjectively report their sleep to be refreshing and adequate.

Disorders of Excessive Sleepiness

In most cases of DOES, the primary symptoms are excessive daytime sleepiness (EDS), irresistable urges to nap, difficulty achieving full arousal after sleep, and decreased cognition and motor performance.

If a condition involving EDS and a tendency to remain in bed for unusually long periods or to return to bed frequently during the day does not persist beyond three weeks, and if that condition can be linked to crisis events like those known to trigger insomnias, then it is diagnosed as transient psychophysiologic hypersomnia. If such a condition persists beyond three weeks, the term "persistent psychophysiologic hypersomnia" is applied. This syndrome is even rarer than its insomnia-related counterpart; it is sometimes found in people who lack a firm sense of purpose or have despairing outlooks, and is marked by a chronic disposition to weariness and napping when the patient is confronting stress-tension or when his coping capacities are overwhelmed [43,44]. All other possible etiologies must be eliminated before this syndrome can be diagnosed.

The chief psychiatric disorders associated with hypersomnias are the affective disorders [45]. Bipolar depressives are especially troubled with excessive sleep; examinations have shown them to have short REM sleep latency, conspicuously reduced amounts of stages 3/4, and subjectively unsatisfying though full-length sleep. As with persistent psychophysiologic hypersomnias, other causes must be ruled out before this diagnosis is possible.

Drug usage is a second major cause of hypersomnias. When central nervous system stimulants like amphetamines or excessife caffeine are involved, the problem arises during withdrawal or with the insidious growth of tolerance. Users of these stimulants may be prepared for the enhanced alertness and performance which the drug provides, but they are unable to cope with the sudden lethargy—either as a series of small sleep attacks or as one major "crash"—when effects of the drug subside. Caffeine too must be suspected, particularly when the patient consumes more than 10 cups of coffee or other caffeinated beverages a day. Diagnosis here is a matter of linking drug habits to sleep disorders.

Central nervous system depressants may also be responsible for excessive somnolence. With intermittent use of depressants we find reduced amounts of REM sleep and increased slow-wave, but among chronic users the amount of both REM and stages 3/4 sleep are diminished.

Another DOES-connected syndrome is sleep apnea, previously mentioned as an occasional cause of insomnia. Apneas are sleep-induced cessations of breathing lasting over 10 seconds. When the episode passes, the patient gasps violently for breath, and consequently suffers a troubled sleep [46]. The three types of apnea are:

1. *Central apnea*—cessation of airflow coupled with cessation of effort.

2. *Upper airway apnea*—cessation of airflow despite continued respiratory effort.
3. *Mixed apnea*—central apnea in the first part of the apneic phase, with renewed respiratory effort in the second part.

In addition to the EDS caused by unsatisfying nocturnal sleep, apneic victims are likely to display a series of secondary symptoms. Abnormal motor activity may occur following the apnea attacks as part of the arousal response; questioning of the patient's bed partner is helpful in this matter. In addition to the apneic attacks, these patients may exhibit a number of daytime symptoms. The patient may experience intellectual decline manifested as loss of wit, humor, and interest. "Automatic behavior syndrome," in which rote chores are performed in a trance-like state and in which initiative or decision-making become impossible, may last from 2 minutes to several hours. Hypnagogic hallucinations, which combine elements of both the real and dream worlds, sometimes occur when the patient is trying to resist sleep attacks. Finally, the patient may experience personality changes (trends toward moodiness and irritability), sexual impairment (decreased libido, impotence, or inability to reach orgasm) and morning headaches which dissipate hours after waking but return following daytime naps.

Laboratory studies reveal that apneic patients have troubled sleep, and their sleep stages are often hard to identify. Apneic episodes usually occur very shortly after sleep onset; in such episodes high-amplitude slow waves develop rapidly (concurrent with sudden chin muscle inhibition) and though sleep spindles are rare, K-complexes occur rather frequently toward the end of NREM sleep apneic phases. Slow-waves are seldom seen. When normal breathing resumes, EEG activities change to theta and/or delta waves, or slow apnea waves resembling those of stage REM. Patients are hard to arouse during apneic episodes, even with painful stimulation.

Narcolepsy, first described by Gelineau in 1880 [47], is now thought to affect 0.03-0.06% of the world's population [48]. Its primary symptoms are the irresistable daytime sleep attacks lasting from 30 seconds to 5-20 minutes (the average is 2-5 minutes) [49]. Attacks vary in number from one to 200 daily. If troubled only with sleep attacks, the patient is diagnosed as monosymptomatic narcoleptic, a group that constitutes 25-30% of all narcoleptic cases. Polysymptomatic narcolepsy involves the secondary daytime symptoms of cataplexy (sudden loss of muscle tone for 5-10 minutes), sleep paralysis (1-10-minute attacks of partial or complete paralysis during sleep-wake transitions), hypnagogic hallucinations, and abnormal, sleep-induced autonomic behavior.

Narcolepsy may be further categorized as idiopathic, in which the disease seems an entity in itself, or symptomatic, in which it is connected with some form of organic brain damage like encephalitis, tumors, or concussions. Secondary symptoms tend to be higher among idiopathic cases, particularly with respect to cataplexy (idiopathic—65-70%; symptomatic—39.2%).

Sleep research has revealed other characteristics of narcolepsy. The most universally acknowledged finding in narcoleptic patients is almost immediate appearance of REM following sleep onset (called "sleep onset REM"), as opposed to the 90 minute REM latency of normal subjects [50-52]. Narcoleptic patients have troubled sleep, with frequent long awakenings and body movements, together with decreased sleep time, decreased slow-wave sleep, and increased amounts of stages 1 and 2, although in most cases there is no substantial REM expansion.

Treatment of narcolepsy usually requires the prescription of stimulants. If cataplexy is present, imipramine is advised.

One noteworthy but rare hypersomnia is the Kleine-Levin syndrome, confined exclusively to adolescent boys. Kleine-Levin cases are marked by hypersomnia, voracious appetites and, less frequently, sexual disinhibition, a craving for sweets following sleep arousal, amnesia during and following attacks, mood swings with depression, euphoria, and weight gain [53,54]. EEG profiles are inconclusive, but there is some evidence that the supposed daytime sleep attacks are not really sleep at all, but merely a form of withdrawal [55-58].

Obesity, hypersomnia and sleep apneas are the prime symptoms of another rare dyssomnia known as the Pickwickian syndrome [59-61]. When EEG evaluation is used for diagnosis, Pickwickians exhibit sleep composed of alternations between apneic phases, EEG arousal (alpha activity or K-complexes), then awakenings. Although Pickwickians may sleep for long periods, those periods are really composed of the apnea, arousal, and awakening cycle.

Disorders of the Sleep-Wake Schedule

As noted previously, the eight-hour sleep period is firmly established within the 24-hour day. The human sleep-wake schedule is integrated with the external light-dark cycle as well as with a number of internal cycles (such as those of temperature and hormone production) known as circadian rhythms. Despite the overall regularity of circadian rhythms, however, the sleep-wake schedule can be disrupted on both a transient and a persistent basis.

Symptoms of rapid time zone change syndrome (jet lag) are familiar to anyone who has crossed multiple time zones by airplane. By forcing oneself to abide by the hours of a new time zone against the dictates of the internal clock, one incurs extreme fatigue and exhaustion [62]. Jet lag symptoms usually abate after 2 days, and the syndrome itself presents no problem in diagnosis, owing to its clear relationship with the circumstances of jet travel.

A change in work shift may also disrupt the sleep-wake schedule, resulting in hypersomnia, insomnia, decreased mental acumen, irritability, lassitude, and gastrointestinal disturbances. Unlike victims of the jet lag syndrome, however, "work shift" cases frequently fail to adjust because of reversion to normal schedules on weekends. Again, the syndrome is recognizable by its circumstances.

Repeated time zone changes or frequently changing hours can lead to persistent disruption of the sleep-wake schedule [63,64]. These cases suffer all the symptoms of work-shift but are prone to even greater mood changes and diminution of cognitive faculties, and have a tendency to develop peptic ulcer disease within a few years of starting shift-work. One curious finding is that shift-workers who scrupulously maintain their day-sleep schedule on weekends are still prone to suffer, albeit to a lesser degree, from sleep disorders.

In the delayed sleep phase syndrome, the actual time of sleep onset grows later and later, even though the structure and 8-hour duration of sleep is unaltered [65]. Despite unvarying total sleep time, though, the victim begins to lose sleep because work and social activities demand rising at regular hours. EDS soon develops. Delayed sleep phase syndrome can be distinguished from sleep-onset DIMS by the presence of EDS, from psychiatric disturbances by the refreshing nature of sleep when allowed to run its full course, and from transient sleep wake schedule disruptions by its lack of unusual circumstances.

There is also an inverse pathology known as advanced sleep phase syndrome, in which sleep onset advances while total sleep time remains unchanged. Advanced sleep phase syndrome is extremely rare.

A third type of abnormal sleep pattern is the non-24-hour sleep-wake syndrome. The sleep-wake schedule becomes asynchronous with the 24 hour day, and the patient develops a 25 hour schedule. Episodes may be intermittent or continuous, but victims are invariably troubled with insomnia and EDS. Blind people [66] and schizoid personalities seem predisposed to the problem. The treatment for this syndrome is to allow the individual's sleep phase to progress naturally until sleep onset time returns to normal hours, and then to maintain a strict 24-hour schedule.

Finally, there is the possibility of an irregular sleep-wake pattern, in which chaotic and unpredictable sleeping and waking behavior disrupt the regular schedule [67]. Victims of this syndrome are prone to frequent daytime naps at odd hours, excessive bedrest, and blocks of sleep time spread out over the 24-hour day. Meal times begin to lose their regularity. Irregular sleep-wake patterns are distinguishable from transient disruptions by their lack of extenuating circumstances.

Dysfunctions Associated with Sleep, Sleep Stages, or
Partial Arousals (Parasomnias)

The parasomnias are a group of undesirable phenomena either restricted to or exacerbated by sleep. Their etiology evidently involves central nervous system activities transmitted into skeletal muscles or autonomic nervous system channels. Parasomnias provide no great challenge to the diagnostician, since each symptom seems a clinical entity in itself, but in a few cases there may be minor diagnostic confusion.

Sleep-walking (nocturnal somnambulism), for example, is not to be confused with either sleep-related epileptic seizure or sleep drunkenness [68,69]. In a sleep-related epileptic fit, the victim demonstrates no responsiveness to the environment, and is likely to experience automatic behavior like hand-rubbing and swallowing. None of these factors are present in sleep-walking. Sleep drunkenness [70], an inability to achieve complete wakefulness, frequently results in confused and aggressive behavior, while the sleepwalker is never aggressive.

Diagnosticians may separate night terrors (pavor nocturnus) from dream anxiety attacks by examining the patient for dream recollection and by EEG evalua tion [71]. Night terrors, sudden fits of screaming which rouse one from sleep, occur almost exclusively in children of ages 4-12, and their singular characteristic is that although the victims can remember sensations of anxiety and terror, they seldom recall a particular dream sequence. EEG evaluations show that the night-terror process begins early in stages 3 and 4 when delta waves become higher than normal, that respiratory and heart rates slow, and that the duration of the attack is proportional to the length of the preceding slow-wave episode. When screaming begins, heart rate may show a two- to fourfold increase, while the EEG assumes an alpha pattern. In contrast, dream anxiety attacks occur during REM, toward the middle and late third of the night, and in most cases specific dream sequences are remembered.

Writers on nocturnal enuresis, or bed-wetting, traditionally ascribed it to psychological disturbances, especially when clear organic pathologies were absent. Speculation on the nature of those supposed disturbances has been provocative and, at times, outlandish. However, children with idiopathic enuresis exhibit no archetypal personality pattern; nor can idiopathic enuretics be linked to psychopathological features [72]. A good diagnostic approach, therefore, is to look for the following traits of idiopathic enuresis before positing psychological etiologies: increased NREM (the stage when enuresis occurs), heavy sleep, presence of daytime stress, and changes in the sleep-wake schedule. In some cases nocturnal enuresis may be confused with urinary incontinence during an epileptic seizure, but if enuresis occurs without seizure, even among known epileptics, then idiopathic enuresis probably co-exists with the epilepsy.

Other parasomnias include bruxism (teeth-grinding), jactatio capitus nocturnus (head-tossing), sleep talking and painful sleep-induced penile tumescence. The first consideration in treatment of parasomnias is to ensure the patient's safety. Sleep-walkers, for example, must be prevented from injuring themselves. Tricyclics are prescribed for idiopathic enuretics, since they reduce the amount of stage 4 sleep, in which the enuresis occurs. For other parasomnias, benzodiazepines may be prescribed for short periods of time.

THE FUTURE OF THE SLEEP CLINIC IN DIAGNOSTIC PSYCHIATRY

Future applications of the sleep clinic technology depend on both sleep researchers and diagnostic psychiatrists. The former must continue to organize and refine their techniques, while the latter must familiarize themselves with the uses of this new diagnostic method. When psychiatrists use sleep clinics more routinely, sleep researchers will profit from the expanded data bank. The psychiatrist, by having available improved methods of diagnosing sleep complaints and impotency, will gain a better understanding of his patients' pathology.

There is much evidence that sleep clinic methods have become recognized as a useful diagnostic tool. First, the public is caught in the uneasy position of becoming more health- and stress-conscious in a society that is in many ways more *unhealthy* and stressful than ever before. For instance, recent evidence suggests that over 50% of the population has sleep complaints [73]. If diagnosticians are to be responsive to this situation, they must avoid automatic prescription of drugs like hypnotics, amphetamines and barbiturates—a practice which medical [74], governmental [75], and public sectors are now decrying. Instead they must provide more systematic psychophysiologic evaluations. Sleep evaluations may be time-consuming and expensive, but this be balanced against the possibilities of years of persistent discomfort, uncertain diagnoses, drug prescription, and drug dependencies?

Secondly, sleep electroencephalography has an important role in the diagnosis of sexual disorders. In conjunction with NPT evaluations, it can help ascertain the etiology of male impotence. Previous methods had diagnosed over 90% of all impotency cases as psychogenic. Now, however, we can demonstrate and treat physiologic factors in many of these cases.

As an example of what sleep research might offer in the future, clinicians should consider the proposals of Dement, who, in speaking before an international symposium [76], cited the following as uppermost on his discipline's agenda:

—More research concerning normative data; again, information discovered in the course of diagnoses can be helpful either by reinforcing or refuting existing norms.
—More research into sleep pathology.
—Inquiry into the sleep of schizophrenics. Despite a lack of positive evidence, there have long been suspicions regarding some connection between REM, dreams, and hallucinations.

Sleep researchers agree that their primary goal is the establishment of a unified and comprehensive theory of sleep [77,78]. Such a theory will facilitate the tasks of research, diagnosis, and treatment. And finally, we may point to the current record of sleep research as some promise of its capabilities: in only three years we have compiled information regarding over 40 different sleep disorders. The discipline therefore seems to hold the promise of many future contributions.

REFERENCES

1. Gayet M: Affection encéphalique (encéphalite diffuse probable) localisée aux étage superiours des pédoneules cérébraux et aux couches optiques, ainsi qúau plaucher du quatrinième vértricule et aux parois latérales du troisième observation recuellie. Arch. Physiol Brown Séquard 7:341-351, 1875
2. Mauthner L: Pathologie und physilogie des schalfes. Wein Klin Weschr 3:445-446, 1890
3. Von Economo C: Schlafttheorie. Ergebn d Physiol 28:312-339, 1929
4. Caton R: The electric currents of the brain (abstract). Br Med J 2:278, 1875
5. Ladd GT: Contributions to the psychology of visual dreams. Mind 1:299-304, 1892
6. Berger H: Uber das electroenkephalogramm des menschen. Arch Psychiatr Nervenkr 87:527-570, 1929
7. Loomis AL, Harvey EN, Hobart G: Further observations on the potential rhythms of the cerebral cortex during sleep. Science 82:198-200, 1935
8. Gibbs FA, Davis H, Lennox WG: The electroencephalogram in epilepsy and in conditions of impaired consciousness. Arch Neurol Psych 34:1133-1148, 1935
9. Diaz-Guerrero R, Gottlieb JS, Knott JR: The sleep of patients with manic-depressive psychosis, depressive type. An electroencephalographic study. Psychosom Med 8:399-404, 1946
10. Aserinsky E, Kleitman N: Regularly occurring periods of eye motility, and concomitant phenomena during sleep. Science 118:273-274, 1953
11. Dement W: The effect of dream deprivation. Science 131:1705-1707, 1959
12. Hawkins DR, Puryeer HB, Wallace CD, et al: Basal skin resistence during sleep and "dreaming." Science 136:321-322, 1962
13. Jouvet M: Recherches sur los structures nervenses et les mèchanismos responsables des différentes phases des sommeil physiologique. Arch Ital Biol 100: 125-206, 1962
14. Oswald I: Sleep Mechanisms: Recent advances. Proc R Soc Med 55:910-912, 1962
15. Oswald I, Priest R: Five weeks to escape the sleeping pill habit. Br Med J 2: 1093-1095, 1965
16. Williams RL, Karacan I, Hursch CJ: Electroencephalography (EEG) of Human Sleep: Clinical Applications. New York, John Wiley & Sons, 1974
17. Rechtschaffen A, Kales A (eds): A Manual of Standardized Terminology, Techniques and Scoring System for Sleep Stages of Human Subjects. Los Angeles, UCLA, Brain Information Service/Brain Research Institute, 1971
18. Dahlstrom WG, Welsh GS, Dahlstrom LE: An MMPI Handbook, Vol 1: Clinical Interpretation. Minneapolis, University of Minnesota, 1977
19. McNair DM, Larr M, Drappleman LF: Manual for the Profile of Mood States. San Diego, Educational and Industrial Testing Service, 1971
20. Spielberger CD, Gorsuch RL, Lushene RE: STAI Manual for the State-Trait Anxiety Inventory ("Self-Evaluation Questionnaire"). Palo Alto, Consulting Psychologist Press, 1970.

21. Carskadon MA: Basics for polygraphic monitering of sleep. In Guilleminault C (ed): Sleeping and Waking Disorders: Indications and Techniques. Menlo Park, CA, Addison-Wesley 1982

22. Borstein SK: Respiratory monitcring during sleep: Polysomnography. In C Guilleminault (ed): Sleeping and Waking Disorders: Indications and Techniques. Menlo Park, CA, Addison-Wesley, 1982

23. Coleman RM: Periodic movements in sleep (nocturnal myoclonus) and restless legs syndrome. In C Guilleminault (ed): Sleeping and Waking Disorders: Indications and Techniques, Menlo Park, CA, Addison-Wesley, 1982

24. Karacan I: Evaluation of nocturnal penile tumescence and impotence. In C Guilleminault (ed): Sleeping and Waking Disorders: Indications and Techniques. Menlo Park, CA, Addison-Wesley, 1982

25. Karacan I, Aslan C, Williams RL: Diagnostic Evaluation of Male Impotence: Problems and Promises (in press)

26. Karacan I, Salis PJ: Diagnosis and treatment of erectile impotence. Psychiatr Clin North Am 3:97-111, 1980

27. Karacan I, Salis PJ, Williams RL: The role of the sleep laboratory in diagnosis and treatment of impotence. In RL Williams, I Karacan (eds): Sleep Disorders: Diagnosis and Treatment. New York, John Wiley & Sons, 1978

28. Hartsa KM: Manual of Standardized Terminology, Techniques and Scoring System for Sleep Stages of Human Subjects. Bethesda, Md, US Department Of Health, Education and Welfare, 1968

29. Association of Sleep Disorders Centers: Diagnostic classification of sleep and arousal disorders. Sleep 2:5-137, 1979

30. Williams RL, Karacan I: Pharmacology of Sleep. New York, John Wiley & Sons, 1976

31. Kales A, Bixley E, Tan T, et al: Chronic hypnotic drug use: Ineffectiveness, withdrawal insomnia and dependence. JAMA 227:513-517, 1974

32. Kales A, Malinstrom EF, Schorf MB, et al: Psychophysiological and biochemical changes following the use and withdrawal of hypnotics. In A Kales (ed): Sleep: Physiology and Pathology. Philadelphia, JB Lippincott, 1969

33. Bonnett MH, Webb WB, Barned G: Effect of flurazepam, pentobarbital and caffeine on arousal threshold. Sleep 1:271-279

34. Oswald I: Sleep and dependance on amphetamine and other drugs. In: A Kales (ed): Sleep: Phsyiology and Pathology, Philadelphia, JB Lippincott, 1969

35. Gross MM, Goodenough DR, Huston J, et al: Experimental study of sleep in chronic alcoholics before, during and after four days of heavy drinking, with a non-drinking comparison. Ann N Y Acad Sci 215:254-275, 1973

36. Johnson LC, Burdick A, Smith J: Sleep during alcohol intake and withdrawal in the chronic alcoholic. Arch Gen Psych 22:406-418, 1970

37. Guilleminault C, Dement WC: Sleep apnea syndromes and related sleep disorders. In RL Williams, I Karacan (eds): Sleep Disorders: Diagnosis and Treatment. New York, John Wiley & Sons, 1978

38. Coleman RM, Pollack CP, Kokkoris CP, et al: Periodic nocturnal myoclonus in patients with sleep-wake disorders: A case series analysis. In MH Chase, M. Mitler, PL Walter (eds): Sleep Research, Vol 8. Los Angeles, Brain Information Service /Brain Research Institute, UCLA, 1975, p 175

39. Zorick F, Roth T, Salis P, et al: Insomnia and excessive daytime sleepiness as presenting symptoms in nocturnal myoclonus. In MH Chase, M Mitler, PL Walter (eds): Sleep Research, Vol 7. Los Angeles, Brain Information Service/ Brain Research Institute, UCLA, 1978, p 256

40. Exbom RA: Restless legs syndrome. Neurol 10:868-873, 1960
41. Frankel BL, Patten BN, Gillen JC: Restless legs syndrome. Sleep electroencephalographic and neurologic findings. JAMA 230:1302-1303, 1974
42. Karacan I, Williams RL, Salis PJ, et al: New approaches to the evaluation and treatment of insomnia (preliminary results). Psychosom 12:81-88, 1971
43. Hartmann EL: The Functions of Sleep. New Haven, Yale University Press, 1974, pp 123-130
44. Murray EJ: Sleep, Dreams and Arousal. New York, Appleton-Century-Crofts, 1965, pp 257-261
45. Kupfer DJ and Foster FG: The sleep of psychotic patients: Does it all look alike? In DX Freedman (ed): Biology of the Major Psychoses: A Comparative Analysis. New York, Raven Press, 1975
46. Lugaresi E: Snoring and its clinical applications. In C Guilleminault, WC Dement (eds): Sleep Apnea Syndromes, New York, Alan R Liss, 1978
47. Gélineau JBE: De la narcolepsie. Gaz Hop Paris 55:626-628, 635-637, 1880
48. Daniels LE: Narcolepsy. Med 13:1-102, 1934
49. Hishikawa Y, Nan'no H, Taclibana M, et al: The nature of sleep attacks and other symptoms of narcolepsy. Electroencephalogr Clin Neurophysiol 24: 1-10, 1968
50. Roth B: Narcolepsy and hypersomnia. In RL Williams, I Karacan (eds): Sleep Disorders: Diagnosis and Treatment. New York, John Wiley & Sons, 1978
51. Roth B: Narcolepsy and Hypersomnia from the Aspect of the Physiology of Sleep. Prague, Státní Zoravotnické Nakkadatelstuí, 1957, p 331
52. Rechstshaffen A, Wolpert EA, Dement WC, et al: Nocturnal sleep of narcoleptics. Electroenceph Clin Neurophysiol 15:599-609, 1963
53. Critchley M: Periodic hypersomnia and megaphagia in adolescent males. Brain 85:627-657, 1962
54. Critchley M, Hoffman HL: The syndrome of periodic somnolence and morbid hunger (Kleine-Levin syndrome). Br Med J 1:137-139, 1942
55. Garland H, Sumner D, Fourman P: The Kleine-Levin syndrome. Some further observations. Neurol 15:1161-1167, 1965
56. Green LN, Cracco RQ: Klein-Levin syndrome. A case with EEG evidence of periodic brain dysfunction. Arch Neurol 22:166-175, 1970
57. Rosenkotter L, Wende S: EEG-befunda beim Kleine-Levin syndrom. Monatsschr Psychiatry Neurol 130:107-122, 1953
58. Thacore VR, Ahmed M, Oswald I: The EEG in a case of periodic hypersomnia. Electroenceph Clin Neurophysiol 27:605-606, 1969
59. Burwell CS, Robin ED, Whaley RD, et al: Extreme obesity associated with alveolar hypoventilation—a Pickwickian syndrome. Am J Med 21:811-818, 1956
60. Kerr WJ, Lagen JB: The postural syndrome related to obesity leading to postural emphysema and cardiorespiratory failure. Ann Intern Med 10:569-595, 1936
61. Schwartz BA, Seguy M, Escande J-P: Correlations EEG, respiratories oculaires et myographiques dans le "syndrome Pickwickien" et autres affections paraissant apparentees: proposition d'ure hypothese. Rev Neurol (Paris) 117:145-152, 1967
62. McFarland RA: Air travel across time zones. Am Sci 63:23-30, 1975
63. Walsh JK, Stock CG, Tepas DI. The EEG sleep of workers frequently changing shifts. In MH Chase, M Mitler, PL Walter (eds): Sleep Research, Vol 7. Los Angeles, UCLA Brain Information Service /Brain Research Institute, 1978, p 314

64. Weitzmann E, Kripke D, Goldmacher D, et al: Acute reversal of the sleeping-waking cycle in man. Arch Neurol 22:483-489, 1970
65. Weitzman E, Czeisler C, Coleman R, et al: Delayed sleep phase syndrome: A rhythm disorder. In MH Chase, M Mitler, PL Walter (eds): Sleep Research, Vol 8. Los Angeles, UCLA Brain Information Service /Brain Research Institute, 1979, p 221
66. Miles LM, Raynal DM, Wilson MA: Blind man living in normal society has circadian rhythms of 24.9 hours. Science 198:421-423, 1977
67. Hauri P: The Sleep Disorders. Kalamazoo, The Upjohn Company, 1977, pp 22-34
68. Broughton R: Sleep disorders: Disorder of arousal? Science 159:1070-1078, 1968
69. Kales A, Jacobsen A, Paulson MJ, et al: Somnambulism: Psychophysiological correlates. Arch Gen Psych 14:586-594, 1966
70. Roth B, Neusimalova S, Rechtschaffen A: Hypersomnia with "sleep drunkenness." Arch Gen Psych 26:456-462, 1972
71. Fisher CJ, Byrne J, Edwards T, et al: A psychophysiological study of nightmares. J Am Psychoanal Assoc 18:747-782, 1970
72. Williams RL, Karacan I: Sleep disorders and disordered sleep. In MF Reisner (ed): American Handbook of Psychiatry, Vol 4: Organic Disorders and Psychosomatic Medicine. New York, Basic Books, 1975
73. Miles L, Dement W: Sleep and aging. Sleep 3:1-150, 1981
74. Solomon F, White CC, Parron DC, et al: Sleeping pills, insomnia and medical practice. N Engl J Med 300:803-808, 1979
75. US Department of Health, Education and Welfare: A Report to the President on Medical Care Prices. Washington DC, US Government Printing Office, 1967
76. Dement WC: Proposals for future research. In The Experimental Study of Human Sleep: Methodological Problems, Proceedings of International Symposium, Bordolino, Italy, April 3-5, 1974. New York, Elsevier Scientific Publishing Company, 1975
77. Dement WC: Forward. In C Guilleminault (ed): Sleeping and Waking Disorders: Indications and Techniques. Menlo Park, CA, Addison-Wesley, 1982
78. Dement WC, Karacan I: Will sleep research survive the 1980's? In I Karacan (ed): Psychophysiological Aspects of Sleep. Proceedings of the Third International Congress of Sleep Research. Park Ridge, NJ, Noyes Medical Publications, 1981

CHAPTER 3

Identification of Melancholia Using EEG Studies of Sleep

MICHAEL FEINBERG

The Greeks observed depressive illness over 2,000 years ago, named it melancholia, and noted that the sufferers had disturbed sleep. Two millennia later, many investigators have used EEG recordings to study the sleep of depressed patients. Kupfer and Foster have reviewed the literature through 1978 and I will discuss only work published since their excellent review [1].

All research in depression is made more difficult by the myriad of diagnostic schemes used to classify the subtypes of depressive disorder. To make things worse, different diagnostic systems use the same term to describe patient groups which are not identical. Our diagnostic system is described more fully elsewhere in this volume [2]. We use the terms melancholia, endogenous depression (ED), and endogenomorphic depression [3] synonymously to refer to a recurrent, episodic illness with a clear biologic basis. This form of depression is not necessarily identical to "Major Depression with Melancholia" as described in DSM-III [4] or with "Major Depressive Disorder, Endogenous Subtype" as described in the RDC [5], although there is considerable overlap in classification. We contrast endogenous depression with nonendogenous ("neurotic") depression (ND). Other investigators have used one or more of these diagnostic schemes and have also used the primary-secondary distinction promulgated by the St. Louis group [6]. The primary-secondary distinction is not equivalent to the endogenous-nonendogenous distinction [7].

Handbook of Psychiatric Diagnostic Procedures, vol. 2, edited by R. C. W. Hall and T. P. Beresford. Copyright © 1985 by Spectrum Publications, Inc.

We make a further distinction among patients with endogenous depression. Unipolar depressives (UP) are those who have never suffered from mania or hypomania, whereas bipolar depressives (BP) have [8]. The bipolar group is further divided into bipolar I (BP I) patients, who have been manic, and bipolar II (BP II) patients, who have been hypomanic but never manic.

Different investigators use different definitions of crucial sleep variables, and may also collect sleep EEG data differently and score the records differently. Although all the researchers follow the guidelines of Rechtschaffen and Kales [9], these allow significant latitude. Knowles et al. [10] have discussed the differences in REM latency arising from using different definitions of sleep variables. The differences in methods of sleep data collection and in diagnosis have hampered replication of any group's work and will make the wide diagnostic use of the sleep EEG far more difficult. Our definitions and methods of data collection are described in the Appendix.

Several investigators have separated endogenous from nonendogenous adults using sleep EEG data. Kupfer et al [11] used the primary-secondary distinction, but all the patients in the primary group were endogenously depressed (Kupfer, personal communication, 1978). Gillin et al [12] separated depressed patients from normal volunteers and from insomniacs, and Rush et al [13] used the RDC [14] to classify patients as primary-secondary and as endogenous (ED)-nonendogenous (ND). Rush et al found that short REM latency was more closely related to the ED-ND distinction than to that between primary and secondary depression. REM latency was significantly shorter in ED patients than in ND patients or normal subjects in all of these studies, giving it a central role in this diagnostic distinction. Kupfer [11] and Feinberg [15] found that a discriminant function using REM latency and REM density was more powerful than REM latency alone in making this diagnostic distinction. Gillin et al [12] showed that measures of sleep disturbance could be used to advantage in separating ED patients from normals; this result was confirmed by Feinberg et al [15]. However, the latter authors found that measures of sleep disturbance were far more powerful in separating UP patients from normals than in distinguishing between BP depressives and normals. This is consistent with earlier work by Kupfer and his colleagues [16,17], who found that BP depressed patients may oversleep, rather than suffer from insomnia.

Akiskal and his colleagues have studied patients with a variety of "nonclassical" depressive syndromes, and have published extensively on sleep EEG findings in these patients [18-20]. They suggest that patients with "subaffective dysthymias" have short REM latencies and respond well to treatment with antidepressants, even though they do not meet the symptom criteria for major depressive disorder [18].

REM latency is a sensitive marker for affective disorder, but not necessarily a specific one. Gillin and his colleagues [21] have recently shown that a group of obsessive-compulsive patients had short mean REM latency but normal REM density. These patients who were significantly (secondarily) depressed had shorter REM latencies than those who were not depressed.

Several groups have studied the sleep of depressed children. Kupfer's group reported shortened REM latency in an 11-year-old depressed girl [22], but later work by this group [23] and by others [24,25] describes no consistent differences between the sleep of depressed and normal prepubertal children.

Kupfer [1,26] found that patients who had a good antidepressant response to amitriptyline in a three-week fixed-dose trial had had a marked increase in REM latency after the first one or two doses of drug, whereas those who failed to respond had had significantly less change in REM latency. This finding was confirmed by Gillin and his colleagues [27]. However, there are several confounding variables in the first study which make premature interpretation risky and make it less certain that the initial sleep response to antidepressant treatment will predict eventual antidepressant response. First, the effect on REM latency may have been a nonspecific anticholinergic response. This possibility is supported by work in rats [28] showing that the effects of imipramine on REM latency are blocked by physostigmine and by work in man showing that an increase in cholinergic function shortens REM latency [29]. The second problem is a "side effect" of a fixed-dose study. Those patients who had higher (and therapeutically effective) blood levels at the end of this study probably had higher blood levels after the first dose of amitriptyline. Kupfer's group [30] has shown that the effects of amitriptyline on REM sleep are significantly correlated with plasma levels of the drug.

The methods recommended here for the diagnostic use of sleep EEG data were derived as described in our earlier publications [7,15]. Gillin generously shared the data from his study of depressed, normal, and insomniac subjects [12], and we used these data to derive several discriminant functions (DFs) for first separating the depressed and normal subjects and then for classifying patients studied in Ann Arbor. Following Kupfer's work [11], we derived a DF using REM latency and REM density, and we found that this consistently classifies the Ann Arbor patients more accurately than other DFs derived from Gillin's data. This DF is:

Sleep DF Score = 0.032894 $\times$ REM latency $-$ 0.28408 $\times$ REM density.

We chose a cutting score of 1.0 for this DF to make specificity = 0.90 at the expense of sensitivity. Our most recent results are shown in Table 1. We now find that the DF is more sensitive in UP than BP depressives ($p < 0.05$; chi-squared test), with most of the difference coming from the low sensitivity in BP II patients. The specificity is unchanged, varying between 0.86 and 0.92 as the sample size increases. The sensitivity has varied between 0.60 and 0.70 for the total ED group, and is 0.91 for the UP patients.

It is important to note that we can draw no diagnostic conclusions if the sleep

Table 1. Clinical Diagnosis

	UP	BP	ED	ND
Sleep DF score < 1.0	28	12	40	10
≥ 1.0	12	15	27	60
N	40	27	67	70
Sensitivity	0.70	0.44	0.60	–
Specificity	–	–	–	0.86

DF score is ≥ 1.0, since many ED patients fall into this group. We can, however, say that a patient whose DF score is < 1.0 is likely to be suffering from an endogenous depression and is, therefore, likely to benefit from somatic treatment.

Both Rush et al [13] and Feinberg et al [31] have shown that sleep EEG data provide useful diagnostic information in patients with normal ("suppressor") responses to dexamethasone [32]. Given the relative ease and expense of the two tests, it makes good clinical sense to use the sleep EEG as a diagnostic test only in those patients with normal DSTs or in whom the DST will be invalid (e.g., patients taking physiologic doses of corticosteroids).

Many workers have shown independently that patients with endogenous depression have abnormalities of sleep which differentiate them from normal subjects and from nonendogenous ("neurotic") depressed patients. No one is certain which methods of gathering and interpreting sleep EEG data will provide the most reliable diagnostic information, and comparison across centers has proved difficult. The methods presented here provide a diagnostic test with good sensitivity and specificity that can be used for the differential diagnosis of depressed patients.

REFERENCES

1. Kupfer DJ, Foster FG: EEG Sleep and Depression. In RL Williams, I Karacan (eds) Sleep Disorders: Diagnosis and Treatment. New York, John Wiley & Sons, 1978, pp 163-204
2. Feinberg—chapter on Diagnostic Criteria
3. Klein DF: Endogenomorphic depression. Arch Gen Psych 31:447-454, 1974
4. American Psychiatric Association: Diagnostic and Statistical Manual of Mental Disorders, 3rd ed. Washington DC, APA, 1980
5. Spitzer RL, Endicott J, Robins E: Research Diagnostic Criteria, 2nd ed. New York, New York State Department of Mental Hygiene, New York Psychiatric Institute, Biometrics Research, 1975
6. Feighner JP, Robins E, Guze SB, et al: Diagnostic criteria for use in psychiatric research. Arch Gen Psych 26:47-63, 1972
7. Woodruff RA, Goodwin DW, Guze SB: Psychiatric Diagnosis. New York, Oxford University Press, 1974

8. Leonhard K: Aufteilung der endogenen Psychosen, 4th ed. Berlin, Aufl Akademie Verlag, 1968
9. Rechtschaffen A, Kales AA: A Manual of Standardized Terminology, Techniques, and Scoring System for Sleep Stages of Human Subjects. Bethesda, MD, National Institute of Neurological Diseases and Blindness, 1968
10. Knowles JB, MacLean AW, Cairns J: Definitions of REM latency: Some comparisons with particular reference to depression. Biol Psych 17:993-1002, 1982
11. Kupfer DJ, Foster FG, Coble P, et al: The application of EEG sleep for the differential diagnosis of affective disorders. Am J Psych 135:69-74, 1978
12. Gillin JC, Duncan W, Pettigrew KD, et al: Successful separation of depressed, normal, and insomniac subjects by EEG sleep data. Arch Gen Psych 36:85-90, 1979
13. Rush AJ, Giles DE, Roffwarg HP, et al: Sleep EEG and dexamethasone suppression test findings in unipolar major depressive disorders. Biol Psych 17:327-341, 1982
14. Spitzer RL, Endicott J, Robins E: Research Diagnostic Criteria for a Selected Group of Functional Disorders, 3rd ed. New York, New York State Psychiatric Institute, 1978
15. Feinberg M, Gillin JC, Carroll BJ, et al: EEG studies of sleep in the diagnosis of depression. Biol. Psych 17:305-316, 1982
16. Detre T, Himmelhoch J, Swartzburgh M, et al: Hypersomnia and manic-depressive disease. Am J Psych 128:123-125, 1972
17. Kupfer DJ, Foster FG, Detre TP: Sleep continuity changes in depression. Dis Nerv Syst 34:192-195, 1973
18. Akiskal HS, Rosenthal TL, Haykal RF, et al: Characterologicl depressions. Arch Gen Psych 37:777-783, 1980
19. Akiskal HS, Lemmi H, Yerevanian B, et al: The utility of the REM latency test in psychiatric diagnosis: A study of 81 depressed patients. Psychiatry 7:101-110, 1982
20. Akiskal HS: Dysthymic disorder: Psychopathology of proposed chronic depressive subtypes. Am J Psych 140:11-20, 1983
21. Insel TR, Gillin JC, Moore A, et al: The sleep of patients with obsessive-compulsive disorder. Arch Gen Psych 39:1372-1377, 1982
22. Kane J, Coble P, Conners CK, et al: EEG sleep in a child with severe depression. Am J Psych 134:813-814, 1977
23. Kupfer DJ, Coble P, Kane J, et al: Imipramine and REM sleep in children with depressive symptoms. Psychopharmacology 60:117–123, 1979
24. Puig-Antich J, Goetz R, Hanlon C, et al: Sleep architecture and REM sleep measures in prepubertal children with major depression. Arch Gen Psych 39:932-939, 1982
25. Young W, Knowles JB, MacLean AW, et al: The sleep of childhood depressives: Comparison with age-matched controls. Biol Psych 17:1163-1168, 1982
26. Kupfer DJ, Foster FG, Reich L, et al: EEG sleep changes as predictors in depression. Am J Psych 133:662-626, 1976
27. Gillin JC, Wyatt RJ, Fram D, et al: The relationship between changes in REM sleep and clinical improvement in depressed patients treated with amitriptyline. Psychopharmacology 59:267-272, 1978
28. Hill SY, Reyes RB, Kupfer DJ: Imipramine and REM sleep: Cholinergic mediation in animals. Psychopharmacology 69:5-9, 1980

29. Sitaran N, Nurnberger JI Jr, Gershon ES, et al: Faster cholinergic REM sleep induction in euthymic patients with primary affective illness. Science 208: 200-202, 1980
30. Kupfer DJ, Hanin I, Coble PA, et al: EEG sleep and tricyclic blood levels: Acute and chronic administration in depression. J Clin Psychopharmacol 2: 8-13, 1982
31. Feinberg M, Gillin JC, Carroll BJ, et al: EEG studies of sleep and the dexamethasone suppression test in the diagnosis of depression. Psychopharmacol Bull 17:20-22, 1981
32. Carroll BJ, Feinberg M, Greden JF, et al: A specific laboratory test for the diagnosis of melancholia. Standardization, validation and clinical utility. Arch Gen Psych 38:15-22, 1981

APPENDIX

Methods for Collecting Sleep EEG Data

1. Electrode placement is exactly as described in Rechtschaffen and Kales [9].
2. We use Grass gold-cup electrodes for EEG, EOG, and EMG leads. The reference electrodes are Beckman bipotential electrodes because these reduce an artifact present when gold-cup electrodes are used. We use Grass electrode paste and Beckman electrode gel as appropriate. EMG, EOG, and reference electrodes are secured with tape; EEG electrodes, with collodion.
3. We use both a Grass Model 7 polygraph with 7P5B pre-amplifiers and 7DA driver amplifiers and a Grass 8-16D EEG machine, and find no significant differences. Paper speed is 1 cm/sec. Pre-amplifier settings are:

Channel	Sensitivity	Half-amplitude frequency Low	High	60 Hz filter
EEG	50 μv/cm	0.3 Hz	35 Hz	In
EOG	50 μv/cm	0.3 Hz	35 Hz	In
EMG	50 μv/cm	5 Hz	70 Hz	In

4. Despite all efforts to standardize the staging of sleep records, differences among centers persist. We will be happy to consult with others who wish to use the sleep EEG data for diagnosis to minimize these differences.

Definitions of Sleep EEG Variables

[a]Awake: Time (minutes) awake between sleep onset[b] and end of sleep.

Delta Sleep: Stages III and IV.

[a]Early Morning Awakening (EMA): Time (minutes) awake between end of sleep and arising (end of recording).

REM Activity (RA): The sum of the eye movement scores during REM sleep for the entire night, based on a score of 0–8 for each minute of REM sleep.

REM Density: REM activity/REM time (RA/RT).

[a]REM Latency: Time (minutes) from sleep onset[b] to onset of stage REM.

REM Latency Minus Awake (RLMA): REM Latency minus any time awake between sleep onset [a] and REM onset (minutes).

REM Percent (REM%): RT/(TS-A) × 100%.

REM Time (RT): Time (minutes) spent in stage REM.

[a]Sleep Efficiency: (TS-A)/TRP × 100%.

Sleep Latency: Time (minutes) from beginning of recording to sleep onset[b].

Time Sleeping (TS-A): Time (minutes) from sleep onset[b] to end of sleep, minus Awake.

[a]Total Recording Period (TRP): Time (minutes) from beginning of recording ("lights out") to end of recording.

---

[a]These variables were used in the five-variable discriminant function separating NIMH normal and depressed groups.

[b]Sleep onset is the first minute of stage II sleep which is followed by nine minutes containing not more than one minute of awake time. Or, sleep may begin with a REM period containing three or more minutes of REM sleep (sleep-onset REM).

CHAPTER 4

Tests of Psychomotor Function

JOHN F. GREDEN

INTRODUCTION

Clinicians historically have considered psychomotor abnormalities as paramount features for the diagnosis of affective disorders. Nelson and Charney [1] reviewed 95 studies to determine distinctive symptoms of major depressive disorder. They found that psychomotor retardation was at or near the top of most lists. Overall and associates [2], Kendell [3], and Paykel and colleagues [4,5], each identified motor retardation as the one symptom most useful for both classification and prediction of treatment responses. More than half a century ago, Adolf Meyer [6] stated that psychomotor acceleration is the most striking feature associated with mania, and this observation is still accepted. Both DSM-III [7] and the Research Diagnostic Criteria [8] list psychomotor retardation and agitation among items necessary for the diagnosis of depression and mania.

Despite such acceptance, clinical assessments of psychomotor functions tend to be subjective, imprecise, and inaccurate [9]. Such poor performance is attributed primarily to lack of objective measuring techniques. This lack of good tests is due to many factors. Psychomotor functions are multifaceted, complex, and difficult to isolate into measurable segments. Accurate instrumentation was not available until recently. Baseline norms were ill-defined. Widespread differences in the classification of affective disorders made it impossible to compare findings

Handbook of Psychiatric Diagnostic Procedures, vol. 2, edited by R. C. W. Hall and T. P. Beresford. Copyright © 1985 by Spectrum Publications, Inc.

from different studies. Some of these problems persist, but three developing tests (facial electromyography (EMG), speech periodicity measures, and limb motility monitoring) show promise for overcoming some of these barriers and for introducing some objectivity and accuracy into psychomotor assessments. In this chapter, I will briefly review psychomotor abnormalities, the background for each of the three tests, and current applicability in clinical or research settings.

CLINICAL DESCRIPTION OF PSYCHOMOTOR ABNORMALITIES

Psychomotor retardation (deceleration) is clinically characterized by slowing of speech, delayed response time, reluctance to answer questions, a preponderance of monosyllabic replies, low, weak or whispered voice, lack of inflection or apparent emotion in voice, labored movements, stooped gait, apathy, apparent indifference, absence of gestures or motionlessness, a fixed or "wooden" facial expression, dull gaze, and occasionally a stuporous demeanor.

Psychomotor agitation (acceleration) in depressed melancholic presents as motor restlessness, difficulty relaxing, inability to sit quietly, continuous pacing, hand wringing, increased muscle tension, an apprehensive facial appearance with contraction of "forehead" muscles, a "fearful" or "pained" gaze, hunched shoulders, staccato or "clipped" speech, often at a higher than normal pitch, and an emphasis upon repetition of certain phrases.

Psychomotor acceleration during manic states differs somewhat from this profile of depressive agitation, as evident from the description by Meyer [6]: "The (manic) patient is all activity, yields irresistibly to every impulse; but in distinction from other forms of motor restlessness, manic restlessness can almost always be traced to some moods or purposes, playfulness, etc. The condition is easily exaggerated, and the ready incitability is perhaps the fundamental trait, together with insensitiveness to fatigue. The part played by speech, the tendency to drift in the direction of alliterations and rhymes, is especially important owing to its influence on the flight of topics in which connection and leading thought are lost. In writing too, the trivial signs of activity get the better of legibility and sense."

Although it does not seem to be widely recognized, components of both "retardation" and agitation may coexist in selected patients. This explains partially why both items are rated separately in clinical rating scales. Unfortunately, it confounds the task of developing tests to measure psychomotor abnormalities.

Although global motor activity can and should be considered in assessments of psychomotor abnormalities, it is notable that virtually every historical description emphasized disturbances in speech, facial expression, and motility. Thus, there is a clear rationale for isolating and emphasizing tests of speech, facial expression, and motility in trying to compile a psychomotor battery.

SPECIFIC TESTS OF PSYCHOMOTOR FUNCTION

Facial Electromyography (EMG) during States of Affective Imagery

People continually monitor the facial expressions of others to obtain feedback, but as Ekman and colleagues [10,11] stated, "The rules of translating a particular set of facial wrinkles into the judgment that a person is angry, afraid, etc. would be very hard for most people to describe." Confirming this judgment, chronic patterns of muscle tension documented by EMG in depressed subjects are not readily visible to the naked eye [12]. For these and other reasons, a quantifiable sensitive measure of facial expression was needed.

Schwartz et al [13,14,15] proposed that use of electromyographic (EMG) patterns of low-level facial muscle activity during states of affective imagery might differentiate clinical states. He and his colleagues placed surface electrodes upon selected muscle regions of the face and recorded EMG activity during states of affective imagery (e.g., happy, sad, angry, "typical day"). The muscle regions studied were: 1) corrugator muscles (located bilaterally above the bridge of the nose; activity is associated with grief, pain, and sadness); 2) zygomatic muscles (located between the angles of the mouth and cheek bones bilaterally; activity is associated primarily with smiling); and 3) perioral muscles, such as the depressor anguli oris, depressor labii inferioris, and mentalis; activity is associated with changes in mouth expressions during affective states of sadness, anger, pain, happiness, and pouting.

These innovative pilot facial EMG studies suggested that: 1) each discrete imagery task produces a distinct EMG profile; 2) depressed patients might be diagnostically differentiated from nondepressed controls on the basis of these EMG profiles; 3) decreases in resting corrugator muscle EMG activity during antidepressant treatment may monitor clinical improvement; and 4) baseline corrugator EMG activity possibly predicts clinical response.

We have measured facial EMG activity during different states of affective imagery in approximately 75 patients and 30 normal controls. We found EMGs to be relatively simple, safe, well tolerated by most patients (except manics), and with no significant complications.

Specific Techniques for Monitoring Facial Electromyography (EMG) Activity During Affective Imagery Prior to EMG testing, to minimize subject bias, no specific reference should be made to any movement of facial muscles. Females should remove facial makeup, and males should shave cleanly. In males with beards, only upper facial muscles can be studied. Subjects should be seated in a comfortable, cushioned chair.

Our approach has been to use eight pairs of miniature Ag/AgCl electrodes, placed bilaterally over the regions of the corrugator, zygomaticus, depressor anguli oris, and depressor labii inferioris. Prior to attaching the electrodes, all skin locations are vigorously scrubbed and gently abraded with alcohol pads until a slight redness appears on the skin surface. Placement procedures are standardized in the following way:

1. Corrugator: This horizontal muscle arises from the frontal bone at the medial end of the supercilliary arch. For placement, we vertically ascend from the nasal corner of the eye to the distal border of the eyebrow and medially 1/2 cm for the first electrode. The second electrode is placed over the eyebrow 1 cm from the first electrode in a horizontal plane.

2. Zygomaticus: This muscle arises from the temporal process of the zygomatic bone, on the lateral surface of the face, with the flat band running downward and forward to the corner of the mouth. For our electrode placement, we vertically descend 2 cm from the lateral corner of the optic orbit and temporally another 2 cm. This is the first electrode placement. The second electrode is placed 2 cm along a line from the first electrode to the corner of the mouth.

3. Depressor anguli oris: This muscle forms a triangular plate with its posterior border, ascending vertically to the corner of the mouth. The muscle bundle becomes thicker at its upper end. Our electrode placement is 5–7 mm, from the vermillion border on a 45-degree angle from the corner of the mouth. The second electrode is placed 1 cm from the first toward the posterior border of the muscle.

4. Depressor labii inferioris: We selected the region of the depressor labii inferioris (DLI) for electrode placement in preference to the mentalis muscle because DLI fibers are known to run vertically, whereas there are wide individual differences in fiber direction of the mentalis muscle. The superomedial portion of this muscle is visible to and above the medial border of the depressor anguli oris. The first electrode is placed 1 cm laterally off the midline and approximately 5–7 mm below the vermillion border. The second electrode is placed 1 cm below and 3–5 mm lateral to the first.

To reduce static charge effects, a single ground connection to the nape of the neck is used. The low level DC bioelectric potential is amplified, full-wave rectified, and integrated.

Reliability of electrode placement over repeated sessions and subject-to-subject reliability are aided by using Polaroid photographs immediately after placement and analyzing these photographs with a transparent grid. Specifically, the grid is placed over the photograph and X-Y coordinates drawn along the nasal corner of the eyes and base of the nasal cartilage as reference markers. This is done for each facial location and for each session, and placements on the grid are compared.

In order to at least partially distract attention from the facial electrodes, we utilize "dummy" electrodes. These are placed on both wrists, on both forearms over the region of the flexor muscles, and below the left clavicle.

Subjects are asked to *sit as quietly as possible with their eyes closed*. We then instruct them: "During this procedure, you will be asked to think about several types of situations. Do the best you can with each of these instructions without actually talking with me. You do not need to tell me what you are thinking. Please try to continue to think about a particular situation until you hear me tell you to relax."

The specific instructions for the various self-generated stimuli were: "Now I want you to think about a particular situation which made you feel _____ (i.e., happy, sad, a typical day, excited, or emotionally painful). While you are thinking about it, please try to re-experience the feeling you had at that time." Instructions for the typical day imagery were further amplified by telling subjects that we wanted them to think about what they did throughout a typical day until the time they went to sleep.

Interpretation of Data Based upon our EMG studies in normal subjects, we agree with previous reports which state that: 1) contrasting imagery states produce different EMG patterns; 2) that these patterns are relatively consistent and reliable over time; and 3) that patients with affective disorders can be differentiated from normals on the basis of these patterns. Such findings are essential if facial EMGs are to ever have diagnostic utility.

EMG Profiles in Normal Subjects When facial EMGs are measured in normal subjects during sadness imagery, there is higher activity in the corrugator muscle. Happy imagery, in contrast, tends to produce higher activity in the zygomatic muscle region. These findings have face validity with known clinical and neuroanatomical patterns. The typical day stimulus is indeed more "neutral" in that there is relative balance between corrugator and zygomatic regions. These distinct profiles are portrayed schematically in Figures 1 and 2. When EMG values are compared for the three imagery states (happy, typical day, sad), significant differences are found.

The test-retest reliability of EMG activity levels is fair. Although variances are large, differences in EMG scores across sessions are small and are not statistically significant.

In order to ... distract the ... primary attention from the facial activities, the ... differ... were drained ... they are placed on both legs ... after tracking ... test function with the ... time interval...

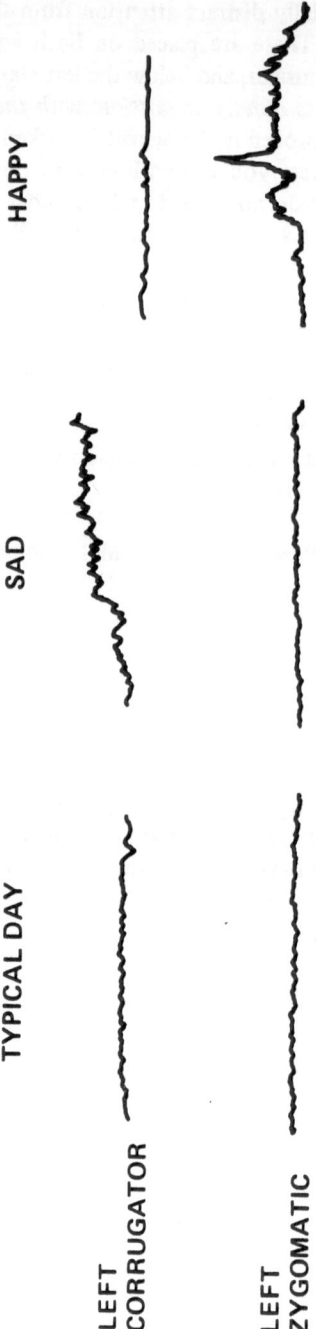

Figure 1. Low-level facial electromyographic recordings from left corrugator and left zygomatic muscle regions drawn from a normal control curing three imagery states ('typical day', 'sad', and 'happy').

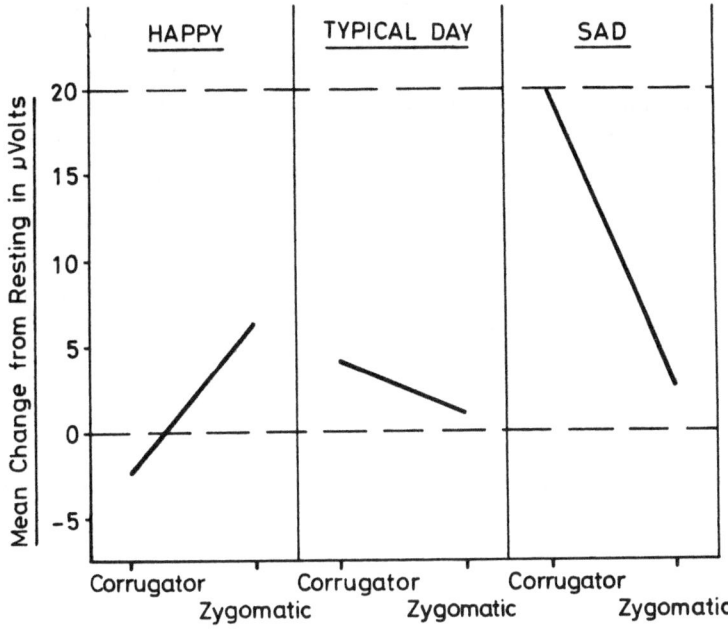

Figure 2.

Comparisons Between Normals and Depressed Patients When normal subjects are compared with depressed patients, different profiles are found. The most obvious finding is for the "happy" profile; normals differ from all subtypes of depressed patients. Specifically, zygomatic activity from depressed patients is lower than from normal individuals. Stated clinically, facial EMGs seem to document that depressed patients have difficulty generating the characteristic happy profile of facial muscle activity.

Serial Monitoring with Facial EMGs Baseline and discharge EMGs have been conducted on a small number of melancholic patients. The most important trend is the suggestion that the sad profile changes with clinical improvement in the hoped-for direction. The hypothesis that serial EMG testing will aid in monitoring treatment progress thus is supported in preliminary findings but needs further study. Pilot data [15,16] also suggest that increased corrugator activity prior to treatment may be associated with good eventual outcome. If so, baseline EMG values might predict treatment response.

Implications of Abnormal Facial EMGs The pathophysiologic mechanism which might underlie abnormal facial EMG patterns during affective imagery are unknown. Depressed patients presumably could be unable to generate happy imagery states. Limbic modulation of nigrostriatal or other CNS-mediated motor function also may be impaired, or some yet unknown network(s) might be dysfunctional. Extensive work is required before speculating further.

Speech Measures

Speed of talking is a constant, stable variable among normal individuals [17, 18]. Slow, delayed speech is traditionally found in patients with "retarded" depressions [19,20] whereas rapid pressured speech is considered symptomatic of mania [21]. Unfortunately, subjective determinations of speech are also known to be imprecise and prone to errors [9].

Recent developments permit more accurate speech analyses [22]. Many speech parameters, such as amplitude, fundamental frequency, latency, and pitch, now can be readily measured from speech recordings. These techniques—once introduced—were soon applied to patients with affective disorders.

In 1976, Szabadi et al. [23] modified a voice-operated relay technique previously designed for measuring speech periodicity in Parkinsonism and studied speech rhythms among unipolar depressives before and after treatment with amitriptyline and among a small number of normal controls. He noted that speech pause time (SPT)—the silent intervals between phonations—was elongated among patients with depression, and shortened with improvement. Phonation time—the audible component of speech—was unchanged. These findings suggested that SPT might be an objective pathophysiologic marker of psychomotor retardation. Concurrent validation was suggested in reports from Leanderson and co-workers [24, 25], who found prolonged EMG latencies between the onset of muscular activity and the corresponding acoustic segment. These latencies decreased with treatment, similar to the decreases in pause times during treatment of depressives noted by Szabadi [23] and Greden et al [26,27].

Specific Techniques for Measuring Speech Values Prior to recording speech measures, we avoid any reference to specific speech characteristics and simply indicate that we wish to record the subject's voice to conduct studies on psychophysiology. On the mornings of data collection, we awaken patients at least 30 minutes prior to speech recordings. Subjects sit in a chair and wear a set of headphones with an attached microphone. This apparatus—similar to those used by television commentators—consistently maintains mouth-to-microphone-distance from session to session. The microphone is connected to a tape recording machine, which transmits prerecorded standardized instructions to the subjects through the headphones. The message requests that patients recite their name, and this is followed by a pause to enable them to do so. A similar arrangement is then used to determine date and time of day. We next ask subjects to recite the alphabet from A to J (10 alphabet phonations), to count forward from one to ten (10 numerical phonations), during "automatic speech". This is the data that we have predominantly analyzed for our studies. We further ask the subject to count backward from ten to one (also 10 numerics, but not "automatic speech"). The tape can then be analyzed for speech pause time, phonation time, fundamental frequency, amplitude, and other speech parameters. Multiple variations of this data collection procedure are obviously possible.

Intrepretation of Data   Expanded sample sizes have enabled comparisons of SPT between subgroups. Melancholic patients have longer SPT than normal subjects or nonmelancholic depressives. Furthermore, there is the suggestion of a descending hierarchy among patient subtypes in the length of SPT (bipolar I > bipolar II > unipolar > nonendogenous depressives > nonaffective psychiatric patients > manic). Thus, bipolar patients have the most speech retardation.

We also studied various different cutting values of morning baseline SPTs [28] to determine how effective each cutting value was in differentiating patients with melancholia from patients with nonendogenous depression or other psychopathologies. These pilot results suggested that SPTs greater than 2600 msec denote relative psychomotor retardation and may provide the best blend of sensitivity and specificity. Because melancholic patients were older than nonmelancholics, we considered that SPTs might be related to increasing age but found little evidence for this.

Serial Monitoring   As reported in our recent publications [26,27] melancholic subgroups have statistically significant decreases in SPT during clinical improvement. This confirms the hypothesis that SPT would decrease with treatment among melancholic patients. We noted also that significant decreases in SPT occurred soon after starting treatment in several patients. Each of these patients had a good final response to treatment, suggesting that prompt decreases of SPT may provide an *early* prediction of outcome.

Validity of SPT as a Marker of Retardation   Concurrent validity of SPT as a measure of psychomotor retardation is suggested in a comparison of 79 patients who were rated as having "no retardation" (0 or 1 on the Hamilton Depression Rating Scale) [29] with 19 patients who were rated as "retarded" (2, 3, or 4 on this item of the HDRS). Retarded patients had an SPT of 3575 ± 2792 msec, compared to 2525 ± 1372 msec for those without retardation (Mann-Whitney U, $p < .05$).

Rapidly cycling bipolar patients, by fluctuating from depressed to euthymic or manic states, also provide good models to assess construct validity of state-related markers. As shown in Figure 3, we monitored longitudinally two BP cycling patients with SPT measures and matched 100 mm visual line scale scores (0 = worst ever; 100 = best ever). We assessed a total of 24 values in one patient and 13 in another, correlating modd ratings with SPTs. Spearman's rho for the first patient was -.76 and for the second patient was -.71. These findings—in addition to supporting the construct validity of SPT as a state-marker of psychomotor retardation associated with depressed mood—suggest that SPT does not automatically decrease as a function of the number of trials (i.e., "practice effect" = minimal).

SPT as an Aid in Selection of Treatment Psychomotor features have been claimed to aid in the selection of specific antidepressant approaches. In treatment lore, for example, amitriptyline was considered more effective for agitated patients and imipramine or desipramine for retarded patients. SPT results do not confirm this. Rather, it appears that SPT decreases significantly (Wilcoxon test, $p < .04$) regardless of the treatment selected as long as the patient clinically improves.

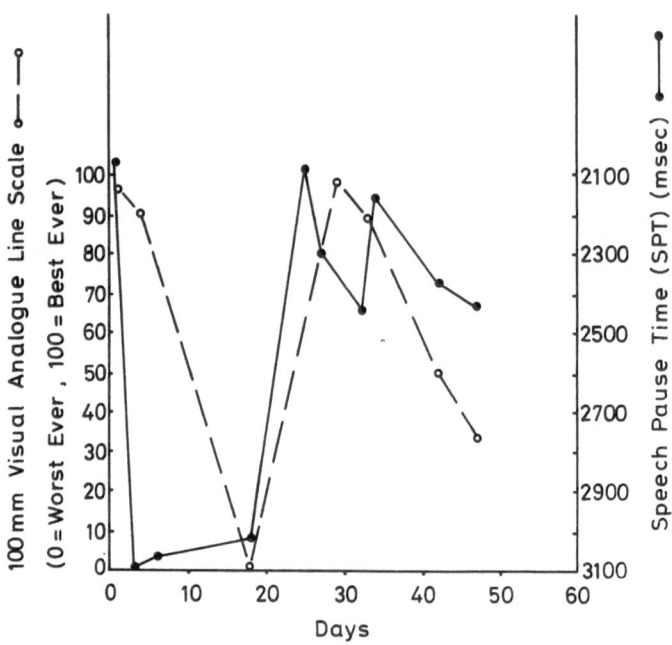

Figure 3. Serial speech pause time in a 32 year-old rapidly-cycling bipolar patient throughout two cycles.

Interaction with Other Laboratory Markers We conducted a preliminary analysis of interactions between SPT and the dexamethasone suppression test (DST) [30]. We tested 54 melancholic patients with both the DST and SPT. Abnormal DST results were found in 37 cases (68.5%). A prolonged SPT was found in 10 of the remaining 17 cases (SPT > 2600 msec). Thus, the two tests in combination (series) improved sensitivity to 47 of the 54 cases (87%). The diagnostic potential of the SPT in conjunction with the DST is hinted at in these results.

Measurement of Motility with Movement Activated Recording Monitors

Carlsson et al [31] demonstrated in 1957 that motor activity was neurochemically mediated. Since then, our knowledge about the neurobiology of movement has grown considerably. Measurement techniques were still deficient until the early 1970's however. Movement-activated-recording monitors were introduced then. Such monitors differ in design [32,33], but a typical monitor resembles a wristwatch, to be worn on the nondominant wrist. Motility monitors still are technologically in an ongoing stage of development but they have been used to evaluate psychomotor activity among patients with affective disorders in a number of studies (34,35,36]. Findings from these early studies revealed that unipolar depressed patients had higher motility counts than bipolar depressives, that motility changed with treatment, and that there were diurnal variations in activity levels. Perhaps most importantly, these pioneering studies documented that motility could be quantified.

Specific Techniques for Monitoring Motility We currently use "Solicorder" motility monitors (Model SA16), manufactured by Ambulatory Monitoring Incorporated, Ardsley, New York. Each monitor consists of a recorder module and a direct computer interface unit for data recovery. The modules are small, wristwatch-sized, self-contained digital data recorders, connected by a cord to a battery worn in a leather pack at the waist. Each module is capable of recording up to 2048 eight-bit data words at intervals which can be adjusted (0.125-16 minutes). The activity monitor uses a counting system which allows the recording of data even when the event rate is as high as four per second. This is possible because the solicorder contains a data compression technique which automatically self-adapts to the number of events occurring during a given recording interval. Each unit is powered by a rechargeable nickel cadmium battery pack, which can operate continuously for up to 300 hours. A battery test switch is provided to indicate the presence of charge. If the indicator light stops glowing, enough power remains for 24 hours to enable data recovery.

At the end of the measuring period, we take the recorder module from the patient and attach it to the direct computer interface unit. Recorded data can be easily transferred to microcomputers and a teletype to produce raw motility count printouts. The entire data dump procedure requires only one half hour for each week of tracing. Thus, a large number of subjects theoretically can be monitored with ease.

Prior to motility monitoring each subject receives explanations about the equipment and provides informed consent. No reference should be made to counting movements per se. The project can simply be described as physiologic monitoring. Despite such attempts to maintain patient "blindness" it is our impression that they are at best "near-sighted," since most of them perceive the general purpose of the instrument. For this reason, we discard first-day data collections to permit subjects to acclimate to the instrument. Compliance has been fair. Patients may complain, for example, about the cord connecting the motility monitor to the battery supply. Thus, it would be an improvement to use a unit with the power supply located within the actual wrist instrument.

Large amounts of data are generated by motility monitoring, and data interpretation in clinical settings would still be a problem. Several approaches are possible. First, the actual number of activity counts recorded might be compared with standard parametric statistics using either matched times of days or total counts from specified time periods. Second, the data could be normalized by expressing each time-interval value point as a percent of the mean count for all time periods during a specified interval (e.g., 24 hours) and these could be compared with parametric tests. Third, cosinor analysis could be employed as described by Crowley et al [33]. The data analysis technique will vary depending upon the clinical purpose of the test.

Interpretation of Results Few patients or controls have been studied with motility monitors. Indeed, single case reports and small sample sizes dominate this literature. Thus, any conclusions are premature. Figure 4 illustrates the motility graph of a 26-year-old patient with bipolar melancholia who simultaneously kept a diary of her routines. Changes in activity (e.g., napping, activities therapy) produce obvious alterations in her motility profile. This confirms reports by other investigators [35] and provides a measure of face validity for the instrument. We have similarly validated patterns in other subjects whom we have studied.

Motility Values as a Serial Marker of Clinical Progress Serial monitoring of motility may document improved psychomotor functioning. We observed a typical pattern in a 33-year-old bipolar melancholic with psychomotor retardation who wore the motility monitor for separate three-day segments at baseline, midway through treatment, and for the last three days prior to discharge. She demonstrated progressive increases in total motility with more sustained activity periods during daylight hours. These changes clearly paralleled diminishing retardation and global clinical improvement.

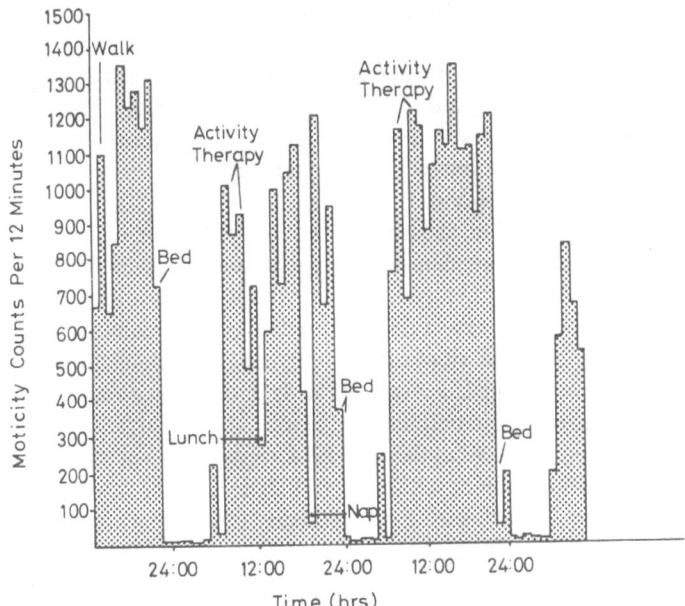

Figure 4. Motility counts per 12 minute segments over three days illustrating changes with circadian routines (face validity).

An intriguing observation occurred when we monitored a 29-year-old bipolar patient. The patient wore the monitor for three days prior to a weekend pass. She was clinically stable when monitoring was initiated and when her pass from the hospital was approved. On her second pass day, however, she switched into a depression. Her Hamilton Depression Rating Scale [29] increased from 8 to 20. When we retrospectively analyzed the three-day segment of motility values, it was apparent that psychomotor deceleration occurred on the last day of monitoring before apparent clinical change, thus perhaps predicting the clinical "switch."

These pilot applications of motility monitoring need to be studied in many more patients before clinical application becomes a reality, but this approach has the potential to be one of the easiest and perhaps most sensitive tests of psychomotor function.

Future Applications of Psychomotor Tests Depression and mania have high incidences, recurrent courses, and severely disabling clinical and economic consequences. If accurate psychomotor testing were available to aid in diagnosis and treatment monitoring, this negative impact could be lessened. Patients with psychomotor deceleration almost certainly have different neurochemical substrates than those with psychomotor acceleration. Objective, sensitive pathophysiologic markers could help in selecting treatments, predicting treatment responses and avoiding premature and expensive shifts from one treatment to another. Outpatient assessments during states of remission might document or suggest impending relapse or confirm continued "biological stability." Most importantly, psychomotor tests by their nature tend to be relatively inexpensive, noninvasive, and readily integrated with other pathophysiologic approaches.

Tests for facial expression, speech, and motility still are in early stages of development. In each area, proposed psychomotor tests show promise, but there is a great need for normal measures and determinations of reliability, validity, sensitivity, specificity, and predictive value. Methodologic shortcomings limit comparisons of previous reports and slow future progress. These include lack of normal controls; the absence of drug-free evaluations; lack of comparisons between differing affective subgroups (e.g., unipolar vs. bipolar; melancholic [endogenous] vs. nonendogenous; primary vs. secondary); small sample sizes; a paucity of longitudinal assessments ("within-subject design"); and little consideration being given to possible confounding factors, such as: 1) laterality effects (e.g., for electrode placement for facial EMGs) [38] ; 2) circadian variations in selecting a time of day for data collection; 3) failure to determine reliability of repeat measures before assigning significance to observed changes; 4) scanty attention to the possible effects of different orders of presentation (e.g., of imagery states) or "practice effects"; 5) differences in self-generated vs. externally-generated imagery (for facial EMGs); 6) lack of drug-free state or failure to consider the effects of drug withdrawal; and 7) the absence of "within-subject" controls. Future testing and clinical applications of psychomotor tests must strive to control for these methodologic problems by studying rigorously diagnosed, operationally defined affective and nonaffective subgroups and matched normal controls, by comparing morning and evening data during drug-free states, by serially monitoring patients over time to compile prospective longitudinal data, and by controlling whenever possible for technical variants (e.g., by using bilateral facial EMG electrode placements and differing orders of stimuli). If such guidelines are followed, then psychomotor measures should assume a significant position in the future repertoire of psychiatric laboratory tests.

ACKNOWLEDGMENTS

The author gratefully acknowledges the contribution of Clinical Studies Unit staff in the careful collection and analysis of psychomotor data, especially H. Laurence Price for facial EMG measures and Wendy Sabbath, Judy Matthews, Robert Gardner, and Henry Shein for speech measures.

This project was supported by NIMH Grant MH-32736 and by the University of Michigan Department of Psychiatry and Mental Health Research Institute.

REFERENCES

1. Nelson JC, Charney DS: The symptoms of major depressive illness. Am J Psych 138:1-13, 1981
2. Overall JE, Hollister LE, Johnson M, et al: Nosology of depression and differential response to drugs. J Am Med Assoc 195:946–948, 1966
3. Kendell RE: The Classification of Depressive Illness. London, Oxford University Press, 1968
4. Paykel ES: Depressive typologies and response to amitriptyline. Br J Psych 120:147–156, 1972
5. Paykel ES, Prusoff BA, Klerman GL, et al: Clinical response to amitriptyline among depressed women. J Nerv Ment Dis 156:149–165, 1973
6. Winters EE (ed): The Collected Papers of Adolf Meyer, Vol. II, Psychiatry. Baltimore, Johns Hopkins Press, 1951
7. Diagnostic and Statistical Manual of Mental Disorders, 3rd ed. American Psychiatric Association, Washington DC, 1980
8. Spitzer RL, Endicott J, Robins E: Research Diagnostic Criteria for a selected group of functional disorders, 3rd ed. New York State Psychiatric Institute, 1977
9. Greden JF, Carroll BJ: Psychomotor function in affective disorders: An overview of new monitoring techniques. Am J of Psych 138:1441–1448, 1981
10. Ekman P, Friesen WV, Ellsworth P: Emotion in the Human Face. New York, Pergamon Press, 1972
11. Ekman P, Friesen WV: Unmasking the Face, Englewood Cliffs, NJ, Prentice-Hall Inc, 1975
12. Whatmore GB, Ellis RM: Some neurophysiologic aspects of depressed states. Arch Gen Psych 1:70–80, 1959
13. Schwartz GE, Fair Pl, Slat P, et al: Facial muscle patterning to affective imagery in depressed and nondepressed subjects. Science 192:489–491, 1976
14. Schwartz GE, Fair PL, Slat P, et al: Facial expression and imagery in depression: An electromyographic study. Psychosom Med 38:337–347, 1976
15. Schwartz GE, Fair PL, Mandel MR, et al: Facial electromyography in the assessment of involvement in depression. Psychosom Med 40:355–360, 1978
16. Carney RM, Hong BA, O'Connell MF, et al: Facial electromyography as a predictor of treatment outcome in depression. Br J Psych 138:485–489, 1981
17. Goldman-Eisler F: Measurement of time sequences in conversational behavior. Br J Psych 42:355–362, 1951
18. Goldman-Eisler F: On variability of speed of talking and on its relation to length of utterances in conversation. Br J Psych 45:94–107, 1954
19. Darby JK, Hollien H: Vocal and speech patterns of depressive patients. Folia Phoniatr 29:279–291, 1977
20. Blackburn IM: Mental and psychomotor speed in depression and mania. Br J Psych 126:329–335, 1975
21. Stoddard FJ, Post RM, Bunney WE Jr: Slow and rapid psychobiological alterations in a manic-depressive patient: Clinical phenomenology. Br J Psych 130:78–82, 1977
22. Darby JK: Speech evaluation in Psychiatry. New York, Grune & Stratton Inc, 1981
23. Szabadi E, Bradshaw CM, Besson JAO: Elongation of pause-time in speech: A simple, objective measure of motor retardation in depression. Br J Psych 129:592–597, 1976

24. Leanderson R, Persson A, Ohman S: Electromyographic studies of facial muscle activity and speech. Acta Otolaryngol 72:361–369, 1971a
25. Leanderson R, Meyerson BA, Persson A: Effects of L-dopa on speech and parkinsonism: An EMG study of labial articulatory function. J Neurol Neurosurg Psych 34:679–681, 1971
26. Greden JF, Carroll BJ: Decrease in speech pause times with treatment of endogenous depression. Biol Psych 15:575–587, 1980
27. Greden JF, Albala AA, Smokler IA, et al: Speech pause time: A marker of psychomotor reatrdation among endogenous depressives. Biol Psych 16:851–859, 1981
28. Galen RS, Gambino SR: Beyond Normality: The Predictive Value and Efficiency of Medical Diagnosis. New York, John Wiley & Sons, 1975
29. Hamilton M: A rating scale for depression. J Neurol Neurosurg Psych 23:56–62, 1960
30. Carroll BJ, Feinberg M, Greden J, et al: A specific laboratory test for the diagnosis of melancholia. Standardization, validation and clinical utility. Arch Gen Psych 38:15–22, 1981
31. Carlson A, Lindquist M, Magnusson T: 3,4-dihydroxy-phenylalanine and 5-hydroxytryptophan as reserpine antagonists. Nature 180:1200–1203, 1957
32. Colburn TR, Smith BM, Gvarini JJ, et al: An ambulatory activity monitor with solid state memory. Int ISA Biomed Sci Instrumentation Symposium, ISA BM 76322, 117, 1976
33. Crowley TJ, Hydinger-MacDonald M: Motility, parkinsonism, and prolactin with theothixene and thioridazine. Arch Gen Psych 38:668–675, 1981
34. Kupfer DJ, Foster FG: Sleep and activity in a psychotic depression. J Nerv Ment Dis 156:341–348, 1973
35. Kupfer DJ, Weiss BL, Foster FG, et al: Psychomotor activity in affective states. Arch Gen Psych 30:765–768, 1974
36. Weiss BL, Foster FG, Reynolds CF, et al: Psychomotor activity in mania. Arch Gen Psych 31:379–383, 1974
37. Foster FG, Kupfer DJ: Psychomotor activity and serum CPK activity. Arch Gen Psych 29:752–758, 1975
38. Schwartz GE, Davidson RJ, Maer F: Right hemisphere lateralization for emotion in the human brain: Interactions with cognition. Science 190:286–288

CHAPTER 5

Evoked Potentials

MAURICE RAPPAPORT

DEFINITION AND OVERVIEW OF THE HISTORY AND DEVELOPMENT OF THE PROCEDURE

Evoked potentials (EPs) are a pattern of electrophysiologic activity recorded from the brain (or spinal cord) shortly after the occurrence of an event, usually a form of sensory stimulation. Because an EP pattern can be obtained under various conditions, even upon the omission of an expected sensory event, the phenomenon is sometimes referred to as an event-related potential response. It is also referred to by other descriptive phrases such as cerebral-evoked potential, cortical-evoked potential, averaged-evoked response (AER) or by the sensory modality eliciting the response. Thus we have the auditory-evoked potential (AEP), visual-evoked potential (VEP) and somatosensory-evoked potential (SEP). Other modalities (i.e., olfactory, vestibular, pain, vibratory, etc.) can be employed but seldom are because of technical difficulties. Details of the methodology and procedures employed to obtain EP patterns are described later in this chapter.

Since the brain is considered the organ of understanding, perception and control, there is a fascination in trying to learn how it performs its functions. Discoveries of the brain's on-going electrophysiologic activities reflecting sensorimotor and sentient events have led to increasingly sophisticated methods of "looking in" on how the brain works. Caldani [1] reported as early as 1784 that electrical stimulation of the brain caused convulsion:. Fritsch and Hitzig [2] in 1870 demonstrated that certain regions of the cortex were excitable by electricity and elicited specific movements. This gave rise to the concept of functional localization. In

Handbook of Psychiatric Diagnostic Procedures, vol. 2, edited by R. C. W. Hall and T. P. Beresford. Copyright © 1985 by Spectrum Publications, Inc.

1875, the idea that the brain had electrical properties of its own arose. Caton [3], when putting two recording electrodes on the surface of the cortex, found that there was a weak waxing and waning of electrical current in the absence of stimulation. He also reported "impressions through the senses were found to influence the currents of certain areas . . ." This may have been the first brain-evoked potential observation. Beck [4], in Poland, at about the same time, showed that he could evoke an electrical potential change in the brain with a light stimulus as well as with a sound stimulus (actually a shout) when one of his electrodes was placed on the temporal cortex. Hans Berger [5], a psychiatrist and "father of the EEG", is well known for his demonstration and report in 1929 that stated that on-going electroencephalographic activity—the EEG—can be recorded through the skull of man. The much smaller electrical potential evoked by sensory stimulation and buried in the EEG was originally clearly demonstrated by Dawson [6] in 1947. He reported a method for detecting cerebral action potentials obtained by peripheral nerve stimulation. He presented EEG patterns in response to sensory stimulation on a cathode ray tube and copied several traces on a photographic record. He was able to show that there was a consistent time relationship between the onset of a sensory event and a repeatable EEG pattern that was different from the background EEG. His use of an averaging process, that is, the averaging of cerebral EEG responses relating to the time of onset of a sensory stimulus presented many times, made use of a known principle of averaging employed by other disciplines such as physics.

Photographic averaging techniques have been described by Calvet and Scherrer [7] and others. Additional techniques for averaging included storage tubes [8] and magnetic tapes [9].

The major impetus to evoked potential work, however, came from the development of specialized digital computers in the 1960s and 1970s. Clark [10] and coworkers designed the Average Response Computer. The Mnemotron Computer of Average Transients (CAT) and the Nuclear Data Enhancetron followed. All-purpose laboratory digital computers, such as those developed by Digital Equipment Corporation (PDP-8, PDP-12, PDP-11 series), made possible signal averaging tasks. In the 1970s and early 1980s specialized digital computers designed for commercial use for obtaining averaged evoked potential patterns appeared with some proliferation. Companies producing such equipment included Nicolet, Grass, Tracor, Caldwell, Teca, Bio-Logic Systems, Disa and others. Some were originally designed to record EEGs or electromyograms. With the establishment of EP testing requirements equipment was modified or completely redesigned. Although there were variations in design, all equipment provided for the application of a common set of procedures. The basic elements of the EP procedure are described below in the fourth section of this paper.

Table 1. Clinical Applications of Evoked Potentials

Area	Purpose: To help assess or detect these conditions	Type of EP[a]
Psychiatry	Malingering	AVS
	Hysteria	AVS
	Organic brain syndrome	AVS
	Alcoholism	AVS
	Psychoses	AVS
	Affective disorder	AVS
	Sensory disorders	AVS
	Drug influence on CNS function	AVS
	Cognitive responsivity	
Industrial injury	Sensory dysfunction complaints	AVS
Developmental disability	Sensory dysfunction	AVS
	Cortical dysfunction	
Neonatology	Hearing impairment	AVS
	Cortical dysfunction	AVS
	Sudden infant death (SID) possibility	A
Neurological disorders	Multiple sclerosis	AVS
	Optic neuropathy	V
	Peripheral neuropathy	S
	Nerve root entrapment	S
	Spinal cord disease	S
	Hemianopsia	V
	Acoustic neuromas	A
	Sensorineural hearing impairment	A
	Retinal impairment in presence of cataract	V
	Optic pathway tumors	V
	Various dystrophies	AVS
	Encephalopathy	AVS
	Stroke	AVS
	Hemispheric lesions	AVS
	Coma	AVS
	Brain death	AVS
Intraoperative monitoring	Spinal cord function	S
	Neurosurgical	
	(Removal of auditory or	A
	visual pathway tumors)	V
Interoperative monitoring	Effects of traction on spinal cord function	S

[a]A – Auditory
V – Visual
S – Somatosensory

With the advent of commercially produced equipment capable of signal averaging, there has been an outpouring of evoked potential research and clinical findings. Within medicine, in general, such utilization [11] is ever-expanding. A list of current clinical applications is presented in Table 1. As discussed below some of these applications at the present time have limited utility and may not be cost-effective. Other applications have immediate and important utility in medicine in general. Current efforts suggest that there may in the future be a considerable clinical payoff as the state of the art advances. There has been a particularly concentrated effort in psychiatry to examine relationships between evoked potential patterns and an individual's mental status and factors affecting mental status such as medication, organic pathology, level of arousal, emotional state, and cognitive abilities.

LITERATURE REVIEW OF EVOKED POTENTIALS IN PATIENTS EXHIBITING DIFFERENT MENTAL CONDITIONS

If evoked potential work has done nothing else, it has emphasized the inseparable mind-body interface and the fact that modern psychiatry, particularly neuropsychiatry, is an integral part of medicine. Some of the following findings may improve diagnosis and treatment in psychiatry as well as improve our understanding of the functioning of the brain. This section will focus on a selected array of mental states and conditions where significant EP findings have been reported. Despite the infancy of the EP literature, the range of findings is impressive.

EP parameters used to differentiate one type of patient or one type of mental condition from another include peak latencies and amplitudes, pattern variability, degree of overall pattern abnormality, pattern replicability, degree of cerebral asymmetry found under different test conditions, and pattern recovery characteristics.

Psychosis and Affective Disorders

Relationships between EP findings and psychosis have been reported in a number of books as well as in numerous articles [12-22] which delineate ways of possibly differentiating psychotics from nonpsychotics and from organic brain syndrome patients; schizophrenic from depressive and manic patients; and chronic from acute schizophrenic patients [23-30].

Findings include the observations that psychotics, in contrast to nonpsychotics, show lower peak amplitudes and greater EP variability [24,25]. In comparisons between schizophrenics and patients with affective disorders, it has been reported that patients with mood disorders show greater asymmetrical responses between the left and right hemispheres, less EP pattern variability, and a more pronounced P300 (cognitive) wave. In addition, Buchsbaum [31] has reported that bipolar patients tend to be augmenters (i.e., show increased peak amplitudes with increasing intensities of light stimuli) in comparison to patients with a unipolar depressive disorder. Later Buchsbaum [32] reported that patients with affective disorders with an augmenting response also showed low monamine oxidase (MAO) activity. If, however, they had high MAO activity, they appeared to be reducers (i.e., they showed decreasing EP amplitudes to visual stimuli of increasing light intensity). Friedman and Meares [33] suggested that the situation may be even more complex. They reported that amplitudes of cortical potentials "may be a function of severity of depression." [16]

The state of the art, however, is such that while results reported to date are of interest they do not warrant routine diagnostic EP testing of schizophrenic patients or patients with affective disorders. Unless there is a suspicion of sensory dysfunction or CNS pathology, clinical observation provides a more cost-effective approach to the diagnosis of major mental disorders at the present time.

Dementia

Reports show that demented patients exhibit delayed latencies of positive-going peaks normally occurring within 300–450 msec after stimulus onset. Squires et al, [14] and Visser et al [34] showed that patients suffering from senile or presenile dementia had longer latencies and larger amplitudes of visual EPs than did normal subjects. Rappaport [35] demonstrated diffuse, undifferentiated, and very abnormal late cortical response patterns to auditory, visual, and somatosensory stimulation in a 59-year-old woman with a severe organic brain syndrome. A summary of other EP findings in patients with chronic brain syndromes is given by Shagass et al [16].

Distinct differences in EP patterns between patients with an organic brain syndrome and patients with either psychosis or an affective disorder or individuals who do not have a major mental disorder, suggest that the EP test, in selected instances, can provide useful additional diagnostic information not otherwise available. This can confirm cortical impairment in those suspected of having an organic brain syndrome.

Dissociative Disorder and Personality Characteristics

There is a dramatic contrast in hysterical patients between their reports of the absence of sensation and their EP patterns. Their EP patterns are generally robust and difficult to differentiate from patterns obtained from normal subjects [35]. Some authors, however, do report differences. Shagass and Schwartz [36] report that hysterics have higher SEP amplitudes and less SEP habituation on the hysterically anesthetic side. Moldofsky and England [37] generally support these observations.

Malingerers, of course, show no pattern abnormality to either auditory, visual, or somatosensory stimulation. Because of the short latencies involved in the electrophysiologic activity measured in evoked potential testing, they have virtually no opportunity to influence test outcome. We had one case of a young male who slipped and fell in a supermarket. He promptly declared himself paraplegic and it was clear there was litigenous intent to recover "damages." After SEP testing was completed, the patient asked about the results. He was told that the patterns looked quite normal. Shortly thereafter he said he was feeling better and walked out of the hospital. One must keep in mind therefore the "curative" power of EP testing in addition to the diagnostic information it can provide.

One way to distinguish analgesic hysterics from analgesic malingerers is to use somatosensory stimuli of increasing intensity. The hysteric will remain relaxed and comfortable even at maximum stimulus intensity (in our laboratory a 500 μsec pulse at 19.9 ma presented two times a second) whereas the malingerer will show marked tension, agitation, and discomfort and will probably request cessation of stimulation before it reaches its maximum level.

Extroverted in contrast to introverted individuals are reported to show larger amplitudes of the late components of the auditory EP patterns [33]. Stelmack et al [38] however, report that when auditory stimuli are presented at relatively low intensity levels, introverts have a greater amplitude of response than extroverts for the negative-positive peaks occurring between about 120–225 msec after stimulus onset.

Reports show insomniacs to be reducers since they show lower evoked potential responses to higher intensity sounds than do normal sleepers [39].

Those who attempt suicide have been reported to be augmenters because they show an augmenting pattern of response to flashing light of increasing intensity as well as low platelet MAO activity [41]. The authors go so far as to suggest "that the combination of low platelet MAO activity and AER augmenting may be associated with a possible genetic vulnerability to psychiatric disorders."

Some studies have examined EP patterns in patients with multiple personalities, but these have yielded few consistent or dramatic findings [41,42].

Differences have been reported to exist between sex and SEP patterns [43]. The group mean for males vs females has a significantly smaller baseline amplitude that shows up to the greatest extent for the negative-positive peaks occurring between about 45 and 165 msec after stimulus onset.

While many of the findings reported above are of considerable interest, most do not appear to have immediate clinical application except for identifying and differentiating instances of either malingering or hysteria.

Childhood Disorders and Learning Disability

Many behavioral, learning, and emotional disorders of childhood are being shown to have a physical basis and are responsive to neurophysiologic changes induced by chemotherapeutic interventions. Evoked-potential testing as an electrophysiologic measure is contributing to our growing understanding of relationships between impairment in cortical function and various clinical disabilities and treatment approaches.

Halliday et al [44] has demonstrated that hyperactive children who respond to methylphenidate hydrochloride show a normalization of their visual EP patterns. Methylphenidate hydrochloride also has been shown to have normalizing effects on hyperactive children's vigilance performance as well as on the late positive components of visual EP patterns [45].

Tanguay et al [46] and Sohmer and Student [47] report that a high percentage of autistic children have significantly delayed brainstem transmission times. Auditory-evoked potential tests calling for selective attention also reveal a severe dysfunction in hyperactive boys compared to controls [48]. It has been shown that AEP patterns reflect maturation and development along brainstem acoustic pathways. Longitudinal AEP analyses, therefore, can help differentiate infants and young children at risk and help identify those who are likely to show developmental problems [49]. Such knowledge ultimately may help differentiate those children with problems stemming from poor family and environmental conditions from others whose problems have more of an organic or genetic basis.

Research on relationships between selected EP (and EEG) parameters and learning, language and psychiatric disorders already has been rewarding in its applicability to the neurometric approach described by John et al [50] which reflects both general and specific learning disabilities. This technique appears to be largely free of cultural, educational, interpersonal, ethnic, socioeconomic, and sex biases [51,52]. It has the potential of enabling us to identify specific electrophysiologic brain dysfunctions associated with a wide variety of psychologic disorders. It focuses primarily on the frequency composition of the electroencephalogram in relation to age within four frequency bands for four bilateral regions of the brain. Preston et al [53] have provided information on visual EP differences between normal and disabled readers. Normal compared to disabled readers showed increased amplitudes for the P200 peak and the late positive component (LPC) on the left side of the brain in response to word stimuli. Wasman and Gluck [54] report that slow learners show less recovery of cortical responsiveness at brief interstimulus intervals. On the other hand, it has been reported that no significant auditory or visual EP findings were discovered in dyslexic members of families where more than one person had a reading problem [55]. Yet it has been demonstrated that conditioning of average-evoked potentials is related to intelligence in children [56].

Saletu et al [57] have reported that in childhood psychosis there is a trend toward shorter latencies and smaller amplitudes in EPs. Also Saletu et al [58] and Itil et al [59] indicated that children with schizophrenic mothers showed latency reductions similar to those found for schizophrenic children. It has been pointed out, however, that levels of significance were "modest" and differences between mean latency values were about 15 msec at about 300 msec. There is some question therefore about whether this represents a real neurophysiologic trait or simply a state of tension, anxiety, and arousal [16]. Other workers, however, report that children at risk for schizophrenia have evoked potentials that are "characterized by low amplitude N150, small LPCs to nonsignal stimuli, large LPCs to signal simuli and high amplitude P240 components—components implicated in mechanisms of selective attention and cognitive processing [60].

Mongoloid children in contrast to normal children are reported to show markedly greater amplitudes and later peak latencies in the late cortical components, uniquely distinctive somatosensory EP patterns, and no significant hemispheric asymmetry [61]. Similar findings have been reported in Down's syndrome subjects by Gliddon et al [62].

The above findings showing relationships between childhood disorders and learning disabilities and evoked-potential patterns are, of course, of great interest and, hopefully, one day can be developed to the point of diagnostic significance. At the present time, however, it would appear that one practical clinical application of EP testing in this population would be to assess the effects of pharmacologic agents in normalizing brain responsivity to sensory stimulation. Perhaps the greatest practical clinical application at the present time is the use of the EP technique to assess sensory functioning, peripherally and centrally, particularly in children who manifest behavioral and psychologic problems and who cannot cooperate adequately in a routine physical assessment process. Since analyses of sensory functioning is relevant to infants, children, and adults, it will be reviewed in the next section on sensory disorders.

Sensory Disorders

Psychiatric evaluations often reveal complaints of sensory dysfunction. Blurring of vision, inability to hear well, somatosensory symptoms of numbness, tingling and pain—to mention just a few symptoms—are frequently reported with little objective evidence to support such complaints. Obviously it would be quite helpful to psychiatrists and to other physicians, as well as to patients, to establish, whenever possible, a physical basis for sensory complaints so that therapy can proceed in as realistic a context as possible. Obviously if a patient has a sensory complaint and there is objective electrophysiologic evidence to support that complaint, then the approach to treatment of that patient will proceed somewhat differently than when such objective evidence cannot be found.

An EP assessment of any sensory modality is possible as long as a discrete short duration, time-locked constant stimulus can be applied a number of times. An evoked central nervous system electrophysiologic response can be picked up by appropriately placed recording electrodes and the signals amplified and averaged. Usually, however, only auditory, visual, and/or somatosensory stimuli are employed. A good overview of some of the sensory applications of the EP technique has been given by Chiappa and Ropper [63,64].

In a clinical psychiatric context Rappaport [35] has reported four cases of interest. In one instance AEPs were used to demonstrate that a suspected case of hysterical deafness in a young man was in actuality a neurophsyiologic rather than a psychiatric problem. In another instance SEPs were used to demonstrate the presence of hysterical hemianesthesia. A third case involved malingering. The fourth case involved a patient with a behavior problem associated with an organic brain disorder. The patient's family was convinced that the patient's behavioral problems were due primarily to psychologic factors until they were shown markedly abnormal auditory, visual, and somatosensory EP patterns.

Notwithstanding the occasional occurrence of dramatic cases such as those described above, EP tests can be quite useful in assessing sensory functioning in some individuals with behavioral, severe psychological, and developmental disability problems, as well as in those who develop problems subsequent to trauma or disease. Sensory deficits can often contribute to abnormal perceptual reports, abnormal psychologic functioning, or abnormal behavior. For example, pattern reversal VEPs can help identify whether neurophysiologic difficulties are anterior to, posterior to, or at the optic chiasm. The means for making this interpretation are discussed below. VEP patterns can sometimes detect optic neuritis or preclinical signs of multiple sclerosis and thereby help explain newly developing personality aberrations. Also, abnormal pattern reversal VEPs may be associated with a number of disease entities having psychiatric manifestations, such as pernicious anemia, Huntington's chorea, and renal disease.

Brainstem AEPs are quite useful in detecting hearing impairments due to multiple causes. For example, it can be used to identify conductive and sensorineural hearing losses or losses associated with tumors such as acoustic neuromas, pontine hemorrhages, or multiple slcerosis. It is particularly useful in testing neonates since 5–15%, depending on certain risk factors, are known to have hearing deficits. Mothers may not become aware of such deficits until the child is one-two years of age or older. Consequently the AEP is an important screening tool, particularly in neonates at risk (i.e., those who are premature, have low Apgar scores, need extended ventilatory assistance, have possible anoxia secondary to various complications such as umbilical cord strangulation, or have hyaline membrane disease etc.).

Loss of adequate contact with the auditory world early in life can have grave consequences for a child's later psychologic and behavioral adjustment. A psychiatrist, particularly a child psychiatrist, may want to recommend AEP testing in young children with developmental and/or behavioral problems if he suspects the presence of either hearing impairment or cortical dysfunction. We have had the opportunity to test an infant that was not showing normal maturational changes and yet no disease process could be identified. Very abnormal cortical AEP patterns suggested extreme cortical dysfunction. This led to a CT brain scan which showed that the infant had virtually no cortex.

SEPs can be quite helpful in differentiating whether patient complaints about impaired sensory functioning have a basis in fact. It can provide information on the integrity of peripheral components, such as the brachial plexus and dorsal roots, as well as whether or not there is impairment in the transmission of somatosensory information within the cord, from the cord through the brainstem to the thalamus and from the thalamus to the cortex. Identification of SEP abnormalities can relieve a patient particularly when their reported dysfunction cannot be identified by less sensitive measuring techniques. Information of this type can contribute to mental well-being particularly when a patient is not assigned erroneously and demeaningly to the "crock" category. One such case involved a 58-year-old man who was referred to us for assessment by a neurosurgeon. The patient had been complaining persistently of loss of sensation and a "strange feeling" on one side of his face. His face did not look asymmetrical, as in Bell's palsy, nor was there any convincing evidence of sensory dysfunction after careful clinical neurologic examination. The patient was described by the referring physician as someone with probably unidentified psychologic problems, hypochondriac tendencies, and "probably was a crock." SEP tests were done involving stimulation of homologous points on each side of his face. A marked asymmetry of patterns was found. This provided firm physical evidence that there was impairment in the transmission of sensory information on the side about which the patient had been complaining. The patient's credibility was restored, a more diligent search for the etiology of his symptoms ensued, and perhaps, most important, the patient was relieved to learn that there was a neurophysiologic basis for his complaints and that it "was not all in my mind."

SEP tests have been found useful in helping to interpret subjective sensory complaints in industrial injury and workman compensation cases. This will be discussed further below in the section on the interpretation of the results of EP testing.

Psychopharmacologic Consideration and Substance Abuse

Pharmacologic effects on EP patterns have been reported by a number of authors [65–70]. Saletu [65] reports that anxiolytics produce SEP profiles characterized by latency increases in early peaks and decreases in late peaks, as well as an attenuation in amplitudes. He records that neuroleptics induce latency increases in all peaks as well as generalized peak attenuation. Stimulatory drugs, on the other hand, produce latency decreases in early peaks as well as in late components of the EP pattern. MAO inhibitors, according to Saletu, induce alterations similar to stimulants. Tricyclic antidepressants produce a latency decrease in early and a latency increase in late SEP components. Saletu mentions that the EP technique can also be used to assess the clinically therapeutic spectrum of a drug. Friedman and Meares [68] found that the amplitudes of VEPs and AEPs were not only significantly greater in depressed patients but they returned towards normal when depression was relieved by antidepressants. This also occurred in placebo responders. Changes were reported as being most evident in the auditory system. Heninger [69] demonstrated that lithium carbonate has an effect on SEP latencies. He reported that prior to lithium treatment there was a longer latency period for depressed patients and a shorter latency period for manic patients. After treatment and patient improvement, both latency periods were more normal.

The effects of major psychotropic medications, overall, have been difficult to demonstrate consistently. Shagass [66] reports that "we were not able to demonstrate significant differences between patients who received some phenothiazines ... and patients who either had not received drugs at all or in whom drug administrations had been stopped for periods longer than one week." Rappaport et al [24] also reported that they could not detect significant differences in VEPs of different intensities among schizophrenics, some of whom received only placebos whereas others received up to 900 mg per day of chlorpromazine. Other investigators, however, do report differences. Saletu et al [71] report that both fluphenazine and thiothixene reduced the amplitude of initial SEP components in schizophrenics whereas 50 mg of chlorpromazine, given in a single dose to nonpatient volunteers, tended to produce an increase in amplitude [72].

The effects of other pharmacologic agents on EP responses have been reported. Lonsdale et al [70] report that thiamine metabolism affects brainstem function. He cites improvement in auditory brainstem responsivity in two infants with apnea after treatment with thiamine. Davis et al [73] report that there is a similarity between morphine effects on EPs of normals and schizophrenic EPs, as well as a similarity between EPs of normals and EPs of schizophrenics on naltrexone. This is cited as presumptive evidence of a role for endorphins in schizophrenia.

Effects of marijuana on EPs reported by Lewis et al [74] revealed no consistent differences between occasional and frequent users. The most prominent finding was a slowed latency of response of evoked peaks with little change in amplitude. It was hypothesized that this reflected increased threshold of cortical and subcortical neurons and neural networks. Unlike alcohol, THC did not alter hemispheric amplitude asymmetry. Shagass [66] concluded that doses of THC sufficient to produce clinical changes do not necessarily produce electrophysiologic changes. Herning et al [75] report that the negative-going component of the auditory EP occurring between 75 and 150 msec after stimulus onset was depressed relatively consistently only when tested during days 1-3 while 180-210 mg/day of THC was administered but not when tested after the chronic administration of THC for 10–14 days of a lower dose involving 70–90 mg/day.

Alcohol has been reported to cause progressive increases in the latencies of brainstem potential peaks III through VII with no changes in amplitudes [76]. This indicates that alcohol has a depressive effect on neural transmisstion within the primary auditory brainstem pathway. It is also known that alcohol causes significant reductions in the amplitude of auditory, visual, and somatosensory cortical potentials. Gross et al, Lewis et al, Begleiter et al [77-79] suggest that chronic alcohol abuse results in possible demyelinization of auditory tracts. Thus this is an additional argument that can be presented to patients to encourage them not to drink excessively. Chu, et al [80] report that brainstem abnormalities are related to age and number of alcoholic neurological diseases, particularly cerebellar degeneration. Also a high correlation was reported between CT scans showing cerebral atrophy in alcoholic patients and abnormal brainstem responses.

Pain and pain relief is another area where the results of EP testing may ultimately prove useful. Buchsbaum et al [82] have shown that SEP testing has been useful in evaluating the effects of various analgesics in relieving pain. In one study they demonstrated that both aspirin and morphine significantly diminished the N120 component at high stimulus intensities. In a related paper they [81] describe a pain assessment technique that shows stability in individuals tested seven months apart. Carmon, Mor and Goldberg [83] using laser-emitted radiant heat to induce cutaneous pain in humans found a late negative-positive component of the EP (130-160 msec) which correlated in amplitude with stimulus intensity and the subjective sensation of pain.

Brain Injury

Relatively recent work has demonstrated that there are significant correlations between the degree of evoked potential pattern abnormalities and both the physical and psychologic disability of severe head injury patients [84-87]. EP patterns also appear to have predictive power with respect to clinical outcome one–two years after head injury if the initial EP patterns are obtained within about sixty days of injury. In addition there is evidence that postconcussion cases, as a group, have latency abnormalities in brainstem auditory EPs [63,88].

Psychiatrists will find that there is a great need to work with head injury patients and that the results of EP testing can be helpful in differentiating organic from functional causes of mental and behavioral disturbances. It is anticipated that progress made so far in showing relationships between EP patterns and cognitive functioning will be extended to head injury patients. This will not only help to assess existing and changing deficits in higher level cognitive functioning but also will help to predict ultimate clinical outcome, particularly among brain-damaged patients who are not adequately assessed by clinical examination or existing neuro-psychologic techniques [82,92]. It is quite likely, for example, that the ability to show a cognitive response in a simple EP conditioning situation will have predictive value in estimating clinical outcome and in determining the need for intensive, extensive and expensive rehabilitation efforts.

Cognition

Psychiatry must continue to look with great interest on any electrophysiologic technique that holds promise for allowing investigation of factors associated with cognitive functioning. Disorders of cognitive functioning are the hallmarks of mental disturbances. EP testing may be able to identify the neurophysiologic correlates of cognitive dysfunction. This supposition is based upon findings already reported in the literature which demonstrate relationships between variations in EP patterns and various higher level cerebral activities. Some of these activities are fundamental to orderly and appropriate thought processes, processes which are disturbed in mental illness. Such processes include detection, selection, and attention to appropriate informative events occurring in one's environment [94-102]; assessment of probability of events and responsivity to instructional sets [103-106]; memory and hemispheric differences in cognitive processing [107,108]; cortical information processing in relation to the handling of sequential events; decision making and factors that interfere with decision making [109-111]; and the assessment of meaning [112-116].

For example, Parasuraman [101] demonstrated in an auditory signal detection task that N100 peak (the negative evoked potential peak occurring 100 msec after stimulus onset) varies only with the certainty or uncertainty of detection of an auditory signal and is not related to recognition of an auditory event that has occurred. This finding has also been reported by other investigators [94,97,99]. N100 also varies in amplitude with attentional set and has been shown to be significantly larger when attention is focused on a given channel [100]. It would appear that the well established attentional deficit problems in certain patients with mental illness could be studied in greater detail using the EP approach.

Duncan-Johnson [106] has demonstrated that the latency of the P300 wave as it reflects stimulus and response processing within the brain is affected by the probability of the stimulus. Further they have demonstrated that the duration of stimulus processing in a complex task (i.e., Stroop color-word task where the subject must name the ink color of a word that spells a conflicting color) remains constant and the delay in making an appropriate response appears to be associated with a response competition condition [111]. It would seem that this type of sophisticated analysis could be refined to study in greater depth how schizophrenic thought and decision making processes deviate from normal. The relationship between the P300 wave and the probability of an actual or expected event has been reported by other investigators [104,105,103].

Being able to recall events from memory is essential for efficient cognitive functioning. Before one can recall information it must be stored in memory. It was been reported that an evoked potential component with a poststimulus peak occurring at about 250 msec after stimulus onset is related to the storage of information in short term memory [107]. Recall was predicted by the magnitude of this storage component. This finding lends itself readily to the study of short-term memory storage capabilities in individuals with different mental disorders of this etiology.

Ritter et al [109] have found an N200 peak which covaried in latency with reaction time such as to support the hypothesis that this peak reflects a decision process which controls behavioral responses in sensory discrimination tasks. They believe that the P300 wave may be more closely related to future events since it often occurs too late to be involved in the behavioral response triggered by the eliciting stimulus. Goodin, et al [116] report a P165 peak that is related to cognitive stimulus processing and that could be differentiated from the N200 and P300 potentials. The nature of the P165 and N200 responses in mentally ill patients has yet to be studied definitively.

Perhaps the most exciting findings that need further study are those that demonstrate that EP patterns can reflect meaning. In 1969 Begleiter and Platz [112] reported that late component amplitudes of the evoked potential pattern were significantly related to whether words were neutral or taboo. Taboo words had greater peak amplitudes between about N96 and P165 and also between P165 and N360 than did neutral words. In 1973 Brown, Marsh and Smith [114] reported that EP wave forms differed according to the context in which the same stimulus word was imbedded. Responses to the word "fire" differed when presented in the phrases "sit by the fire" and "ready, aim, fire." Scalp electrodes were over Wernicke's and Broca's areas and over homotopic points on the nondominant hemisphere. "Waveform differences were significantly greater for left hemisphere than for right hemisphere loci." In 1974 Johnston and Chesney [113] demonstrated that late components (beyond 160 ms) of frontal EP patterns reflected changes of meaning. Subjects were given an instructional set to respond to either letters or numbers. One ambiguous visual stimulus could be called either a "B" or "13." EP patterns to these different stimuli were analyzed and pattern differences were found. Reaction time was not affected, ruling out possible differences in arousal level and attention. In 1980 Kutas and Hillyard [115] discovered a late negative component (N400 but beginning at about 250 msec) which was elicited by a semantically inappropriate word. For example, a sentence might be presented such as "I take coffee with cream and *cement*." The N400 is a "double take" or "second look" electrophysiologic response of the brain to the word cement which suggests there is "reprocessing" of semantically anomalous, unexpected or inappropriate information. This wave does not occur if there is semantic congruity. It is suggested that this wave has promise as a clinical tool in the evaluation of reading impairment and language disorders. Obviously it is a tool that also can be used in studying deficits in the capabilities of mentally ill individuals to detect and evaluate incongruities in semantic information. Implications of these findings for future advances in understanding mental disorders are discussed briefly later.

CURRENT INDICATIONS FOR USE WITH PSYCHIATRIC PATIENTS

Psychiatry is a part of medicine. At the medical-psychiatric interface there are a number of indications for the use of EP testing. Before a psychiatrist or other physician reaches a conclusion about the presence of a psychiatric condition it may be prudent to look at the results of EP testing in selected situations.

EP testing should be considered whenever psychologically disturbed individuals complain of persistent sensory problems, the causes of which have not been identified previously by adequate physical examinations, diagnostic procedrues, and tests of a nonelectrophysiologic nature.

Auditory and Vestibular System Symptoms

The eighth nerve should be assessed by means of the auditory nerve and brainstem auditory evoked response test (BAER) if the patient complains of hearing difficulties, tinnitus, dizziness, loss of balance, pressure in the ear or other symptoms relating to possible dysfunction of the auditory or vestibular systems. Each ear should be tested independently. While the BAER test does not measure directly the functioning of the vestibular system, an abnormal eighth nerve, of course, does not preclude a deficit in the functioning of the vestibular component. While it has been demonstrated that a vestibular component in the BAER pattern can be elicited, the technical difficulties are such that it is not feasible to do this test routinely, particularly since a precisely calibrated centrifuge device may be required.

The cortical AEP also has utility when there is need to document that behavioral and psychologic abnormalities may be associated with cerebral dysfunction due to various causes such as physical trauma, anoxia, toxic substance effects, tumors, tissue or cavity swelling, infectious processes, vascular aberrations, or congenital or maturational defects.

Visual System Symptoms

The third nerve should be tested by means of visual evoked-potential (VEP) tests whenever a patient complains of otherwise undocumentable visual problems. It may be useful also when a patient complains of pain behind the eyes, headaches, or if there is suspicion that emotional problems may be related to a physical disorder such as optic neuritis or a demyelinating process as incipient multiple sclerosis. Each eye should be tested independently. The presence of a pituitary tumor or a craniopharyngioma, as well as other hard to document space-occupying lesions, may also cause visual and other physical symptoms that might be attributed erroneously to psychologic problems. Pressure of these lesions on the optic nerve, the optic chiasm, or the optic tract can show up as abnormal patterns. Interpretations of abnormal VEP patterns with such lesions are discussed later.

When working with retarded, severely schizophrenic, head injured, stroke, or other patients who cannot cooperate adequately with an examiner, the VEP test can also be used to refract eyes in order to fit a patient with corrective lenses. This technique has been reported to give results at least as good as reading the Snellen chart [117].

The VEP test can have value also in working up patients reporting blindness suspected to be of an hysterical nature. In occipital blindness associated with brain trauma, however, VEP patterns may occur in the presence of functional blindness. Caution therefore must be used in interpreting findings when this condition is suspected.

Stimuli consisting of reversing black and white checkerboard patterns (usually with 1° or 20' check sizes) yield the most definitive information. Using two sizes of check is recommended since in our experience abnormalities may show up with one but not with the other. In other words, it does not always follow that an abnormal VEP pattern to a 1° check size leads to an abnormal pattern for a 20' check size, or vice versa. The reasons for this are not known.

It is quite possible to use simple light flash stimuli and obtain information on whether a patient's visual pathway is at least transmitting light to the cortex and whether the cortex is responding in a normal or grossly abnormal manner. The latter type of information can be helpful in establishing whether or not an organic brain problem is present. The flash stimulus technique is not as useful as the pattern reversal technique, but nevertheless it can provide significant information particularly for patients who are not able to cooperate adequately in the pattern reversal testing situation that requires sustained attention and visual fixation.

Somatosensory System Symptoms

SEP testing is indicated whenever a patient complains of any one of a number of limb or body symptoms or sensations that cannot be documented by other means. These symptoms include complaints of numbness, tingling, formication, hypersensitivity or hyposensitivity to light touch or vibration, or other unusual sensations that can reasonably be assumed to be transmitted through the dorsal column pathways of the spinal cord. Each limb or area needs to be tested independently. Homologous points on the left and right sides should be tested and results compared. SEP testing can be particularly useful in helping to distinguish real from imagined or feigned sensory impairments or impairment associated with an hysterical condition. SEP testing can also help identify whether sensory problems are peripheral, within the cord, or at subcortical or cortical levels.

Cortical Related Symptoms

Cortical responsivity may be obtained upon stimulation of any sensory modality but usually is restricted to auditory, visual and somatosensory channels. One condition where cortical evoked potentials (CEPs) are useful is in the differentiation of an organic brain syndrome from a functional disorder. Other conditions where CEP patterns are useful are in instances of severe head injury or severe developmental disability. CEP information in these cases is helpful in judging the extent and severity of CNS dysfunction. The degree of abnormality of EP patterns is known to be related to the degree of clinical, physical, and cognitive disability in some patients [84,85]. Early after brain damage, it also has a relationship to clinical outcome one-two years after injury. Soon after injury it may be helpful in identifying psychologic deterioration associated with worsening organic problems such as developing hydrocephalus, metabolic deficiencies, or toxic conditions. In general, it can be useful in distinguishing between physiologic and functional causes of psychologic deterioration. CEPs are also useful as mentioned earlier in helping to identify cases of malingering and hysteria and in ruling out gross organic deficits in individuals displaying personality and behavioral disorders.

Depression, schizophrenia, autism, mental deficiency and drug effects are areas where interesting findings have been found as reported above. CEP pattern interpretations may be helpful at times but, in light of current knowledge, application of EP technology in these areas must be considered of secondary importance. Much work needs to be done before EP testing done on a routine basis will have practical utility in the aforementioned areas.

It is also premature to consider using CEPs to help assess intelligence and higher level cognitive functioning. As mentioned subsequently, however, there seems to be a good possibility that CEPs in conjunction with other special electrophysiologic indices may indeed have the potential of being able to evaluate deficits in certain higher level cognitive activities.

THE EVOKED POTENTIAL TESTING PROCEDURE

To carry out the evoked potential testing procedure successfully, careful attention must be paid to six elements that are part of the testing situation: the patient, the testing environment, the equipment, the technique, artifacts, and the interpretation of results. The first five elements are discussed in this section and the sixth, interpretation, is discussed in the next section.

The Patient

Patients of any age can be tested. The condition of the patient, however, can affect results. There should be as little agitation or muscle movement as possible and the patient should remain relaxed throughout the testing session. The patient should be made physically comfortable. A soft recliner chair is helpful. More complete relaxation can be obtained if the patient is supine but this is not essential. For psychiatric patients, particularly those with paranoid tendencies or those who have received electroconvulsive therapy, reassurance and explanations should be provided to make sure they understand that the wires and electrodes employed are primarily for recording electrical signals normally generated by the body. Significant others in a patient's milieu should also be given clear explanations of the procedure lest they transmit their apprehension and anxiety to the patient. Ratings of patient's cooperativeness, degree of movement throughout the testing session, and level of arousal (fully alert, drowsy, asleep) should be recorded since this information is helpful in interpreting EP patterns accurately. Information on medication that a patient is taking should also be recorded as well as any pathologic condition such as impairment in hearing, vision, or sensation, history of brain or spinal cord trauma, or substance abuse tendencies. The mental status of the patient should be described including any recent history of cognitive or psychologic dysfunctioning.

The Testing Environment

For psychiatric patients more than for other patients, care should be taken to make the testing environment reasonably pleasant and relaxing. There should be as little distraction as possible. Equipment not needed for testing should not clutter the room. Sources of distracting visual, auditory, and other sensory stimuli should be removed or minimized. This includes electromechanical devices of all sorts, telephones, and, or course, sounds of people talking and moving about or interrupting testing sessions.

Equipment

A number of companies, such as those mentioned previously, manufacture reliable signal averaging equipment designed for evoked potential testing. The cost of the equipment varies with its capabilities. Equipment that can be programmed and that has a larger information storage capacity costs more than equipment that does not have these capabilities. All EP testing equipment, however, must have the following basic components. There must be suitable scalp recording electrodes (i.e., silver-silver chloride, gold, etc.) for detecting small electrical signals evoked in the brain (or in the spinal cord) by sensory stimulation. There must be stimulating electrodes or electromechanical devices for controlling and delivering suitable discrete, short duration sensory inputs to selected sensory channels and/or portions of the body (i.e., eyes, ears, arms, legs, torso, face, etc.). Visual input devices are needed which allow the presentation of flash and patterned stimuli such as reversing black and white checkerboard patterns where the check sizes can be varied. An auditory input capability is needed. Usually this requires high quality earphones which can deliver independently to each ear or to both ears simultaneously click or tone stimuli as well as white masking noise.

There is a need for stimulus control capability which allows the tester to specify for the stimulus its duration, intensity, rise time to peak value, fall time, interstimulus interval, number of presentations per trial, rate of presentation, and to which side (left or right) or body site the stimulus is to be presented. In special cognitive testing situations, there should be control over the presentation of two or more stimuli where the probability of occurrence of each stimulus can be specified.

Amplifiers to amplify the small (millionths of a volt) evoked brain signals from each of the scalp or other recording electrodes are required. Various electronic control devices to adjust signal outputs are needed including those which allow: 1) adjustment of low and high frequency bandpass cutoff limits, 2) adjustment of signal sensitivity level; 3) adjustment of display gain and 4) rejection of signal artifacts (viz., muscle activity, 60 Hz and other unwanted electromechanical interference). There is also a need for a computer capability which can sense the time of onset of each sensory stimulus that is presented and record a varying evoked potential pattern over pre-specified lengths of time (viz., 10, 50, 100, 500 or 1000 or more msec after stimulus onset). There is a need for the equipment to be able to digitize and record voltages (usually in microvolts) at different instants in time during the recording epoch (e.g., equipment should be able to record 512 voltage values evenly spaced over a 10–1500 msec recording epoch). In addition, the equipment must be able to average digitized evoked potential voltages for the number of trials (sensory stimulations) presented and be able to present the overall averaged evoked potential patterns in a way that permits accurate measurement of peak latencies and amplitudes. Computer-curve smoothing and addition and subtraction capabilities are useful but not essential. A display capability which allows presentation of the averaged evoked potential pattern at different display gains and cursors which can be used to identify and display absolute and interpeak peak latencies (in msec after stimulus onset or between two peaks, respectively) and amplitudes (in microvolts) is essential. There must also be an EP pattern recording capability so a permanent record of the pattern can be retained for charts, future comparisons, and for various clinical and research uses. The above components and capabilities are available in an integrated fashion in many commercial signal averaging systems now on the market.

Technique

After the patient has been properly oriented to the procedure and feels as relaxed and comfortable as possible, the following steps are taken.

Site of Attachment of Recording Electrodes

Two scalp recording sites are usually adequate unless there are plans to study in detail the topographic distribution of EP patterns over the scalp or to study in detail subtle changes at specific cortical locations. The two recording sites can vary somewhat without grossly affecting EP recordings or their interpretability. Scalp electrode positions are specified using the international 10-20 system of Jasper [117]. The C3 and C4 positions (over the left and right hemispheres, respectively, about 2 cm lateral to and slightly behind the vertex, Cz, the midpoint of the scalp in a line drawn from the top of one ear lobe to the other) are adequate for most EP recordings for auditory, visual, and upper extremity somatosensory stimulation. For lower extremity stimulation the Cz site is preferred. C3, C4 and Cz are considered active electrode recording sites. EP recordings are considered bipolar if the voltage between two active scalp electrodes are compared (e.g., the Cz-Oz [occipital] comparison during visual stimulation). They are considered unipolar if the voltage between an active electrode and a reference electrode is compared (e.g., Cz-Al, vertex to left ear lobe). The reference electrode may be at one of several places. It may be at the ipsilateral ear lobe or mastoid process or it may be at Fpz (in the central midforehead hairline area). There is also a need for a ground electrode. It may be located on the ear lobe or mastoid process contralateral to the side being stimulated or at any other electrically relatively "neutral" site. This, for example, may be the tip of the nose, linked ear lobes, or mastoid processes when Fpz is used as a reference site, or the wrist or knee.

Attachment of Recording Electrodes

The areas where electrodes are to be placed must first be cleaned (with alcohol or other appropriate skin cleansing agents). These areas should then be abraded and electrode gel applied. The electrode should then be fixed firmly to the site wih tape, collodion, or an electro-cap. These four acts—cleansing, abrading, applying electrode gel, and firmly fixing the electrode to the scalp—serve to reduce impedance, the electrical resistance at the interface between the person and the recording electrode. The impedance is generally kept below five Kohms to insure good EP recordings. Needle electrodes can be employed subcutaneously, if this is acceptable to the patient, or in surgery. As with any invasive process that penetrates the skin proper sterile technique should be employed.

Polarity of Recordings

In auditory brainstem EP recordings positivity is generally in the upward direction. In other EP recordings whether positivity or negativity is up is arbitrary but polarity direction must be specified to prevent confusion in interpretation. In our laboratory positivity is up.

Technical Set-Ups

In Table 2 are the values of different stimuli and recording parameters that can be employed when setting up for auditory, visual, and somatosensory evoked potential testing. With experience the skilled technician learns to vary these parameters somewhat in order to enhance recordings. For example, by making adjustments in the low and high bandpass filter settings, unwanted electrical interference may be minimized or eliminated. Or, in the case of suspected organic or brain damaged patients, a slower stimulation rate may be used to more completely define impairment in cortical responsivity to stimulation. Signal amplification is not shown in the table but usually the first order amplification is 10,000 times. The amplitude value of identifiable peaks in EP patterns will vary from tenths of a microvolt for brainstem recordings to several microvolts (up to about 15 μv) for visual EP peaks.

Normative Data

Each laboratory should have its own normative data base. There is, however, a general consistency of values across laboratories, particularly for brainstem auditory EP patterns. Typical auditory, visual, and somatosensory EP patterns are presented in Figure 1.* In Tables 3 through 11 are representative normative latency and amplitude values obtained in our laboratory for three sensory modalities—auditory, visual (flash and pattern reversal), and somatosensory (median, posterior tibial, and sural nerves).

Factors Affecting EP Recordings

There are many factors that can interfere with accurate interpretations of EP patterns. These include artifacts, variations in stimuli, patients, and equipment. A number of these factors will be described and should be kept in mind particularly for the discussion in the next section on the interpretation of EP findings.

---

*Figure 1 and Tables 3–6 and 8–11 are reprinted with permission from the journal Clinical EEG [84].

Table 2. Evoked Potential Stimulus and Recording Parameters

Stim[a]	Stimulus parameters			No. of avgs	CNS level	Recording epoch (msec)	Fil Lov
	Intensity	Duration	Rate/sec				
A	80db[b]	100 μs (click) 5 msec (tone)	10.1 or 20.1	2000	Aud. nerve and brainstem	10 (15 msec for infants)	150 l
A	80db	100 μs (click)	1.1	200	Cortex	500	1
V_f	Variable[c,d]	10 ms	1.1	200	Cortex	500	1
V_{pr}	Variable[c,d,e]		1.88	120	Cortex	300	1
S_m	Twitch[f] level	300– 900 μs	2.1	200	Cord, subtex and early subcortical	60g	5 Hz 30 H:
			2.1 or 0.7	100	Cortex	500	1
S_{pt}, sural or peroneal	Twitch level	300– 900μs	5.3	200	Cord, subcor- tex and early subcortical	100g	5 or :
			2.1 or 0.7	100	Cortex	500	1

[a]A–Auditory; V_f Visual flash; V_{pr}–Visual pattern reversal; S_m–Somatosensory, median nerve; S_1 Somatosensory, posterior tibial nerve (or sural or peroneal nerve).
[b]If threshold or intensity latency curves are needed, intensity may be varied from 0 to 100 db, usu: in 10 or 20 db steps.
[c]Must be established for each laboratory.
[d]Bipolar leads are used at times (C3–03; C4–04; Cz–Oz).

Artifacts can include stimulus-generated electrical potentials. These show up as brief spikes at the onset, usually within 1-3 msec of the onset or termination of the stimulus. Muscle-generated potentials are other frequent artifacts that distort the EP pattern. Thus efforts are made at the beginning of testing to make sure that the patient is comfortable and relaxed. When a patient is very tense and agitated the use of anxiolytics (rather than barbiturate sedatives which can affect cortical EP patterns) should be considered.

Reflex responses to stimuli also introduce unwanted signals. For example, auricular and temporalis muscle responses occur respectively 8-12 msec and 20-35 msec after auditory stimulation, mostly when the patient is in an awake state. Eye

| | Recording parameters | | | Sensitivity in μv per full scale | | Gain | |
| settings | Electrode placement | | | | | | |
High	Active	Reference	Ground	Range	Usual	Range	Usual
3000 Hz	C3, C4 or Cz	Fpz or ipsilateral ear lobe or mastoid	Contralateral ear or mastoid or other "inactive" site (shoulder, knee, etc.)	25, 50 or 100 μv per full display depending upon presence of artifact and size of pattern envelope	50	Arbitrary to yield best display	64
100	C3 and C4				100		32
100	C3 and C4[d] or O3 and O4				100		16
100	C3 and C4				100		16
250 Hz	C3 and C4[h] and/or Erb's point	Fpz or ipsilateral ear lobe or mastoid	Linked ear lobes or other "inactive site"	25, 50 or 100 μv per full display depending upon presence of artifact and size of pattern envelope	100	Arbitrary to yield best display	16
100	C3 and C4				50		16
250	Cz[d]	"	"		100		16
100	Cz	"	"		100		16

[e]Check sizes must be standardized for each laboratory. A $1°$ check size is used typically.
[f]If a muscle twitch at the site of stimulation is not obtainable a constant current of 19.9 ma is usually employed, if tolerated.
[g]150 msec under anesthesia in surgery.
[h]Recording electrodes in certain cases are placed at L1-L5 and C7 or other sites to evaluate further the transmission of somatosensory information through the spinal cord.

movements, eye blinks, and tongue movements also inject artifactual responses into recordings. EKG responses also intrude at times. Beyond body generated electrophysiologic responses there are other electrical artifacts such as ever present 60 Hz "noise" or other uncontrolled electro-mechanical events occurring in the nearby environment. 60 Hz signals frequently are controlled by a notch filter which eliminates or suppresses a narrow frequency band around 60 Hz. Most modern equipment should have an artifact rejection mode to exclude large unwanted signals.

Stimulus parameters also can account for variations in EP patterns. The type of stimuli needed to activate different sensory modalities yields different patterns. Thus distinctive responses are associated with auditory, visual, somatosen-

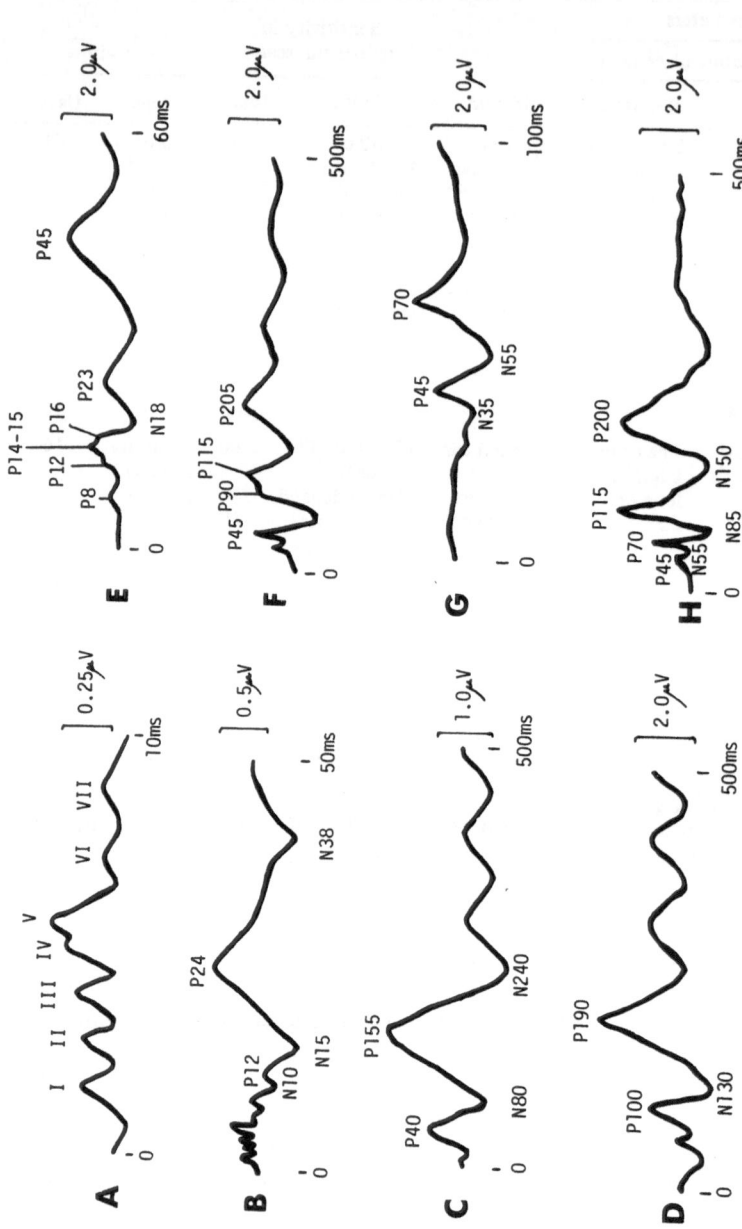

Figure 1. Typical normal auditory (AEP), visual (VEP), and somatosensory (SEP) evoked potential patterns. A. AEP short latency (0–10 msec): auditory nerve and brainstem responses; B. AEP intermediate latency (0–50 msec): auditory myogenic reflex and early cortical responses; C. AEP long latency (0–500 msec): auditory cortical responses; D. VEP long latency (0–500 msec): visual flash cortical responses; E. SEP intermediate latency (0–60 msec): somatosensory pre-cord, cord, subcortical, and early cortical responses to median nerve stimulation; F. SEP long latency (0–500 msec): somatosensory cortical responses to median nerve stimulations; G. SEP intermediate latency (0–100 msec): early cortical responses to sural nerve stimulation; H. SEP long latency (0–500 msec): late cortical responses to sural nerve stimulation.

Table 3. Auditory Evoked Potentials: Mean Peak Latencies in Msec after Stimulus Onset and Mean Amplitudes in Microvolts for Short Latency (Auditory Nerve and Brain Stem) Responses (0-10 msec)

		Ia	II	III	IV	V	VI	VII	I-Vb
Latencies	M	1.62	2.65	3.72	4.93	5.55	7.06	8.65	3.93
	SD	.13	.16	.18	.21	.23	.33	.42	.21
	Nc	36	36	36	27	36	24	27	35
Amplitudesd	M	.29	.22	.24	.30	.35	.11	.11	
	SD	.14	.12	.09	.11	.17	.07	.07	
	N	34	34	34	27	34	31	27	

[a]Roman numerals refer to peaks whose electrophysiological activity is thought to be generated primarily in or near the following: I–Auditory Nerve; II–Cochlear nucleus (medulla); III–Superior olivary complex (pons); IV–Ventral nucleus of the lateral lemniscus (pons); V–Inferior colliculus (midbrain); VI–Possibly the medial geniculate (thalamus);VII–Possibly auditory radiations (thalamocortical).
[b]Central conduction time between Peaks I and V.
[c]Ns vary because all peaks are not always seen.
[d]Amplitude measured peak-to-peak from identified positive-going peak to preceding negative trough, except for Peak 1 where the succeeding negative trough was used. Each number is the mean value of C3 and C4 electrode placements.

Table 4. Auditory Evoked Potentials: Mean Peak Latencies in Msec after Stimulus Onset and Mean Amplitudes in Microvolts for Intermediate Latency (Myogenic and Early Cortical) Responses (0-50 msec)

	Latencies					Amplitudes	
	N10	P12[a]	N15	P24[b]	N38	P12	P24
M	10.3	12.5	15.3	24.3	37.8	.59	1.13
SD	2.73	2.61	1.96	3.61	3.88	.94	.44
N	20	20	32	32	27	20	32

[a]P12 Possibly postauricular myogenic reflex response.
[b]P24 Possibly temporalis myogenic reflex response (multilobed except when patient is asleep).
[c]Amplitude measured peak-to-peak from identified positive–or negative-going peak to pre-ceding negative–or positive-going peak. Each number is the mean value of C3 and C4 electrode placements. P–Positive-going peak; N–Negative going peak.

sory and other types of stimuli. In addition, physical parameters of the stimulus and the stimulus conditions such as intensity, duration, number of presentation, rate of presentation, interstimulus interval, rise and fall time to and from the peak value of the stimulus, spatial localization, probability of occurrence, meaningfulness and special or unique characteristics of the stimulus all have an influence on the configuration of the EP pattern. These must be considered when absolute and com-parative EP analyses are undertaken.

Patient parameters can influence the form of the EP pattern. Factors that play a role include age [119,120], sex [43], state of arousal, level of awareness and direction or focus of concentration, attention and expectation. Cognitive require-ments also affect EP responses. Neurophysiologic responsivity and variability and neuropsychologic status as well as level of motor activity during testing also influ-ence results. And, of course, the existence of pathology can seriously affect EP

Table 5. Auditory Evoked Potentials: Mean Peak Latencies in Msec after Stimulus Onset and Mean Amplitudes in Microvolts for Long Latency (Cortical) Responses (0-500 msec)

	Latencies				Amplitudes
	P40	N80	P155	N240	P155
M	39	82	153	238	2.7
SD	13.7	13.4	17.7	29.3	.86
N	17	28	30	29	28

Amplitude measured peak-to-peak from identified positive–or negative-going peak to preceding negative–or positive-going peak. P–Positive-going peak; N–Negative-going peak. Each number is the mean value of C3 and C4 electrode placements.

Table 6. Flash Visual Evoked Potentials: Mean Peak Latencies in Msec after
Stimulus Onset and Mean Amplitudes in Microvolts for Long Latency
(Cortical) Responses (0–500 msec)

	Latencies				Amplitudes	
	P70	P100	N130	P190	P100	P190
M	68	102	131	186	2.8	5.9
SD	9.81	13.6	12.9	21.2	1.56	2.30
N	26	27	28	28	27	28

Amplitude measured peak-to-peak from the identified positive–or negative-going peak to the
preceding negative–or positive-going peak. P–Positive-going peak; N–Negative-going peak.
Each number is a mean value of C3 and C4 electrode placements. Flash based upon a 10 msec
exposure of a light intensity of 37 footcandles emitted by a cluster of five small yellow light
diodes (MV5352, Monsanto).

recordings as can the presence in the blood of anesthetic agents, barbiturates,
neuroleptics, or certain other drugs as described earlier.

Equipment variables represent another set of factors which can influence EP
patterns. Electrodes may vary by type (viz., silver-silver chloride, gold, needle, etc.),
by method of attachment (collodion, electrode paste, adhesive, mechanical pressure, subcutaneous insertion), by montage arrangement and by sites of placement
of the active, reference, and ground electrodes. Other equipment factors that can
influence EP recordings in major ways include the method and amount of amplification of signals, filter band pass settings, number of stimulations that are averaged,
method of averaging and method of recording patterns including the sensitivity
setting for signal detection, and the display gain employed. The reliability of
the equipment and its components as well as its design and serviceability also
should be considered.

Table 7. 1° and 15′ Pattern Reversal Visual Evoked Potentials: Mean Peak
Latencies in Msec after Stimulus Onset and Mean Amplitudes in Microvolts
for Long Latency (Cortical) Responses (0–300 msec)

		Latencies			Amplitudes[a]
		P50	N70	P90	P70
15′	M	51.7	68.7	90.2	7.081
Checks	SD	4.42	3.75	4.35	3.095
	N	17	17	17	17
1°	M	46.3	59.1	90.1	7.014
Checks	SD	3.32	3.10	3.94	5.144
	N	16	17	17	17

[a]Amplitude measured peak-to-peak from the identified positive-going peak to the preceding
negative trough. P–Positive-going peak; N–Negative-going peak.

Table 8. Somatosensory Evoked Potentials (Median Nerve); Mean Peak Latencies in Msec after Stimulus Onset and Mean Amplitudes in Microvolts for Intermediate Latency (Cord, Subcortical and Early Cortical) Responses (0-60 msec)

	Latencies						Amplitudes		
	P8	P12	P14-15	N18	P23	P45	P14-15	P24	P45
M	8.4	12.6	14.8	18.5	23.2	44.3	0.73	1.71	3.85
SD	.87	1.15	.84	2.06	2.20	4.18	.37	1.09	2.02
Nc	12	11	14	15	15	15	13	15	16

aPossible sources of electrophysiological activity: P8—Brachial plexus; P12—Dorsal column nuclei and medial lemniscus; P14-15—Thalamus; N18—Thalmo-cortical radiations; P24—Primary somatosensory cortex contralateral to side of stimulation; P45—Cortex, source unknown.
bAmplitude measured peak-to-peak from identified positive- or negative-going peak to preceding negative- or positive-going peak.
cNs vary because not all peaks are not always seen. P—Positive-going peak; N—Negative-going peak.

Table 9. Somatosensory Evoked Potentials (Median Nerve): Mean Peak Latencies in Msec after Stimulus Onset and Mean Amplitudes in Microvolts for Long Latency (Cortical) Responses (0-500 msec)

	Latencies				Amplitudes			
	P45	P90	P115	P205	P45	P90	P115	P205
M	45	87	116	206	3.0	2.9	2.2	4.0
SD	4.18	8.82	14.10	34.30	1.82	1.43	1.04	2.49
N	14	12	14	14	16	12	14	14

Amplitude measured peak-to-peak from identified positive-going peak to preceding negative-going peak. P—Positive-going peak; N—Negative-going peak.

Table 10. Somatosensory Evoked Potential (Sural Nerve): Mean Peak Latencies in Msec after Onset and Mean Amplitudes in Microvolts for Intermediate Latency (Early Cortical) Responses (0-100 msec)

	Latencies				Amplitudes	
	N35	P45	N55	P70	P45	P70
M	36	44	56	68	1.7	2.4
SD	3.04	3.97	5.90	7.94	0.91	1.5
N	20	22	21	17	19	15

Amplitude measured peak-to-peak from identified positive—or negative-going peak to preceding negative—or positive-going peak. P—Positive-going peak; N—Negative-going peak.

INTERPRETATION OF EP PATTERNS

Peak latencies in msec after stimulus onset are the primary means of determining whether EP patterns are normal or abnormal. Amplitudes in microvolts are considered "soft" data and are usually neither consistent nor reliable indices of abnormality. Yet, they do have value, especially if they are very large, very small, very inconsistent, or vary markedly from side to side. Under anesthesia, peak amplitudes sometimes have been found to vary more than peak latencies. Values for peak latencies and amplitudes in terms of their means and standard deviations in our laboratory are given in Tables 3-11. Again it must be mentioned that each laboratory should develop its own normative data base. If values are more than three (and sometimes two) standard deviations from the mean, they are considered abnormal. This hard data approach is suitable for auditory nerve and brainstem responses occurring between about 1.5-6 msec after stimulus onset; for relatively early cortical visual responses occurring between about 60-250 msec after flash stimulus onset and between about 50-150 msec after the presentation of reversing black and white checkerboard pattern stimuli; and for root and spinal cord, subcortical and early cortical, and later intermediate cortical responses to somatosensory stimulation occurring, respectively, between about 8-13, 14-22, and 23-150 msec after stimulus onset. When there is a need to employ EPs to evaluate higher level cortical activities or general brain dysfunction, then recording epochs may be extended to 500 or 1000 msec or more and additional criteria must be employed. For example, to evaluate brain function in schizophrenics, depressives, developmentally retarded, and those who are known or suspected of having brain injury either from trauma, anoxia, circulatory disturbances, space-occupying lesions, infections, or from toxic substances, one must also employ these additional criteria: 1) the absence of major peaks; 2) the degree of overall (Gestalt) pattern abnormality in terms of "noisiness" and irregularity in the shape and size of the pattern envelope and diffuseness or other irregularities in specific EP peaks; 3) the degree of pattern dissimilarity for recordings obtained simultaneously from the left and right hemispheres; and 4) pattern replicability upon repeat stimulation. Rappa-

Table 11. Somatosensory Evoked Potentials (Sural Nerve): Mean Peak Latencies in Msec after Stimulus Onset and Mean Amplitudes in Microvolts for Long Latency (Cortical) Responses (0–500 msec)

	P45	N55	P70	N85	P115	N150	P200
			Latencies				
M	45	57	68	84	114	146	201
SD	4.2	5.5	8.8	9.8	13.3	15.9	32.3
N	22	18	19	22	23	19	23
			Amplitudes				
M	2.42		2.30	2.91	4.13	3.08	3.19
SD	1.64		1.50	2.54	2.06	1.42	1.52
N	17		19	18	20	17	20

Amplitude measured peak-to-peak from identified positive–or negative-going peak to preceding negative–or positive-going peak. P–Positive-going peak; N–Negative-going peak.

port et al [84] have demonstrated the utility of these criteria in evaluating the clinical condition of head injury patients with psychologic impairments as well as in schizophrenics [24].

Whenever possible, interpretations should be made using a patient as his own control. This means comparing results obtained from the left and right sides whether the data be the results of auditory, visual, or somatosensory stimulation. Such information, used in conjunction with normative data tables, provides not only absolute values but also information on abnormal EP pattern differences between the left and right sides peripherally, subcortically, and at the cortical level. Normative data should be available for individuals in different age categories. Somatosensory stimulation data should also be available for individuals with different lenghts of arms, legs, and torsos.* These data make it possible in some instances to distinguish whether sensory deficits reported by patients do in fact have a neurophysiologic basis or are more likely to have a psychogenic basis. Of course any interpretations of EP patterns must consider the influence of various artifacts, such as those described earlier, which can influence patterns recorded.

EP data can also be used to determine the possible presence of medical disease entities that masquerade or manifest themselves as emotional or cognitive disturbances. Subclinical multiple sclerosis (MS) is an example. Findings of EP abnormalities, particularly in the visual and in at least one other sensory modality, especially when left-right side differences are detected, may be important diagnostic and treatment clues for identifying the presence of MS. The effects of cortical atrophy on cortical EP patterns are such that one can see, particularly in severe cases, diffuse, delayed and sometimes absent peaks, diminished ampli-

---

*Measurement of interpeak latencies remains relatively constant regardless of limb and torso lengths, and therefore is a good measure of function or dysfunction.

tudes, and markedly irregular and noisy configurations. In individuals suspected of chronic alcoholism, there may be abnormally delayed brainstem responses upon auditory stimulation. Distorted visual EP patterns are known to be associated with renal dysfunction. Other abnormal VEP patterns are associated with various space occupying lesions that also may cause behavioral and psychologic problems that mask the underlying pathology. Different VEP patterns can help localize such lesions. For example, prechiasmatic lesions may be detected when abnormal VEP patterns are associated with only one eye. In this type of situation an electroretinogram (ERG) can be useful to rule out the retina as the primary site of difficulty. If the ERG is normal, then the EP has helped localize the lesion in the optic nerve of the affected eye. If bitemporal hemianopsia is present, there is likely to be pressure on the central portion of the optic chiasm. If homonymous hemianopsia is present, there may very well be postchiasmatic problems, such as a lesion affecting the optic tract.

In considering diagnoses in young children such as autism, childhood schizophrenia, and developmental disability, it can be quite helpful to check the functioning of the various sensory channels by EP testing to make sure observed behavioral and psychologic problems are not associated with sensory deficits. In children and adults where behavioral and psychologic aberrations may be associated with developing hydrocephalus (particularly the normal pressure type) or pressure from space occupying masses, cortical EP findings may prove helpful. It has been found that electrophysiologic abnormalities may be seen in EP recordings when CT scans, skull films, and other laboratory diagnostic procedures all report negative findings.

SEP tests may be useful in interpreting subjective complaints in industrial injury cases. Workers will complain of a variety of symptoms such as low back pain, decreased sensation in a limb, motor weaknesses, loss of hearing, tinnitus, dizziness, or visual impairment that they believe are associated with some incident that occurred in the work place or simply thought to be due to "exposure" to certain occupational conditions. If complaints are unilateral, patients can be used as their own control and results of EP testing of the left and right sides can be compared. Caution in interpreting SEP results, however, must be used since SEP testing involves primarily the dorsal pathways of the spinal cord, pathways mediating the senses of light touch, two-point threshold, vibration, and proprioception. SEP results do not provide a direct or good basis for assessing pain or motor dysfunction, conditions which are mediated primarily by lateral and ventral spinal cord pathways. There is the supposition, however, that, if impairment is found in the transmission of somatosensory information through the dorsal pathways, then it is more likely, though by no means certain, that efferent pathways may also be affected. Changes in peak latencies and EP pattern configurations over time can be used to monitor changes in a patient's condition and can help predict outcome. Such cases are usually limited to conditions where a patient has suffered dynamic changes following the acute onset of a pathologic conditions such as in traumatic brain injury, stroke, hydrocephalus, anoxia, drowning, and sometimes drug overdose. The rate of change of peak latencies and pattern configurations towards normal or away from normal is indicative of whether a patient is moving towards remission or towards relapse. Noting whether the left or right cerebral hemisphere is more affected can be helpful in predicting residual sensory and motor dysfunctions, in reaching diagnosis, and in developing appropriate treatment and rehabilitation plans [84,86]. In many of the aforementioned pathologic conditions, clinical and radiologic findings may be equally or more definitive in certain instances. Clinical observations, particularly if they are clear cut and unequivocal, are likely to be more efficient and cost-effective diagnostic approaches than EP testing. If they are not unequivocal then EP testing can be quite useful. Essentially, the current state of the art is such that EP recordings can provide a relatively gross reflection of the electrophysiologic condition of the CNS. The EP technique, however, is still wanting in its ability to reflect reliably, consistently, and sensitively subtle neuropsychologic and higher cognitive impairments associated with altered mental conditions. Although it can be used to identify in a gross way the severity and extent of impairment in cortical and subcortical responsivity to sensory stimulation, the relationship between such observations and intellectual functioning, mood, and specific psychiatric disorders is equivocal at best at the present time. Nevertheless, as mentioned above, it can be helpful for assessing the presence of certain medical disease entities and for ruling out strictly functional etiologies as explanations of various psychologic and behavioral disturbances reported in the psychiatric evaluation.

FUTURE APPLICATIONS

Any electrophysiologic technique that can reflect the processing of information in the brain has the potential to increase our understanding of how the brain performs when it is functioning normally and when it is functioning abnormally. As one examines the literature and notes the thrusts of research efforts, it appears possible to identify future applications of the EP technique which will have special significance for and be of benefit to psychiatry. Such applications include objective assessment of intellectual and cognitive functioning, as well as of level of awareness and ability to attend; identification and classification of learning disabilities and related information processing problems that are reflected in variations in electrophyisologic activity in the central nervous system; measuring responsiveness to various treatment efforts, particularly chemotherapeutic interventions likely to affect disordered neurophysiologic functioning of the brain associated with various mental disorders. Monitoring and predicting clinical outcome psychologically as well as physiologically and physically after insults to the brain have occurred as has already been demonstrated and is likely to be refined to become more useful in the future. Improved differentiation of sensory deficits originating with organic or psychogenic causes is another area where future progress can be expected. The EP technique is also likely to contribute to the early identification of those at risk for developing serious mental disturbances and to lead to improved methods of diagnosing mental dysfunctions and evaluating the effects of different treatment approaches.

One approach that appears to show particular great promise in identifying electrophysiologic manifestations of brain dysfunction associated with a wide range of abnormal neuropsychologic and neurobehavioral disorders is the neurometric approach described by John et al [50] and John and Ahn et al [52]. The existing data base already permits specifying the probability of brain dysfunction in children with general and specific learning disabilities. It can be anticipated that further research will identify combined EEG and EP patterns associated with a wide range of other neuropsychiatric impairments. Flitter and Lieber in a personal communication, for example, report that for about 100 depressed patients with abnormal DST and TRH laboratory findings there is a significant correlation with abnormal neurometric Z-score values (M Flitter and A Lieber, Neurometric Laboratory, St. Francis Hospital, Miami Beach, Florida, personal communication, December 1982). With the array of ways for studying various kinds of cognitive functioning described earlier it would appear more than likely that we shall see in the not too distant future further reports on correlations between abnormalities in EP pattern and abnormalities in the mental processes observed in those suffering cognitive dysfunctions associated with mental illness.

A number of potentially useful studies are warranted based upon EP findings in normal subjects under conditions where attention and cognition were investigated. For example, now that it has been established that the amplitude of the peak occurring at N100 appeats to be an index of attention [94,97,99,101], it would seem quite reasonable to study in schizophrenics who have attentional deficits how various therapeutic interventions may or may not be able to normalize their attentional responses. Similarly now that we appear able to identify deficits in short-term memory storage we can examine how this phenomenon varies in patients with different mental disorders and how various treatment approaches may affect memory storage impairments [107].

Perhaps most exciting, however, is the prospect of using EP patterns to evaluate in mentally ill individuals deficits in their ability to analyze the congruity or incongruity of semantic messages and how this ability changes over time or with various therapeutic interventions [115]. With the array of ways for studying various kinds of cognitive functioning described in the literature review section it should appear more than likely that we shall see in the not too distant future further reports on correlations between abnormalities detected in EP patterns and abnormalities in the mental processes observed in those suffering cognitive dysfunctions associated with mental illness. An even newer electrophysiologic technique on the horizon that may prove to have great utility is the BEAM (Brain Electrical Activity Mapping) technique developed by Duffy, which analyzes both EEG and EP results [121].

REFERENCES

1. Caldani L: Institutiones Physiologicae et Pathologicae. Luchtmans, 1784.
2. Fritsch G, Hitzig E: Uber die elektrische Erregbarkeit des Grosshirns. Arch Anat Physiol 37:300-322, 1870
3. Caton R: The electric currents of the brain. Br Med J 2:278, 1875
4. Beck A, Cybulski N: Fizyologia Czlowieka (The Physiology of Man), vol 2. Krakow, 1915
5. Berger H: Uber das Elektrenkephalogramm des Menschen. Arch Psych 87: 527-570, 1929
6. Dawson GD: Cerebral responses to electrical stimulation of peripheral nerve in man. J Neurol Neurosurg Psych 10:134-140, 1947
7. Calvet J, Scherrer J: Des certaines limites et possibilites nouvelles en electrophysiologie. In Actes des Journees Mesure et Connaissance, Rev Metrologie, Paris, 1955, pp 289-293
8. Walter WG: The convergence and interaction of visual, auditory and tactile responses in human nonspecific cortex. Ann NY Acad Sci 112:320-361, 1964
9. Rosner BS, Allison T, Swanson E, et al: A new instrument for the summation of evoked responses from the nervous system. Electroenceph Clin Neurophysiol 12:745-747, 1960
10. Clark WA: Digital techniques in neuroelectric data processing. Electroencephalogr Clin Neurophysiol. 20 (suppl):75-78, 1961
11. Rappaport M: Brain evoked potentials: Clinical applications. Medical Electronics 84-89, (June) 1983
12. Desmedt JE: Clinical Uses of Cerebral, Brainstem and Spinal Somatosensory Evoked Potentials. New York, S Karger, 1980
13. Desmedt JE: Cognitive Components in Cerebral Event-Related Potentials and Selective Attention. New York, S Karger, 1979
14. Squires K, Goodin D, Starr A: Event related potentials in development, aging and dementia. In D Lehmann, E Callaway (eds): Human Evoked Potentials. New York, Plenum Press, 1979
15. Sutton S, Tueting P: Evoked potentials and diagnosis. In RL Spitzer, D Klein (eds): Critical Issues in Psychiatric Diagnosis. New York, Raven Press, 1978
16. Shagass C, Ornitz EM, Sutton S, et al:.Event related potentials and psychopathology. In E Callaway, P Tueting, SH Koslow (eds): Event-Related Brain Potential in Man. New York, Academic Press, 1978
17. Begleiter H: Evoked Brain Potentials and Behavior. New York, Plenum Press, 1977
18. Desmedt JE: Progress in Clinical Neurophysiology, Vol. 2. Auditory Evoked Potentials in Man. Psychopharmacology Correlates of Evoked Potentials. New York, S Karger, 1977
19. Callaway E: Brain Electrical Potentials and Individual Psychological Differences. New York, Grune & Stratton, 1975
20. Shagass C: Evoked Brain Potentials in Psychiatry. New York, Plenum Press, 1972
21. Donchin E: Data analysis techniques in average evoked potential research. In E. Donchin, DB Lindsley: Average Evoked Potentials. NASA SP-191, 199-217. Washington, DC, US Government Printing Office, 1969

22. Shagass C: Psychiatric diagnostic correlates of evoked potentials. In J Obiols, C Ballus, E Gonzalez, et al (eds): Biological Psychiatry Today. New York, Elsevier/North-Holland, 1979

23. Pfefferbaum A, Horvath T, Walton R, et al: Auditory brain stem and cortical evoked potentials in schizophrenia. Biol Psych 15:209–223, 1980

24. Rappaport M, Hopkins K, Hall K, et al: Schizophrenia and evoked potentials: Maximum amplitude, frequency of peaks, variability, and phenothiazine effects. Psychophysiol 12:196–207, 1975

25. Shagass C, Roemer RA, Straumanis JJ, et al: Temporal variability of somatosensory, visual, and auditory evoked potentials in schizophrenia. Arch Gen Psych 36:1341–1351, 1979

26. Saletu B, Itil TM, Saletu M: Auditory evoked response, EEG, and thought process in schizophrenics. Am J Psych 128:336–344, 1971

27. Heninger G, Speck LB: Visual evoked responses and mental status of schizophrenics. Arch Gen Psych 15:419–426, 1966

28. Begleiter H, Projesz B, Gross MM: Cortical evoked potentials and psychopathology. Arch Gen Psych 17:755–761, 1967

29. Cobb WA, Morocutti C (eds): The evoked potentials. Electroencephalogr Clin Neurophysiol Suppl. 26, 1967

30. Bergamini L, Bergamasco B: Cortical Evoked Potentials in Man. Springfield, IL, Charles C Thomas, 1967

31. Buchsbaum M, Goodwin F, Murphy D, et al: AER in affective disorders. Am J Psych 128:19–25, 1971

32. Buchsbaum MS, Davis GC, Goodwin FK, et al: Psychophysical pain judgments and somatosensory evoked potentials in patients with affective illness and in normal adults. In C Perris: Clinical Neurophysiological Aspects of Psychopathology. New York, S Karger, 1980

33. Friedman J, Meares R: Cortical evoked potentials and extraversion. Psychosom Med 41:279–286, 1979

34. Visser SL, Stam FC, Van Tilburg W, et al: Visual evoked response in senile and presenile dementia. Electroencephalogr Clin Neurophysiol 40:385–392, 1976

35. Rappaport M: Brain evoked potentials as a tool in psychiatric assessment. J Clin Psych 43:465–467, 1982

36. Shagass C, Schwartz M: Cerebral responsiveness in psychiatric patients. Arch Gen Psych 8:87–99, 1963

37. Moldofsky H, England RS: Facilitation of somatosensory average-evoked potentials in hysterical anesthesia and pain. Arch Gen Psych 322:193–197, 1975

38. Stelmack RM, Achorn E, Michaud A: Extraversion and individual differences in auditory evoked response. Psychophysiol 14:368–374, 1977

39. Coursey RD, Buchsbaum M, Frankel BL: Personality measures and evoked responses in chronic insomniacs. J Abnorm Psychol 84:239–242, 1975

40. Buchsbaum MS, Haier RJ, Murphy DL: Suicide attempts, platelet monoamine oxidase and the average evoked response. Acta Psychiatr Scand 56:69–79, 1977

41. Coons PM, Milstein V, Marley C: EEG studies of two multiple personalities and a control. Arch Gen Psych 39:823–825, 1982

42. Ludwig AM, Brandsma JM, Wilbur CB, et al: The objective study of a multiple personality: Or, are four heads better than one? Arch Gen Psych 26:298–310, 1972

43. Ikuta T, Furuta N: Sex differences in the human group mean SEP. Electro-enceph Clin Neurophysiol 54:449–457, 1982

44. Halliday R, Rosenthal JH, Naylor H, et al: Averaged evoked potential predic-tors of clinical improvement in hyperactive children treated with methyl-phenidate: An initial study and replication. Psychophysiol 13:429–440, 1976

45. Michael RL, Klorman R, Salzman LF, et al: Normalizing effects of methyl-phenidate on hyperactive children's vigilance performance and evoked poten-tials. Psychophysiol 18:665–677, 1981

46. Tanguay PE, Edwards RM, Buchwald J, et al: Auditory brainstem evoked responses in autistic children. Arch Gen Psych 39:174–180, 1982

47. Sohmer H, Student M: Auditory nerve and brain stem evoked responses in normal, autistic, minimal brain dysfunctioned and psychomotor retarded children. Electroenceph Clin Neurophysiol 44:380–388, 1978

48. Loiselle DL, Stamm JS, Maitinsky S, et al: Evoked potential and behavioral signs of attentive dysfunctions in hyperactive boys. Psychophysiol 17:193–201, 1980

49. Salamy A, Mendelson T, Tooley Wh, et al: Differential development of brain-stem potentials in health and high-risk infants. Science 210:552–555, 1980

50. John ER, Karmel BZ, Corning WC, et al: Neurometrics. Science 196:1393–1410, 1977

51. Baird HW, John ER, Ahn H, et al: Neurometric evaluation of epileptic chil-dren who do well and poorly in school. Electroenceph Clin Neurophysiol 48:683–693, 1980

52. John ER, Ahn H, Prichep L, et al: Developmental equations for the electro-encephalogram. Science 210:1255–1258, 1980

53. Preston MS, Guthrie JT, Kirsch I, et al: VERs in normal and disabled adult readers. Psychophysiol 14:8–14, 1977

54. Wasman M, Gluck H: Recovery functions of somatosensory evoked responses in slow learners. Psychophysiol 12:371–376, 1975

55. Weber BA, Omenn GS: Auditory and visual evoked responses in children with familial reading disabilities. J Learning Dis 10:153–158, 1977

56. Lelord G, Laffont F, Jusseaume PH: Conditioning of evoked potentials in children of differing intelligence. Psychophysiol 13:81–85, 1976

57. Saletu B, Saletu M, Simeon J, et al: Fluphenazine treatment in the psychotic child: Clinical-evoked potential correlations. Compr Psych 16:265–278, 1975

58. Saletu B, Saletu M, Herrmann WM, et al: Are hormones psycho-active? Evoked potential investigations in man. Arzneimittel-Forsch 25:1321–1327, 1975

59. Itil TM, Hsu W, Saletu B, et al: Computer EEG and auditory evoked potential investigations in children at high risk for schizophrenia. Am J Psych 131:892–900, 1974

60. Friedman D, Vaughan Jr. HG, Erlenmeyer-Kimling L: Event related potential investigations in children at high risk for schizophrenia. In D Lehmann, E Callaway (eds): Human Evoked Potentials Applications and Problems. New York, Plenum Press, 1979

61. Bigum HB, Dustman RE, Beck EC: Visual and somato-sensory evoked re-sponses from mongoloid and normal children. Electroenceph Clin Neuro-physiol 28:576–585, 1970

62. Gliddon JB, Busk J, Galbraith GC: Visual evoked responses as a function of light intensity in Down's syndrome and nonretarded subjects. Psychophysiol 12:416–422, 1975

63. Chiappa KH, Ropper AH: Evoked potentials in clinical medicine, Part 1. N Engl J Med. 306:1140–1150, 1982
64. Chiappa KH, Ropper AH: Evoked potentials in clinical medicine Part 2. N Engl J Med 306:1205–1211, 1982
65. Saletu B: Cerebral evoked potentials in psychopharmacology. In JE Desmedt (ed): Progress in Clinical Neurophysiology. Auditory Evoked Potentials in Man Psychopharmacology; Correlates of Evoked Potentials, Vol 2. New York, S. Karger, 1977
66. Shagass CL: Evoked potentials in psychopathology and psychiatric treatment. IN N Burch: Behavior and Electrical Activity. New York, Plenum Press, 1975
67. Hall RA, Rappaport M, Hopkins HK, et al: Tobacco and evoked potential. Science 180:212–213, 1973
68. Friedman J, Meares R: The effect of placebo and tricyclic antidepressants on cortical evoked potentials in depressed patients. Biol Psychol 8:291–302, 1979
69. Heninger GR: Lithium carbonate and brian function. Arch Gen Psych 35: 228–233, 1978
70. Lonsdale E, Nodar RH, Orlowski JP: The effects of thiamine on abnormal brainstem auditory evoked potentials. Cleveland Clinic Quarterly 46:83–88, 1979
71. Saletu B, Saletu M, Itil TM, et al: Somatosensory-evoked potential changes during thiothixene treatment in schizophrenic patients. Psychopharmacologia 20:242–252, 1971
72. Saletu B, Saletu M, Itil TM, et al: Effect of stimulatory drugs on the somatosensory evoked potential in man. Pharmakopsych Neuropsychopharm 5:129–136, 1972
73. Davis GC, Buchsbaum MS, Naber D, et al: Effect of opiates and opiate antagonists on somatosensory evoked potentials in patients with schizophrenia and normal adults. In C Perris (ed): Clinical Neurophysiological Aspects of Psychopathology. New York, S Karger 1980
74. Lewis EG, Dustman RE, Peters BA, et al: The effects of varying doses of Δ^9-tetrahydrocannabinol on the human visual and somatosensory evoked response. Electroenceph Clin Neurophysiol 35:347–354, 1973
75. Herning RI, Jones RT, Peltzman D: Changes in human event related potentials with prolonged Delta A tetrahydrocannabinol (THC) use. Electroenceph Clin Neurophysiol 47:556–570, 1979
76. Squires KC, Chu NS, Starr A: Acute effects of alcohol on auditory brainstem potentials in humans. Science 201:174–176, 1978
77. Gross MM, Begleiter H, Tobin M, et al: Changes in auditory evoked response induced by alcohol. J Nerv Ment Dis 143:152–156, 1966
78. Lewis EG, Dustman RE, Beck EC: The effects of alcohol on visual and somatosensory evoked responses. Electroenceph Clin Neurophysiol 28:202–205, 1970
79. Begleiter H, Porjesz B, Chou CL: Auditory brainstem potentials in chronic alcoholics. Science 211:1064–1066, 1981
80. Chu NS, Squires KC, Starr A: Auditory brain stem responses in chronic alcoholic patients. Electroenceph Clin Neurophysiol 54:418–425, 1982
81. Buchsbaum MS, Davis GC, Coppola R, et al: Opiate pharmacology and individual differences. II. Somatosensory evoked potentials. Pain 10:367–377, 1981

82. Buchsbaum MS, Davis GC, Coppola R, et al: Opiate pharmacology and individual differences. II. Somatosensory evoked potentials. Pain 10:367–377, 1981
83. Carmon A, Mor J, Goldberg J: Evoked cerebral responses to noxious thermal stimuli in humans. Exp Brain Res 25:103–107, 1976
84. Rappaport M, Hall K, Hopkins HK, et al: Evoked potentials and head injury. 1. Rating of evoked potential abnormality. Clin Electroenceph 12:154–166, 1981
85. Rappaport M, Hopkins HK, Hall K, et al: Evoked potentials and head injury. 2. Clinical applications. Clin Electroenceph 12:167–176, 1981
86. Rappaport M, Hall K, Hopkins HK, et al: Evoked brain potentials and disability in brain-damaged patients. Arch Phys Med Rehabil 58:333–338, 1977
87. Greenberg RP, Becker DP, Miller JD, et al: Evaluation of brain function in severe human head trauma with multimodality evoked potentials. Part 2: Localization of brain dysfunction and correlation with posttraumatic neurological conditions. J Neurosurg 47:63–177, 1977
88. Rowe MJ, Carlson C: Brainstem auditory evoked potential in postconcussion dizziness. Arch Neurol 37:679–683, 1980
89. Sutton S, Braren M, Zubin J, et al: Evoked potential correlates of stimulus uncertainty. Science 150:1187–1188, 1965
90. Sutton S, Tueting P, Zubin J, et al: Information delivery and the sensory evoked potential. Science 155:1436–1439, 1967
91. Hillyard SA, Courchesne E, Krausz HI, et al: Scalp topography of the P3 wave in different auditory decision tasks. IN WC McCallum, JR Knott (eds): The Responsive Brain. Bristol, John Wright & Sons, 1976
92. Hillyard SA, Picton TW: Event-related brain potentials and selective information processing in man. In J Desmedt (ed): Cerebral Evoked Potentials in Man. New York, S. Karger, 1979
93. Hillyard SA, Picton TW, Regan DM: Sensation, perception and attention: Analysis using ERPs. In E Callaway, P Tueting, SH Koslow (eds): Event-Related Brain Potentials in Man. New York, Academic Press, 1978
94. Wastell DG, Kleinman D: Evoked potential correlates of visual selective attention. Acta Psychologica 46:129–140, 1980
95. Broadbent DE: Stimulus set and response set: Two kinds of selective attention. In DI Mostofsky (ed): Attention: Contemporary Theory and Analysis. New York, Appleton-Century-Crofts, 1970
96. Donchin E, Cohen L: Averaged evoked potentials and intramodality selective attention. Electroenceph Clin Neurophysiol 22:537–546, 1967
97. Hillyard SA, Hink RF, Schwent VL, et al: Electrical signs of attention in the human brain. Science 182:177–180, 1973
98. Naatanen R: Selective attention and evoked potentials in humans—a critical review. Biol Psychol 2:237–307, 1975
99. Picton TW, Hillyard SA, Galambos R: Habituation and attention in the auditory system. In WD Keidel, WD Neff (eds): Handbook of Sensory Physiology V/3. Berlin, Springer-Verlag, 1976, pp. 343-389
100. Parasuraman R: Auditory evoked potentials and divided attention. Psychophysiol. 15:460–465, 1978
101. Parasuraman R, Beatty J: Brain events underlying detection and recognition of weak sensory signals. Science 210:80–83, 1980
102. Becker DE, Shapiro D: Directing attention toward stimuli affects the P300 but not the orienting response. Psychophysiol 17:385–389, 1980

103. Ruchkin DS, Sutton S, Tueting P: Emitted and evoked P300 potentials and variation in stimulus probability. Psychophysiol 12:591–595, 1975
104. Johnston VS, Holcomb PJ: Probability learning and the P3 component of the visual evoked potential in man. Psychophysiol 17:396–400, 1980
105. Ruchkin DS, Sutton S, Stega M: Emitted P300 and slow wave event-related potentials in guessing and detection tasks. Electroenceph Clin Neurophysiol 49:1–14, 1980
106. Duncan-Johnson CC: Young psychophysiologist award address, 1980. P300 latency: A new metric of information processing. Psychophysiol 18:207–215, 1981
107. Chapman RM, McCrary JW, Chapman JA: Short-term memory: The "storage" component of human brain responses predicts recall. Science 202:1211–1214, 1978
108. Shucard DW, Shucard JL, Thomas DG: Auditory evoked potentials as probes of hemispheric differences in cognitive processing. Science 197:1295–1298, 1977
109. Ritter W, Simson R, Vaughan Jr. HG, et al: A brain event related to the making of a sensory discrimination. Science 203:1358–1361, 1979
110. Squires KC, Wickens C, Squires NK, et al: The effect of stimulus sequence on the waveform of the cortical event-related potential. Science 193:1142–1146, 1976
111. Duncan-Johnson CC, Kopell BS: The stroop effect: Brain potentials localize the source of interference. Science 214:938–940, 1981
112. Begleiter H, Platz A: Cortical evoked potentials to semantic stimuli. Psychophysiol 6:91–100, 1969
113. Johnston VS, Chesney GL: Electrophysiological correlates of meaning. Science 186:944–946, 1974
114. Brown WS, Marsh JT, Smith JC: Brief report: Contextual meaning effects on speech-evoked potentials. Behav Biol 9:755–761, (abstract 3173), 1973
115. Kutas M, Hillyard SA: Reading senseless sentences brain potentials reflect semantic incongruity. Science 207:203–205, 1980
116. Goodin DS, Squires KC, Henderson BH, et al: An early event-related cortical potential. Psychophysiol 15:360–365, 1978
117. White CT: The visual evoked responses and patterned stimuli. In G Newton, AH Riesen (eds): Advances in Psychobiology, Vol 2. New York, John Wiley & Sons, 1974
118. Jasper HH: The ten-twenty electrode system of the international federation. Electroenceph Clin Neurophysiol 10:371, 1958
119. Klorman R, Thompson LW, Ellingson RJ: Event-related potentials across the life span. In E Callaway, P Tuetin, SH Koslow (eds): Event-Related Brain Potentials in Man. New York, Academic Press, 1978
120. Roth WT, Ford JM, Pfefferbaum A, et al: Event related potential research in psychiatry. In D Lehmann, E Callaway (eds): Human Evoked Potentials applications and problems. New York, Plenum Press, 1979
121. Duffy FH, Bartels PH, Burchfield JL: Significance probability mapping: an aid in the topographic analysis of brain electrical activity. Electroenceph Clin Neurophysiol 51:455–462, 1981

CHAPTER 6

Special Electrophysiological Tests: Brain Spiking, EEG Spectral Coherence

BERNARD SALTZBERG

INTRODUCTION

Largely as a consequence of advances in computer technology, the use of time series analysis methodology to investigate correlations of brain electrical activity with clinical disorders has become an area of intense effort in many EEG Research laboratories. The primary objective of many of these investigations is the detection of EEG time series properties which offer a quantitative basis for aiding diagnosis of mental illness or brain injury. This chapter describes the special electrophysiologic tests we have been developing at the Texas Research Institute of Mental Science (TRIMS) for use in research concerned with detecting EEG properties which correlate with particular abnormalities such as uncontrolled violent behavior, learning disabilities, and epilepsy.

BRAIN SPIKING

Intermittent deep brain electrical spiking as well as scalp EEG spiking have been implicated in certain brain and behavioral disorders such as epilepsy [1] and uncontrolled violent behavior. The correlation of abnormal deep brain elec-

Handbook of Psychiatric Diagnostic Procedures, vol. 2, edited by R. C. W. Hall and T. P. Beresford. Copyright © 1985 by Spectrum Publications, Inc.

trical spiking activity with violent behavior has been demonstrated in nonhuman primate studies [2] by employing invasive methods which involve the surgical implantation of electrodes and subsequent analysis of the electrical activity recorded from the implanted deep brain structures. In light of these results, a significant advancement in the diagnosis of abnormal brain activity, especially that deep brain activity associated with persons exhibiting uncontrolled violent behavior, would be achieved by the development of detection methods that are noninvasive and therefore applicable in ordinary clinical EEG settings.

Our EEG research on noninvasive detection was stimulated primarily by the initial finding of complex patterns of consistent waveshape in scalp EEG which were time-locked to spikes recorded from electrodes implanted in deep brain structures of rhesus monkeys. These studies [2] have also shown that such scalp correlates of deep spiking can be detected even in severe EEG noise backgrounds by the application of digital filters appropriately designed to minimize the effects of unwanted EEG background activity, or by special application of cepstral methods in cases where digital filters for pattern recognition are not suitable because the pattern to be detected is not known a priori. The analytical methods and their potential applications are described in references [3-6].

DETECTION METHODS

The digital filtering procedures developed for detecting scalp correlates of deep spiking were based on an analysis of monkey and human scalp EEG data obtained from research projects where simultaneous recordings from deep brain structures were available. Using the deep spike as the trigger for averaging scalp EEG activity, it was observed that transient slow-wave activity frequently appeared in scalp activity at the same time that a spike occurred at depth. The waveshape of this transient activity was usually distorted by the presence of noise; therefore averaging procedures were used to achieve a better estimate of the transient waveshape. The power spectral density of the scalp EEG background activity was also estimated in order to appropriately weight the spectral components in the transient waveshape obtained by averaging. The digital filter derived from the spectral estimates of both the transient waveshape and the noise was employed as a detector which looks at scalp activity and reports on the presence or absence of transient patterns which match the characteristics of the digital filter. It is interesting to note that this coincidence of deep spiking and transient EEG slowing implies that pathologic sharp spiking activity at depth produces slow wave activity at the surface. This is consistent with clinical EEG criteria which consider focal slow activity to be an abnormal indication.

The procedure for evaluating candidate digital filters was based on the number of spikes detected in normal subjects as compared to the number of spikes detected in the recording of mentally ill subjects. In the initial evaluation a comparison was made of the incidence of spikes in normals and in violent subjects, based on a Poisson model for random spiking. In this model the number of spikes detected over a given length of recording is compared with the expected number derived from data on normals. The normal control is used to test the hypothesis that a given record represents the EEG of a normal subject under the assumption that spikes in normal subjects are uniformly randomly distributed. The methods of analysis underlying these evaluation procedures depend on the performance characteristics of the digital filter as a detector, as well as on the statistical model for evaluating the significance of the number of spikes detected. These methods are described in the next section.

COMPUTER IMPLEMENTATION

By virtue of our computer configuration, Fourier series methods (rather than matrix inversion methods) were used to design as well as evaluate the digital filter. The Fourier methods for the design of the optimum filter proceed as follows:

1. Obtain (a) the complex Fourier series of the candidate transient patterns and, (b) the power spectral density of the signal plus noise, i.e., the background EEG signal.
2. Divide the conjugate complex Fourier series of the transient pattern by the power spectral density of the signal plus noise.
3. Take the inverse transform of the Fourier series obtained in Step 2 which gives a discretely sampled time function that is the desired template or matched filter.

In addition to the above operations, the computer in our laboratory is also capable of performing running convolution. This allows continuous digital filtering of the scalp EEG to rapidly evaluate the performance characteristics of a candidate digital filter as a detector of abnormal transient activity.

The above analytical procedures refer to the detection of spike induced events, but it is necessary to assign some significance to the number of events detected in terms of background activity and artifacts that produce false spike indications. The major difficulty which presents itself in physiologic signal studies of this type arises from the fact that any given signal characteristic such as a spike can and usually does appear due to random background effects. The problem then becomes one of determining whether the appearance of this signal characteristic is due to background effects or to some inherent neurophysiologic abnormality in the EEG being analyzed. The analysis and evaluation rationale are straightforward if it is assumed that the timer interval between spike indications is random and uniformly distributed due to background activity in the normal EEG. With the foregoing assumptions, the analysis proceeds as follows:

let $p_n(t)$ = probability of exactly n spikes occurring in time t due to EEG background activity in normal subjects and,

$p_n(t + \Delta t)$ = probability of exactly n spikes occurring in time $t + \Delta t$ due to EEG background activity in normal subjects and,

λ = averate rate at which spikes occur in the EEGs of normal control subjects;

then

$$p_n(t + \Delta t) = p_n(t)(1 - \lambda \Delta t) + p_{n-1}(t)\lambda \Delta t. \tag{1}$$

Equation (1) states (a) that the probability of exactly n spikes occurring over $t + \Delta t$ is equal to the probability that n spikes occur over time t and none in Δt, plus the probability that exactly $(n - 1)$ spikes occur over time t and exactly one in Δt and that the time increment Δt is so small that (b) the probability of two or more spikes occurring during Δt is zero, and (c) that the probability of one spike occurring at Δt is $\lambda \Delta t$. Rearranging terms in Equation (1), and passing to the limit as $\Delta t \to 0$ gives:

$$\frac{dp_n(t)}{dt} + \lambda p_n(t) = \lambda p_{n-1}(t). \tag{2}$$

The solution of this difference-differential equation is the Poisson probability density:

$$p_n(t) = \frac{(\lambda t)^n}{n!} e^{-\lambda t}. \tag{3}$$

The average or expected number of spike occurrences, $\overline{n}$, during time t is given by:

$$\overline{n} = \lambda t.$$

The variance of spike occurrences is also equal to λt, so:

$$\sigma^2 = \overline{n}.$$

If the actual number of spikes detected in an EEG record of length t is N, then to test significance we need to determine the likelihood that N or more spikes could occur in a normal EEG record. This is given by the cumulative distribution:

$$P_n(t) = \sum_{n=N}^{\infty} \frac{(\lambda t)^n}{n!} \, e^{-\lambda t}$$

$$= 1 - \sum_{n=0}^{N-1} \frac{(\lambda t)^n}{n!} \, e^{-\lambda t}. \tag{4}$$

If N is large compared to $\bar{n}$ (= λt), then the likelihood computed from Equation (4) is small. If this likelihood is sufficiently small, then we reject the hypothesis that an EEG record containing N spikes in a time t is a normal record.

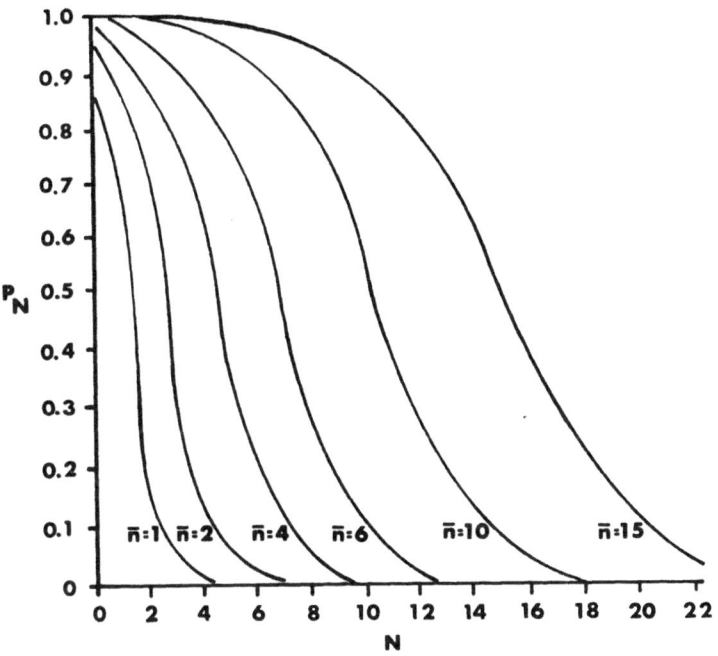

Figure 1. Probability criterion for the significance of N spike indications given $\bar{n}$ (Poisson Model). N = the actual number of spike indications in a given EEG recording, P_N = the probability of N or more spike indications, and $\bar{n}$ = the expected number of spike indications in a normal or control record of the same length.

For several values of spike-count expectation, the level of significance associated with this hypothesis for a record with N spike indications can be obtained from plots of the cumulative distribution shown in Figure 1. For example, if the expected number of spikes over a given length of a normal record is 6, then the plot shows that the probability of 18 spikes occurring in a normal record is 0.0001. Therefore, the hypothesis that an EEG in which 18 spikes are detected represents a normal subject is rejected at the 0.0001 level. The detection of 12 spikes would allow rejection of the hypothesis at the 0.02 level.

It should be pointed out that such statistical modeling of multiple detections over long EEG records is essential because of the false signals, artifacts, and the many uncontrollable sources of physiological interference that plague the evaluation of EEGs. These statistical procedures follow and supplement the digital filtering procedures used in designing the detector, as outlined in the previous sections and described in our publications.

DETECTION OF SPIKE CORRELATED SCALP TRANSIENTS
OF UNKNOWN WAVESHAPE

An alternate approach to the deep spike noninvasive detection problem is required when the recurring scalp EEG transient pattern is of unknown waveshape. Since averaging methods for visualizing a recurrent waveshape in noisy EEG require that the averaging process be synchronized by the deep spike event which can be detected only by invasive methods, the waveshape of the recurrent transient is frequently unknown. Under these conditions, the methodology for detecting the presence of a recurrent complex transient in scalp recorded brain electrical activity is based on the application of deconvolution procedures as described below.

A recurrent transient waveform in the EEG can be represented as follows:

$$E(t) = \sum_{k=0}^{n} A_k X(t - \tau_k) + N(t) \tag{5}$$

Alternatively, (5) may be written as a convolution product:

$$E(t) = X(t) * \sum_{k=0}^{n} A_k \delta(t - \tau_k) + N(t) \tag{6}$$

where * designates convolution, and

$X(t)$ = intermittent pattern; i.e., waveshape of recurrent transient
$N(t)$ = EEG background activity
$\delta(t - \tau_k)$ = Dirac delta function at τ_k

The deconvolution of the convolution factors in equation (6) is accomplished in several steps. First, the Fourier transform of (6) gives the algebraic product of the individual Fourier transforms of the intermittent pattern and the set of delta functions. This suggests the use of cepstral analysis which involves computation of the logarithm of the Fourier transform as a second step and, as a third step, computation of the inverse Fourier transform of this result to produce a function called the cepstrum. The properties of the cepstrum will reveal the presence of a recurrent pattern in the EEG by virtue of spikes which will appear in the cepstrum when two or more recurrences of the pattern are embedded in the EEG epoch analyzed.

If the waveform characteristics are of interest, then this methodology can also be used to determine the shape of the transient pattern. This is accomplished by smoothing the cepstrum to eliminate the spikes, and then reversing all the transformations used to produce the cepstrum. However, this is a difficult computational problem and it is possible to circumvent these procedures if one is not interested in ascertaining the shape of the pattern, but simply in detecting whether a recurrent pattern is contained within the time epoch analyzed. If at least two pat-

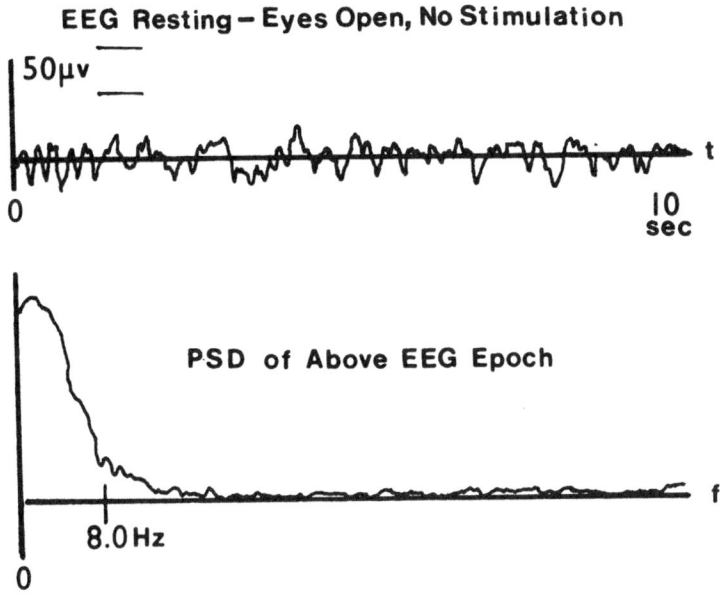

Figure 2. Resting—eyes open EEG without stimulation, and corresponding Power Spectral Density.

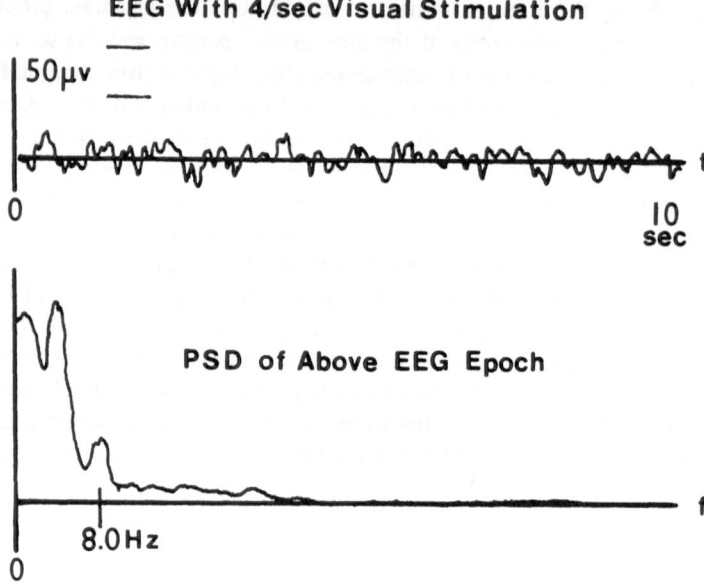

Figure 3. Resting—eyes open EEG with 4/sec visual stimulation, and corresponding Power Spectral Density.

terns are captured in the data epoch, then analysis shows that the power spectral
density (PSD) will contain ripples which are attributable to the presence of the
recurring pattern. The assumption underlying the utility of this approach is that
the background EEG, in the absence of a recurrent transient pattern, will possess
a smooth or unrippled PSD. Figures 2 and 3 demonstrate that this assumption
holds for the EEG data recorded under "eyes open" conditions from occipital
leads during an experiment in which transients were introduced into the background EEG by intermittent visual stimulation. The figures show that the PSD
for the no stimulus condition is smooth (Figure 2), whereas the PSD for the stimulus condition exhibits ripples (Figure 3) whose peaks are separated by the recipro-
cal of the stimulus interval.

In summary, the above results demonstrate that PSD analysis of sufficient
frequency resolution to resolve ripples may provide a tool for noninvasively diagnosing illnesses in which deep brain electrical spiking may be a factor. More generally, the analytical methods described in this section provide a basis for investigating the clinical implications of weak recurrent transients which are embedded
in EEG background and therefore usually not discernible by visual inspection of
the EEG time series.

EEG SPECTRAL COHERENCE

Spectral coherence analysis of the EEG provides a frequency dependent measure of shared* electrophysiologic activity. Thus, if linearly related (i.e., coherent) electrophysiologic activity between two EEG channels is present in a restricted portion of the frequency spectrum while the remainder of the spectrum contains activity which is linearly independent (i.e., incoherent) then the spectral coherence function by virtue of its frequency dependence, can detect coherent activity even in situations where intense levels of incoherent activity dominate the energy spectrum. Since differences in shared EEG activity may reflect differences in neural connectivity (i.e., communication between brain regions) this measure (coherence) has been adopted by several investigators [7] as a logical approach to the study of brain function in projects dealing with EEG correlates of cognition and learning disability.

PROBABILITY DISTRIBUTION OF COHERENCE ESTIMATES

The coherence function (i.e., spectral coherence) is defined in terms of the normalized cross-spectrum of two time series. The cross-spectrum is defined as the Fourier transform of the cross-correlation function, viz.:

Denote, $S_1(t), S_2(t) \equiv$ different time series
$\phi_{1,2}(\tau) \equiv$ cross-correlation function of $S_1(t), S_2(t)$

where τ is the variable time shift between S_1 and S_2, and $\phi_{1,2}(\tau)$ is defined by the integral equation (7)

$$\phi_{1,2}(\tau) = \frac{1}{T} \int_0^T S_1(t)S_2(t + \tau)dt \tag{7}$$

Then denote, $P_{1,2}(f)$ = cross-spectrum of $S_1(t)$, $S_2(t)$ where $P_{1,2}(f)$ is defined by (8), using the exponential form of the Fourier transformation.

$$P_{1,2}(f) = \int_{-\infty}^{+\infty} \phi_{1,2}(\tau)e^{-i2\pi f\tau}d\tau \tag{8}$$

(where f is frequency in hertz and τ is time shift in seconds). By substituting equation (7) into equation (8) and appropriately factoring the resulting double integral it can be shown that

---

*In this context shared electrophysiologic activity among brain regions is defined as that activity at a recording site that is related to the activity at another recording site through a linear transformation.

$$P_{1,2}(f) = \bar{S}_1(f)\bar{S}_2^c(f) \ (c \text{ denotes complex conjugate}) \tag{9}$$

where: $\bar{S}(f)$ is the Fourier transform of $S_1(t)$ and $\bar{S}_2^c(f)$ is the conjugate Fourier transform of $S_2(t)$. Note that $\bar{S}_1(f)$ and $\bar{S}_2^c(f)$ are complex numbers in general and therefore so is $P_{1,2}(f)$. We may represent them in polar form, as follows:

$$\bar{S}_1(f) = r_1 e^{i\theta}1 \tag{10}$$

$$\bar{S}_2^c(f) = r_2 e^{-i\theta}2 \tag{11}$$

Substituting (10) and (11) into (9) gives the cross-spectral density in polar form:

$$P_{1,2}(f) = r_1 r_2 e^{i(\theta 1 - \theta 2)} = r_1 r_2 e^{i\theta} \tag{12}$$

(where $\theta = \theta_1 - \theta_2$)

While not explicitly shown, note that the r's and θ's are functions of f. Now to arrive at the spectral coherence function we normalize equation (12) by dividing by $r_1 r_2$ and then averaging over a number of frequencies and/or averaging over a number of time epochs of the two time series being analyzed.

Thus if the average is taken over $2N + 1$ discrete frequencies we may write the spectral coherence as

$$C(f_0) = \frac{1}{2N+1} \sum_{k=-N}^{N} e^{i\theta(f_k)} \tag{13}$$

where f_0 is the center of the spectral window and uniform weighting is used in the window. If the average is taken over M time epochs (ensemble averaging) we may write the spectral coherence as

$$C(f_k) = \frac{1}{M} \sum_{m=1}^{M} e^{i\theta m(f_k)} \tag{14}$$

If a combination of frequency and ensemble averaging is used then spectral coherence may be written

$$C(f_0) = \frac{1}{M(2N+1)} \sum_{m=1}^{M} \left(\sum_{k=-N}^{k=N} e^{i\theta m(f_k)} \right) \tag{15}$$

Again, these expressions assume the use of uniform weighting in the spectral window.

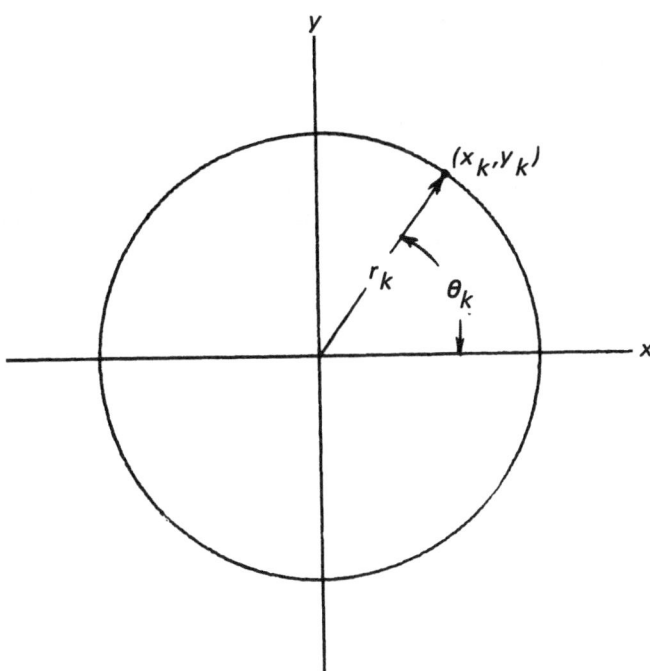

Figure 4. A coherence sample as a point on the unit circle in the complex plane. A coherence estimate is the average of such samples over a specified number of frequencies and/or a specified number of time periods.

It should be noted that for linearly independent signals the phase difference θ ($= \theta_1 - \theta_2$) is a random function over both frequency and ensemble and therefore the expected value of coherence averaged over frequency and/or time (ensemble averaging) is zero.

Thus, when coherence deviates significantly from zero, one may conclude that the two signal processes in question are related through a linear transformation over the spectral region where such significant deviation occurs.

The statistical measure of significance of a particular coherence estimate depends on the number of independent samples of coherence which are used in arriving at the coherence estimate, and upon the probability distribution function of these coherence estimates as described below.

A coherence estimate is the average computed from independent samples of the normalized cross-spectrum. These samples can be represented as points on the unit circle in the complex plane, as illustrated in Figure 4. If these points are uniformly distributed over the unit circle, it is clear that the expected value of coherencies at the origin $(\bar{x} = \bar{y} = 0)$. The normalized samples of cross-spectrum may be written:

$$x_k + iy_k = e^{i\theta k} = \cos\theta_k + i\sin\theta_k$$

The distribution shown in Figure 4 is equivalent to stating that the relative phase values between S_1 and S_2 at frequency f_0 are uniformly randomly distributed over an ensemble of time epochs and/or over a number of frequencies in a spectral window centered at frequency f_0. The complex value of coherence may be written:

$$\text{coh}(f_0) = \frac{1}{N} \sum_{k=1}^{N} x_k + i\frac{1}{N} \sum_{k=1}^{N} y_k \tag{16}$$

Since x_k and y_k lie on the unit circle

$$x_k = \cos\theta_k$$

$$y_k = \sin\theta_k$$

the PDF (Probability Distribution Function) of both x and y (given that θ is a uniformly distributed random variable) have the same form and are given by:

$$D(x) = \frac{1}{\pi\sqrt{1-x^2}} \quad , \quad D(y) = \frac{1}{\pi\sqrt{1-y^2}} \tag{17}$$

The corresponding means, $(\bar{x}, \bar{y})$ and variances (σ_x^2, σ_y^2) are given by

$$\bar{x} = \bar{y} = 0 \tag{18}$$

$$\sigma_x^2 = \sigma_y^2 = \frac{1}{2N} \tag{19}$$

where N = number of samples
From (18) and (19) it follows that the mean and variance of the coherence magnitude $(|\text{coh}(f_0)| \equiv r)$ is given by:

$$\bar{r} = 0 \tag{20}$$

$$\sigma_r^2 = \frac{1}{N} \tag{21}$$

Thus, to test the hypothesis that $S_1(t)$ and $S_2(t)$ are linearly independent time series, one examines the probability that the empirically-obtained mean, computed from N samples, deviates from the expected value (zero in this case). The number of standard deviations by which the empirical value exceeds the expected value determines the level of significance.

For example when the coherence magnitude, r, is obtained by a combination of ensemble averaging over 20 epochs and frequency averaging over 5 spectral components then

$$N = 20 \times 5 = 100$$

and the resulting standard deviation of the estimate is

$$\sigma_r = \frac{1}{\sqrt{N}} = \frac{1}{\sqrt{100}} = 0.1$$

Thus an empirically obtained value of coherence magnitude which exceeds 0.2 would be more than two standard deviations from the expected value for independent signals. Therefore it would be statistically reasonable to conclude that the signals in question are not independent, but rather that they are linearly dependent or coherent over the spectral region where the coherence magnitude exceeds 0.2. At TRIMS this method of coherence analysis has been applied to a pilot study of reading disabled children and normal controls. Our initial findings suggest that bilateral EEG coherence at frequencies above 20 hz is significantly lower in reading disabled children than in normal readers, which may be attributable to reduced sharing or communication between hemispheres at these frequencies. In any event this EEG measure provides a basis for comparing activity which visual examination of the EEG is incapable of discerning because the lower frequency energy which dominates both channels conceals the coherent relationship at high frequencies. The application of coherence analysis to problems in electrophysiology is likely to grow in importance because of the need to examine the relationships among multiple channel activity which may reveal abnormalities that cannot be found in analysis of single channel properties of the EEG.

REFERENCES

1. Saltzberg B, Kellaway P, Burton W, et al: Epilepsy: A heuristic model for relating nocturnal sleep EEG spike distributions to the risk of seizure. J Bio Med Comput 12:9–16, 1981
2. Saltzberg B, Lustick L, Heath R: Detection of focal depth spiking in the scalp EEG of monkeys. Electroencephalogr Clin Neurophysiol 31:327–333, 1971

3. Saltzberg B: Parameter selection and optimization in brainwave research. In N Burch, HL Altshuler (eds): Behavior and Brain Electrical Activity.New York, Plenum Press, 1975
4. Saltzberg B: A model for relating ripples in the EEG power spectral density to transient patterns of brain electrical activity induced by subcortical spiking. IEEE Trans Biomed Eng 23:225–256, 1976
5. Saltzberg B: The potential role of cepstral analysis in EEG research in epilepsy. In P Kellaway, I Petersen (eds): Quantitative Studies in Epilepsy. New York, Raven Press, 1976
6. Saltzberg B, Lustick L: Digital filters in neurological research. In Proceedings of the 1971 Imperial College of Science & Technology Symposium on Digital Filtering. London, England, Aug 31–Sept 2, 1971
7. Sklar B, Hanley J, Simmons WW: A computer analysis of EEG spectral signatures from normal and dyslexic children. IEEE Trans Biomed Eng 20:20–26, 1973

Radiologic Tests

CHAPTER 7

The Role of X-Ray Computed Tomography (CT)

DANIEL R. WEINBERGER

Computed tomography (CT) is a radiologic technique used to visualize gross anatomic structure of the brain in living persons. Since no consistent relationship between brain structure and psychiatric diagnosis has been established, CT does not help to "rule in" a psychiatric illness. It is not, strictly speaking, a diagnostic procedure in psychiatry. However, the CT scan does occupy an important place in the clinical armamentarium of the psychiatrist, who must frequently consider whether structural brain disease exists in his patients. Major psychiatric symptoms such as personality change, depression, and psychosis are nonspecific, clinical descriptors that in some cases represent early manifestations of remediable intracranial pathology. CT may be indicated in the search for such pathology. Furthermore, patients with symptoms of confusion, delirium, and dementia are increasingly being referred for psychiatric evaluation and treatment. The CT scan is an essential ingredient in the "work-up" of such patients.

In this chapter several aspects of the CT scan in clinical psychiatry are considered. First will be a review of the technical aspects of the procedure. Second is a review of structural central nervous system (CNS) disorders observable with CT that may masquerade as psychiatric illness. And finally, the rationale for ordering a CT scan on a psychiatric patient is discussed.

Handbook of Psychiatric Diagnostic Procedures, vol. 2, edited by R. C. W. Hall and T. P. Beresford. Copyright © 1985 by Spectrum Publications, Inc.

HOW CT WORKS

Although CT was introduced only ten years ago, it is now the single most important diagnostic technique in clinical neurology and neurosurgery. The method is revolutionary. It is an outgrowth more directly of computer technology than of traditional roentgenology. Image production does not involve exposure of photographic film as in traditional x-ray procedures. Instead, images are reconstructed mathematically from information derived about the distribution of radiodense tissue in a cross-section of the body, a tomographic slice. The level and angle of cross-section are determined by the plane at which a thin (collimated) x-ray beam scans or traverses the body. The x-rays transmitted through the tissue slice strike scintillation detectors (instead of x-ray film) which produce "counts" inversely proportional to the radiodensity of the tissue lying in the path of the x-ray beam. Because the beam scans from numerous directions in each plane, a two-dimensional map of radiodensity can be mathematically derived for each slice. The more opaque a region of the slice is to x-rays, the higher is its x-ray attentuation coefficient or "CT number" and the more dense it appears on the CT image. CT numbers are linked to a grey scale for imaging. Relatively radiolucent densities, such as water or cerebrospinal fluid (CSF), appear black, whereas radiopaque structures such as bone, appear white.

WHAT THE CT SHOWS

Anatomic detail shown by CT is a result of variation in neighboring structural densities. For example, since grey matter is more radiodense than white matter and thus has a lighter shade of grey on the CT image, the basal ganglia stand out from the surrounding subcortical white matter. In similar fashion, the cortical sulci and ventricular system are well visualized because the CSF that fills these spaces contrasts dramatically in density with the adjacent soft tissue of the brain.

CT abnormalities reflect pathologic deviations from the normal pattern of neighboring densities. For example, increases in the size of the CSF spaces, either because of hydrocephalus or reduction in brain size, appear as characteristic increases in the amount of CSF density. Focal CT abnormalities typically reflect variation in the tissue density of the brain parenchyma. Most focal brain pathology, including neoplastic, degenerative, and inflammatory conditions, involve varying degrees of necrosis, edema, and sometimes cavitation, all of which lead to an overall increase in the water content of the affected region. The result is a relative reduction in structural density and a region of hypodensity or greater blackness on the CT image. Edema may also cause gyral enlargement and consequent obliteration of normal sulci cisterns. Chronic brain lesions, on the other hand, may calcify and appear as a hyperdense area on the scan.

Extravasated blood from subarachnoid, subdural, or intracerebral hemorrhage produces a striking alteration in structural density. Fresh hemorrhage typically appears hyperdense relative to brain tissue and, though less dense than bone, may mimic bone density on a routine CT image. Other deviations from normal anatomic relationships include congenital abnormalities and spatial shifts in normal intracranial contents. One example of the former is the configuration of the ventricular system seen in association with agenesis of the corpus callosum. Mass lesions that produce changes in intracranial pressure usually cause normal structures to shift their location; thus, the lateral ventricles or the basal ganglia may be distorted and pushed to one side.

Radiodense iodine compounds are frequently administered as contrast agents to enhance the resolving power of a CT study. Normally, these compounds do not cross the blood-brain barrier but remain diluted in the intravascular compartment where they pass quickly through the brain. Central nervous system pathology often involves local derangements in the blood-brain barrier permitting extravasation of these iodine compounds into the extravascular compartment. A compromised area appears "enhanced" following contrast injection. This technique is especially useful in identifying areas of active CNS pathology that may not produce major changes in tissue radiodensity. So called "isodense" lesions, pathology with the density of normal brain, may only become obvious following contrast injection. A contrast study is also helpful in identifying abnormal vasculature such as arteriovenous malformations (AVM), which may be invisible in a noncontrast study. In such instances the contrast agent reaches sufficient concentration in a mass of overlapping vessels to appear as an abnormal area of hyperdensity.

Abnormalities that appear hypodense on both the precontrast and postcontrast scan usually reflect relatively static, degenerative conditions. Examples include leukoencephalopathies, such as non-acute multiple sclerosis (MS) lesions, progressive multifocal leukoencephalopathy (PML), primary degenerative dementias, old posttraumatic or postoperative conditions, postinfectious lesions, noninflammatory cysts, and low-grade gliomas. Abnormalities that are hypodense before contrast but then "light up" or show contrast enhancement include primary or metastatic tumors, abscesses, inflammatory diseases, such as encephalitis, acute multiple sclerosis, vascular malformations, leukemic infiltrations, contusions, and some recent infarctions. Finally, some meningiomas, some vascular maliformations, calcified structures or lesions, occasional metastatic tumors (e.g., melanoma), and intracranial hemorrhages appear hyperdense on both pre- and postcontrast studies.

CENTRAL NERVOUS SYSTEM DISEASE AND
PSYCHIATRIC SYMPTOMS

The more classical neurologic manifestations of brain disease, such as head-ache, visual symptoms, alterations in motor and sensory function, and seizures, rarely lead directly to psychiatric consultation. However, brain disease is fre-quently a cause of changes in mood and behavior. In fact, as is well known, psy-chiatric symptoms such as a change in personality, depression, or psychosis may be the earliest signs of CNS pathology or other systemic disease. It is important, therefore, for the psychiatrist to keep the possibility of an organic disorder near the top of the list of initial diagnostic possibilities when evaluating patients with nonspecific behavioral and/or emotional symptoms. This point is emphasized in the DMS-III, the current diagnostic nosology of the American Psychiatric Associ-ation. The CT scan is probably the single most conclusive procedure in ruling in or out structural CNS disease. Most structural disorders that may be associated with psychiatric symptoms can be excluded, diagnosed, or suggested by a CT scan. Before considering when it is reasonable for the psychiatrist to recommend this procedure, we will first review those disorders than can be discerned with CT.

It is important to emphasize that most of the disorders discussed below have characteristic clinical pictures that rule out a primary psychiatric diagnosis. While psychiatric symptoms may be the first manifestations of structural CNS pathology in some cases, only rarely will a neurologic disorder be diagnosed in the context of solely psychiatric symptoms. More frequently, the psychiatrist is called upon to evaluate psychiatric symptoms that appear in the context of a known brain disease.

Psychosis

Psychosis is frequently seen in the context of neurologic illness [1]. Although other clinical signs are usually present, this is by no means invariable. Table 1 lists some structural CNS disorders that may present initially with psychosis as the only manifestation. Huntington's disease has long been associated with psychotic symp-toms in young adults [1-3]. It is not uncommon for schizophreniform episodes or for a chronic psychosis to predate by several years the development of chorea or intellectual decline. Although spontaneous mutation occurs and family histories may be difficult to reconstruct in some cases, most patients will have a parent with a similar disorder. On CT scan, caudate atrophy is seen as a loss of the usual con-vex lateral border of the frontal horns of the ventricles. Ventricular dilatation and cortical atrophy may be present but are less specific than is caudate atrophy in patients under forty years old. Whether patients with only psychiatric symptoms show caudate atrophy is not known, as most studies have scanned patients because

Table 1. Structural Brain Disease Associated with Psychosis

Huntington's disease	Metachromatic leukodystrophy
Encephalitis	Wilson's disease
Lupus	Kuf's disease
Tumor, granuloma, abscess	Idiopathic cerebral ferrocalcinosis (Fahr's disease)
Trauma	

they have chorea. It is known, however, that the CT scan is normal in patients at risk for Huntington's disease who are clinically asymptomatic [4].

Among the hallmarks of Wilson's disease, an inherited disorder of copper metabolism, are personality change, dementia and/or psychosis [5]. As with Huntington's disease, the relationship of the psychopathology to the disorder is rarely appreciated before the onset of typical neurologic symptoms. The CT scan shows atrophic changes in the basal ganglia, cortex, and cerebellum.

Metachromatic leukodystrophy, an autosommal recessive disorder of sulfatide metabolism, occasionally begins in late adolescence as a psychotic disorder indistinguishable from schizophrenia [6]. With time, however, more traditional neurologic symptoms appear, including hemiplegia, as well as gait and movement disorders. Although this is a rare condition, cases with neurologic symptoms show characteristic, though nonspecific, appearance on CT scan. Patchy areas of decreased density appear in the subcortical white matter. It is not known whether these lesions predate the appearance of neurologic symptoms and are also seen in patients whose only manifestation of the disease is psychosis. Such patients have, unfortunately, not been considered for CT until after the development of more typical neurologic manifestations. Finally, Kuf's disease, a rare form of lipofuscinosis, is associated with psychosis in its early stages [7], and diffuse cerebral atrophy would be expected on CT.

Encephalitis, particularly that caused by herpes simplex virus, may present as a schizophreniform psychosis. While more characteristic symptoms, including headache, fever, delirium, and seizures, will become dominant within a few days, psychosis may be the earliest evidence of CNS infection [8,9]. Since herpes encephalitis is a usually devastating yet potentially treatable illness, early diagnosis is crucial. In patients with herpes simplex encephalitis irregular, often asymmetric areas of decreased density are seen in the temporal lobes. These areas may enhance with contrast injection. Because the necrotizing effects of the infection sometimes lead to local hemorrhages, small areas of hyperdensity may also be seen. While such findings are not diagnostic, in the proper clinical context, they are highly suggestive. Of course, it would be incorrect to initiate antiviral chemotherapy on the basis solely of psychotic symptoms and a nonspecifically abnormal CT scan. It would, however, be grounds for vigorous diagnostic efforts to rule out encephalitis (e.g., a lumbar puncture and possibly brain biopsy).

Psychosis, often indistinguishable from schizophrenia, may be the only manifestations of CNS lupus (SLE), though accompanying nonneurologic abnormalities should exist (e.g., kidney disease, arthritis, etc.). While the CT scan cannot be used to diagnose CNS lupus, it may support the possibility. Patients with psychosis as a manifestation of lupus are more likely to show focal or generalized cerebral atrophy than are lupus patients who do not have CNS involvement [10,11]. CNS tumors, granulomas, subdural hematomas, and other effects of trauma, as well as other space occupying lesions are associated with psychotic symptoms [1,12]. While it is unusual for psychosis to be the only sign, it is not impossible, particularly if the frontal or limbic lobes are involved [12]. Such lesions are well visualized and usually diagnosed with CT scan.

Affective Disorder

Affective disorder, particularly depression, is associated with many forms of structural CNS disease (Table 2). Space occupying lesions, such as tumors and subdural hematomas, often go undiagnosed until either a more dramatic change in level of consciousness or focal symptoms develop. In the elderly, slow growing tumors such as meningiomas as well as chronic subdural hematomas may be associated with depression long before other signs appear [13]. How these lesions cause depressive symptoms is unclear, but improvement in some cases is linked to treatment. So called normal or low pressure hydrocephalus is a potentially remediable cause of dementia that may initially present as depression [14]. Gait disturbances and urinary incontinence may appear later. The CT scan shows dilatation of the entire ventricular system, classically with relatively little atrophy of the cortex.

Table 2. **Structural Brain Disease Associated
with Depression**

Subdural hematoma

Tumor, granuloma, abscess

Normal pressure hydrocephalus

Lupus

Cerebral infarction

Trauma

Multiple sclerosis

Arnold–Chiari malformation

Cortical atrophy may be prominent, however. Depression and mania may be the only manifestations of CNS lupus, and cerebral atrophy is often seen on CT. Contrary to clinical lore, depression is associated with multiple sclerosis much more frequently than is euphoria [15]. Diffuse atrophy and/or focal areas of hypodensity are usually seen in patients with multiple sclerosis. The Arnold-Chiari malformation may rarely present in young adults, and depression can be an early sign [16]. The CT scan shows obstructive hydrocephalus and structural anomalies in the posterior fossa. Finally, cerebral infarction, especially that involving the left hemisphere, appears to play an etiologic role in the depression frequently observed in patients recovering from stroke [17-19].

Movement Disorders

Patients with abnormal movements are increasingly referred for psychiatric evaluation to consider whether the movements are drug-induced or the result of a conversion disorder. Table 3 lists some of the disorders of movement associated with CT abnormalities. The characteristic chorea-like movements of tardive dyskinesia and the stereotypic movements of chronic schizophrenia resemble abnormal movements associated with disorders of the basal ganglia and cerebellum. In both Huntington's disease and Wilson's disease choreoathetoid movements arise; these illnesses must be considered in a neuroleptic-treated patient with psychosis who appears to have tardive dyskinesia. Psychosis and movement disorder have been associated with cryptogenic calcification of the basal ganglia and cerebellum ("Fahr's disease") [20]. Other cases of choreoathetoid movement disorders that can be observed with CT include ischemic infarction of the basal ganglia, carbon monoxide-

Table 3. Structural Brain Disease
Associated with Movement Disorder

Huntington's disease
Idiopathic cerebral ferrocalcinosis (Fahr's disease)
Wilson's disease
Basal ganglia infarct
Olivopontocerebellar atrophy
Carbon monoxide manganese poisoning
Hallovorden–Spatz disease
Tumor, granuloma
Lupus
Multiple sclerosis

induced basal ganglia infarction, and poisoning with manganese. Reduced structural density of the basal ganglia and cerebral atrophy is also seen in Hallovorden-Spatz disease, a rare disorder that presents usually in young adolescents with rigidity, personality change, and choreoathetosis. Finally, bizarre disorders of gait may be early signs of cerebellar degenerations, visualized on CT as cerebellar and/or pontine atrophy.

Other Psychiatric Syndromes

Two psychiatric syndromes—catatonia and anorexia nervosa—are particularly noteworthy because they may be the only manifestations of CNS structural pathology. Although rare, catatonia with muteness may result from basal ganglia infarction or from a CNS tumor [21]. Because of the overwhelming nature of the syndrome, more typical neurologic signs may be obscured. Rare cases of typical anorexia nervosa secondary to hypothalamic and third ventricle tumors have been reported [22]. Since these tumors are deep and in the midline, they may not produce neurologic symptoms until they have achieved considerable size.

Dementia

Table 4 lists some dementing disorders with characteristic appearance on CT. All patients with dementia, confusion, or intellectual decline of unknown etiology should undergo CT scanning if systematic causes have been excluded. This is not because dementia is diagnosed from a CT scan. Since dementia is a clinical diagnosis, it is based on history, mental status, and cognitive assessment. Nevertheless, because dementia may result from numerous structural brain diseases, the CT scan can often narrow the diagnostic possibilities and even define the etiology.

Primary degenerative dementia, or Alzheimer's disease, is a degenerative disorder of the cerebral cortex and various subcortical nuclei. Consistent with the neuropathologic changes found in Alzheimer's disease, the CT scan usually shows diffuse cortical atrophy and secondary ventricular enlargement ("hydrocephalus *ex vacuo*"). A number of studies have investigated whether the degree of atrophy on a CT scan is predictive of the extent of intellectual impairment. In general, the more atrophy and especially ventricular enlargement, the more cognitive impairment exists [23-27]. However, since many exceptional cases occur, the CT scan cannot be used to predict intellectual impairment or to diagnose dementia [28, 29]. Furthermore, cerebral atrophy is a concomitant of normal aging [30], and this form of atrophy looks qualitatively identical on a CT scan to the atrophy of Alzheimer's disease. The CT scan, therefore, has two purposes in the work-up of the patient with presumed Alzheimer's disease: First to rule out another cause for dementia (see below) and second to confirm that cerebral atrophy has occurred. While dementia and even Alzheimer's disease may exist despite a normal CT scan,

Table 4. Structural Brain Disease Associated with Dementia

Alzheimers disease	Lupus
Picks disease	Metachromatic leukodystrophy
Multi-infarct dementia	Kuf's disease
Normal pressure hydrocephalus	Binswanger's disease
Abscess	Arnold–Chiari malformation
Tumor	Subdural hematoma
Spongiform encephalopathology	

the absence of atrophy means that reversible causes (e.g., hypothyroidism, hepatic disease, drug intoxication) must be more vigorously pursued. Pick's disease, an uncommon form of cortical dementia, is differentiated from Alzheimer's disease by a preponderance of frontal lobe deficits in the former and possibly by subtle neuropathologic differences. CT may help distinguish between the two disorders, because in patients with Pick's disease, cortical atrophy is restricted primarily to the prefontal and anterior temporal lobes.

In multi-infarct dementia, scattered cortical and subcortical areas of decreased density, indicative of old infarction, are seen on CT scan. Such patients usually have a history of recurrent stroke and multifocal clinical signs. A variant of multi-infarct dementia is Binswanger's disease, a subcortical ischemic dementia that may be related to multiple small vessel occlusion. Patients with this uncommon illness may also seem markedly depressed [31]. The CT scan will show diffuse attenuation of subcortical white matter density. In transmissible spongiform encephalopathy (Creutzfeldt–Jacob disease) marked cortical and subcortical atrophy is seen. Dementia occurs in association with CNS lupus, and the CT scan may show diffuse and or focal atrophic changes.

Various rare metabolic disorders associated with dementia in young adults (e.g., Wilson's disease, MLD, Kuf's disease) show nonspecific atrophy as already mentioned. Normal pressure hydrocephalus and space occupying lesions (especially chronic subdural hematomas and meningiomas) can present as dementia. The CT in these disorders have been discussed above.

It is clear from the foregoing discussion that cerebral atrophy is a nonspecific finding consistent with numerous brain disorders. As Table 5 shows, cerebral atrophy is also seen in association with disorders or intoxications that do not present as typical dementia. These include epilepsy, alcohol abuse, psychiatric disorders, and chronic migraine. Cerebral atrophy is, by definition, a final common pathway that indicates loss of brain tissue at some previous date. In addition, several cases of apparent reversible atrophy have been seen in patients following chronic alcohol abuse, steroid administration, and anorexia nervosa [32-34].

Table 5.   Conditions Associated with Diffuse
Atrophy on CT

Aging
Intoxications: Alcohol, heavy metals, organic solvents
Nutritional deficiencies
Head injury
Radiation exposure
Steroid administration*
Multiple sclerosis
Lupus
Anorexia nervosa*
Dementia
Schizophrenia
Affective disorder
Epilepsy
Chronic migraine
Post-encephalitis
Parkinson's disease

*See text

These cases of "reversible atrophy" indicate that all atrophy on a CT scan is not true atrophy of the brain in the neuropathological sense. The etiology of this reversible picture is unclear, but it does not appear to result from acute dehydration [35].

Since cerebral atrophy is nonspecific, its diagnostic importance is easily misunderstood. While it is not strictly normal, it does not necessarily indicate the presence of a cognitive or behavioral deficit. Nevertheless, it probably means that some pathologic process has occurred in the brain. To that extent, it provides the clinician with a clue. In certain clinical settings, this clue may be pivotal, while in others it may be, at most, a curiosity. This situation is analogous to the value of many clinical laboratory tests in medicine. Ultimately, it is up to the clinician to judge which data are relevant.

COMPUTED TOMOGRAPHY IN PSYCHIATRIC RESEARCH

In addition to its primary role as a diagnostic tool in clinical medicine CT has opened a new chapter in psychiatric research. Using quantitative analysis of scans, rather than impressionistic "readings," investigators have shown that structural brain abnormalities are associated with some of the psychiatric syndromes generally regarded as "functional." Nonspecific signs of cerebral atrophy, e.g., ventricular enlargement and dilatation of cortical sulci, had been reported in schizophrenic patients earlier in this century using pneumoencephalography. The results with CT confirm these earlier observations. When compared to normal individuals, schizophrenic patients as a group, have larger cerebral ventricles and, to a lesser extent, wider cortical sulci. In addition, there is a small percentage (from 5–30% depending on the study) of patients whose ventricular size exceeds the upper limit of normal [36]. Whether this latter group is a unique subpopulation or simply the upper tail of a continuous distribution is not clear.

It is clear, however, that psychiatric treatment, e.g., ECT and/or neuroleptic drugs, are not the primary etiology of the findings. Patients with large ventricles have been found among schizophrenic patients who have never received somatic therapies and among patients at the onset of their illness. It is also of interest that evidence of a genetic factor predisposing to larger ventricles has been reported in families containing an individual with schizophrenia. In monozygotic twins discordant for schizophrenia, however, the schizophrenic twin has larger ventricles than his unaffected co-twin [37].

Because of the numerous other disorders associated with cerebral atrophy and the fact that the majority of patients with schizophrenia have normal ventricular size, the CT findings in schizophrenia have no diagnostic or clinical application. From a research perspective, however, they are intriguing signs that a neuropathologic process has occurred in the brains of at least some patients with schizophrenia. Since the process appears to exist even at the onset of the illness, it may be related to the etiology of the disorder. Furthermore, the CT findings offer some clue as to where investigators might look for neuropathologic confirmation. Ventricular enlargement, the most common finding, if indicative of focal pathology, implicates the limbic system for which the lateral and third ventricles form part of the perimeter. One recent controlled postmortem study has reported pathological changes in the limbic periventricular regions of patients with schizophrenia [38].

In addition to providing an impetus for rekindling interest in neuropathologic studies, the CT findings may offer a means of subdividing patients with schizophrenia into more clinically and biologically homogeneous sub-groups. For example, patients with the largest ventricles tend to differ from patients with small ventricles by having greater neuropsychological deficits, poorer premorbid social histories, minor neurological signs, a poorer response to treatment and, perhaps, lower concentrations of biogenic amine metabolites and cyclic nucleotides in CSF [36].

These findings suggest that a neuropathologic process reflected in mild ventricular enlargement is a factor in the pathogenesis of at least some forms of schizophrenia. There is also preliminary evidence that some patients with affective disorders, especially those with a chronic form of illness, have signs of cerebral atrophy. These leads will be the subject of considerable future research. It is important to emphasize that the CT findings and their clinical correlations are statistical group tendencies and not consistent individual characteristics. They do not at the present time provide a rationale for CT scanning psychiatric patients with schizophrenia or affective disorder.

INDICATIONS FOR CT IN PSYCHIATRIC PATIENTS

When should a psychiatrist order a CT scan? There are few generally accepted guidelines to answer this question. For the patient with dementia of unknown etiology, a CT is mandatory. At the other extreme are patients with long-standing characterologic diagnoses or with problems in living for whom a CT scan is clearly not indicated. Between these two groups, are patients with discrete syndromes such as personality change, affective disorder, psychosis, and disorders of movement. Whether to order a CT scan in the initial evaluation of such patients is controversial. Proponents argue that neurologic conditions diagnoseable by CT may masquerade as psychiatric syndromes. Opponents claim that the cost is too high for the minimal yield and that in the absence of neurological signs, the yield is virtually nil.

There is no disagreement about the need in psychiatry for a reliable triage or screening tool for CNS disease. CT has most of the characteristics of the ideal screening procedure. It is reliable, quick, painless and harmless. There are virtually no unmangeable artifacts and the frequency of false negatives is negligible. Furthermore, the entire procedure (with the exception of contrast administration and scan interpretation) can be completed by a technician. The disagreement, therefore, reduces to a cost-benefit analysis.

The only real cost is money. Radiation dose, in the range of 2-3 rads to the head, is not a meaningful concern for adults. The adult brain is highly radiation insensitive and exposure from a CT scan is insignificant. By comparison, radiation therapy for brain tumors is in the range of 5000-6000 rads. Although the lens of the eye is the most radiation sensitive tissue exposed during a head CT scan, it is not adversely affected by this exposure. The cost of a CT scan in dollars is high. In most institutions, a precontrast study costs from $150-300, while contrast adds an additional $150-200. This price is difficult to explain considering the minimal physician involvement required to complete the procedure. It reflects less the cost of the machine than the dependence of radiology departments on CT to generate income. It is doubtful that a CT scan would cost over $100 if a reasonable profit margin were applied. Nevertheless, in assessing the yield from this procedure, the drain on the current health care dollar must be weighed.

The crucial questions are how high is the yield and how useful are the findings. In a retrospective study of 123 diagnostically heterogeneous psychiatric patients scanned to "rule out" CNS disorder, Larson et al [39] found 43 cases (35%) of atrophy and 12 cases of focal CNS disease. While the atrophy findings did not lead to changes in management, in six of the 12 cases with focal pathology, the findings were either diagnostic or led to definitive treatment. The authors minimized the implications of their study by emphasizing that all patients with what they called "true positive" CT findings had focal abnormalities on neurologic examination. They concluded that a CT scan was unnecessary unless focal neurological signs were observed clinically. This conclusion is difficult to accept on the basis of their study. In the first place, it contradicts the clinical experience of many practicing neurologists. After a few years in practice, it is not uncommon to see at least one patient with a brain tumor who had been treated for depression several months before the onset of neurological symptoms. It is reasonable to assume that at some point depression was the sole manifestation of the lesion. This raises an interesting paradox. Patients with acute psychiatric symptoms may be more likely to have positive scans than are chronic patients, because in patients with structural lesions, neurological symptoms soon overshadow the psychiatric ones. An interesting example of this is a recent case record of the Massachusetts General Hospital [40]. Four weeks before neurologic evaluation for a seizure, the patient was seen for depression "ascribed to recent loss of job." In fact, the patient had a cerebral abscess diagnosed by CT scan. It is virtually certain that a CT abnormality would have been appreciated at the time of initial psychiatric evaluation. The patients in the study by Larson et al were already hospitalized on a psychiatric unit, meaning their psychiatric symptoms were probably chronic or at least severe. Some of the patients with "true positive" findings may have had only psychiatric symptoms in a few months earlier without neurological signs. Another problem with this study is their use of the phrase, "true positive." These cases were the six patients for whom the CT findings were considered responsible for their illness. Six other cases, two of whom lacked focal neurologic signs, were called "incidental positives" because their CT findings were not considered relevant to their illness. This is a questionable conclusion, given our limited knowledge about the relationship of CNS pathology to behavior. One of the incidental positive findings was a pituitary adenoma in a patient with psychosis. Pituitary tumors are one of the most common neoplasms associated with psychosis [1]. Finally, Larson et al failed to place any value on the importance of a negative scan in reassuring both patient and physician.

In contrast, Holt et al [41] emphasized the reassurance value of a negative CT scan. In reviewing 99 general hospital psychiatric consultations, they found that in 25% of the cases the CT scan "played a major role in clarifying the patients' problem with respect to psychiatric concerns and thereby facilitated clinical decision making." Slightly more than half of these cases had negative scans. Although this study appears to support a less restrictive approach to ordering CT scans, it is difficult to interpret because the indications for scanning were not clear. Also, the clinical diagnoses for which the scan results were valuable was not specified.

Owens and colleagues [42] report the only study of nondemented psychiatric patients scanned unselectively. Of 136 chronic schizophrenic patients, 10 had findings on CT that were either potentially remediable or that influenced diagnosis. In seven cases (5%), the findings had clear diagnostic implications. Finally, in a retrospective study of 135 CT scans of diagnostically heterogeneous patients from a psychiatric hospital in Iowa studied because of a suspicion of "organic brain disease," only three cases had focal, diagnoseable lesions [43]. In each case other clinical evidence, e.g., abnormal neurological exam of EEG, existed. It was not stated whether the findings explained the psychiatric illness.

In summary, the available studies are only marginally helpful in defining guidelines for CT scanning of nondemented psychiatric patients. More data are needed. The studies suggest that approximately 2-20% of hospitalized patients in primarily psychiatric treatment have diagnoseable structural brain disease other than diffuse atrophy. This is an alarmingly high fraction. It may be misleading, however, because of unclear selection factors. Certain groups such as the elderly are probably overrepresented in this fraction. Furthermore, the yield of positive scans is clearly greater if clinical neurological signs exist. The yield for young patients (less than 40) is not known but is probably much lower. The limited studies available do not provide sufficient data to establish clear guidelines for CT scanning of nondemented psychiatric patients.

In the clinical neuropsychiatry section at NIMH we advocate a CT scan for all first episode patients with psychosis of unknown etiology. To avoid the minimal risks of a reaction to the contrast agent, we administer contrast only if a suspicious area is seen on the non-contrast scan or if focal clinical signs are present. It should be noted, however, that structural lesions such as AVM's and infiltrating gliomas may be invisible without contrast. Since we view schizophrenia as a debilitating, usually chronic illness that is difficult to treat, we feel that the CT scan is justified, not only to search for the unlikely causes mentioned above but also to reassure the patient, family, and physician that all reasonable diagnostic possibilities have been considered. We also advocate scanning all patients with anorexia nervosa and with catatonia, because of the gravity of these disorders and the fact that CNS lesions associated with these syndromes tend to be neurologically occult.

We have no clear guidelines for scanning patients with affective disorder. In patients under 50-years-old, the clinician must maintain a high level of suspicion and consider a scan if atypical features exist. For individuals over 50, a CT scan seems advisable for a first episode of major affective disorder unless psychologic or other factors (e.g., family history) are very compelling. This is an age group at maximum risk for brain tumor and degenerative CNS disease. Again, we reserve contrast for cases with suspicious or abnormal plain scans or other clinical signs.

ACKNOWLEDGMENT

The author would like to thank Charles Citrin, M.D. for his helpful review of the manuscript and Ms. Denise Ondrish for her patience in preparing it.

REFERENCES

1. Davison D, Bagley CR: Schizophrenic-like psychoses associated with organic disorders of the central nervous system. In RN Herrington (ed): Current problems in Neuropsychiatry. Br J Psych 4:113–184, 1969
2. Brothers CRD: Huntington's chorea in Victoria and Tasmania. J Neurol Sci 1:405–420, 1964
3. James WE, Mefford RB, Kimbell I: Early signs of Huntington's chorea. Dis Nerv Syst 30:556–559, 1969
4. Neophytides AN, DiChiro G, Barron SA et al: Computed axial tomography in Huntington's disease and persons at risk for Huntington's disease. In TN Chase, NS Wexler, A Barbeau (eds): Huntington's Disease. Adv Neurol 23: 185–191, 1979
5. Beard AW: The association of hepatolenticular degeneration with schizophrenia. Acta Psychiat Neurol Scand 87:411–428, 1959
6. Manowitz P, Kling A, Kohn H: Clinical course of adult metachromatic leukodystrophy. J Nerv Ment Dis 166:500–506, 1978
7. Adams RD, Lyon G: Neurology of Hereditary Metabolic Disease of Children. New York, McGraw-Hill, 1982
8. Misra PC, Hay GG: Encephalitis presenting as acute schizophrenia. Br Med J 1:532–533, 1971
9. Wilson LG: Viral encephalopathy mimicking functional psychosis. Am J Psych 133(2):165–170, 1976
10. Bilaniuk LT, Patel S, Zimmerman RA: Computed tomography of systemic lupus erythematosis. Radiol 124:119–121, 1977
11. Gonzalez-Scarano Lisak RP, Larisa TB, Zimmerman RA, et al: Cranial computed tomography in the diagnosis of systemic lupus erythmatosis. Ann Neurol 5:158–165, 1979
12. Thompson GN: Cerebral lesions simulating schizophrenia: Three case reports. Biol Psych 2:59–64, 1970
13. Lishman WA, Organic Psychiatry. London, Blackwell, 1978, pp 262–294
14. Rice E, Gendelman S: Psychiatric aspects of normal pressure hydrocephalis. JAMA 223:409–412, 1973
15. Whitlock FA, Siskind MM: Depression as a major symptom of multiple sclerosis. J Neurol Neurosurg Psych 43:861–865, 1980
16. Banerji NK, Millar JHD: Chiari malformation presenting in adult life: Its relationship to syringomyelia. Brain 97:157–185, 1974
17. Robinson RG, Szetela B: Mood change following left hemispheric brain injury. Ann Neurol 9:447–453, 1980
18. Ross ED, Rush J: Diagnosis and neuroanatomical correlates of depression in brain-damaged patients. Arch Gen Psych 38:1344–1354, 1981
19. Finkelstein S, Benowitz LI, Baldessarini RJ, et al: Mood, vegetative disturbance and dexamethasone suppression test after stroke. Ann Neurol 5:463–468, 1982

20. Francis AF: Familial basal ganglia calcification and schizophreniform psychosis. Br J Psych 135:360–362, 1979
21. Gelenberg AJ: The catatonic syndrome. Lancet 1:1339–1341, 1976
22. Weller RA, Weller EB: Anorexia Nervosa in a patient with an infiltrating tumor of the hypothalamus. Am J Psych 139:824–825, 1982
23. Huckman MS, Fox J, Topel J: The validity of criteria for the evaluation of cerebral atrophy by computed tomography. Radiol 116:85–92, 1975
24. Earnest MP, Heaton RK, Wilkinson WE et al: Cortical atrophy, ventricular enlargement and intellectual impairment in the aged. Neurol 29:1138–1143, 1979
25. Kaszniak AW, Garron DC, Fox JH et al: Cerebral atrophy, EEG slowing, age, education, and cognitive functioning in suspected dementia. Neurol 29:1273–1279, 1979
26. Wu S, Schenkenberg T, Wing SD, et al: Cognitive correlates of diffuse cerebral atrophy determined by computed tomography. Neurol 31:1180–1184, 1981
27. Soininen Puranen M, Riekkinen PJ: Computed tomography findings in senile dementia and normal aging. J Neurol Neurosurg Psych 45:50–54, 1982
28. Fox JH, Kaszniak AW, Huckman M: Computed tomography scanning not very helpful in dementia—nor in craniopharyngioma. N Engl J Med 300:437, 1979
29. Wilson RS, Fox JH, Huckman MS, et al: Computed tomography in dementia. Neurol 32:1054–1057, 1982
30. Zatz LM, Jernigan TL, Ahumada AJ: Changes on computed cranial tomography with aging: Intracranial fluid volume. Am J Neurorad 3:1–7, 1982
31. Burger PC, Burch JG, Kunze V: Subcortical arteriosclerotic encephalopathy (Binswanger's disease). Stroke 7:626–631, 1976
32. Heinz R, Martine ZJ, Haenggeli A: Reversibility of cerebral atrophy in anorexia nervosa and Cushing's syndrome. J Comput Assist Tomogr 1:415–418, 1977
33. Carlen PL, Wortzman G, Holgate RC, et al: Reversible cerebral atrophy in recently abstinent chronic alcoholics measured by computed tomographic scans. Science 200:1076–1078, 1978
34. Rodeck CH, Campbell S: Reversible cerebral atrophy caused by corticotrophin. Lancet 1:1246–1247, 1979
35. Mellanby AR, Reveley MA: Effects of acute dehydration on computerized tomographic assessment of cerebral density and ventricular volume. Lancet 2:874, 1982
36. Weinberger DR, Wagner RW, Wyatt RJ: Neuropathological studies of schizophrenia. A selective review. Schiz Bull (in press)
37. Reveley AM, Reveley MA, Clifford CA, et al: Cerebral ventricular size in twins discordant for schizophrenia. Lancet 1:540–541, 1982
38. Stevens JR: Neuropathology of schizophrenia. Arch Gen Psych 39:1131, 1982
39. Larson EN, Mack LA, Watts B, et al: Computed tomography in patients with psychiatric illnesses: Advantage of a "rule-in" approach. Ann Int Med 95:360–364, 1981
40. Case records of the Massachusetts General Hospital. Case 6, 1983. N Engl J Med 308:326–332, 1983
41. Holt RE, Rawat SR, Beresfort TP, et al: Computed tomography of the brain and the psychiatric consultation. Psychosom 23:1007–1019, 1982
42. Owens DG, Johnston EC, Bydder GM, et al: Unsuspected organic disease in chronic schizophrenia demonstrated by computed tomography. J. Neurol Neurosurg Psych 43:1065–1069, 1980
43. Tsai L, Tsuang M: How can we avoid unnecessary CT scanning for psychiatric patients? J Clin Psych 42:452–454, 1981

Laboratory Evaluation for Special Groups of Patients

CHAPTER 8

The Alcoholic Patient

DENNIS G. LOW,
THOMAS P. BERESFORD, and
RICHARD C. W. HALL

The section on alcoholism in Sir William Osler's *Principles and Practice of Medicine,* published in 1892, covered the acute and chronic sequelae, as well as the withdrawal syndromes of alcoholism in less than five pages. In it he states "The diagnosis is not difficult, yet mistakes are frequently made." [1]. His spare pages are rich in detailed signs and symptoms to help avoid misdiagnosing the medical consequences of alcoholism. The current plethora of blood tests, radiological exams, and urinalysis were not available less than 100 years ago. These tests have contributed to the improved medical care of those suffering from alcohol dependence. Their appropriate application, however, requires the skill and knowledge of the dedicated clinician.

The laboratory examination of the patient with alcoholism begins with an assessment of the seriousness of the patient's physical impairment. This allows the physician to tailor the ordering of tests to the individual and to avoid both needless overuse as well as underuse which might result in missing significant complications. In a patient not known to suffer from alcoholism, an incidental laboratory abnormality, on occasion, may lead one to suspect occult alcoholism. However, routine use of most tests for screening purposes is inefficient. Clinical skills are paramount; we will miss the diagnosis often if we rely solely on the laboratory [2].

Handbook of Psychiatric Diagnostic Procedures, vol. 2, edited by R. C. W. Hall and T. P. Beresford. Copyright © 1985 by Spectrum Publications, Inc.

SENSITIVITY AND SPECIFICITY

The value of a technically valid laboratory test is tempered by whether it is sensitive or specific. The sensitivity of a test is defined as the ratio of true positives to the total number of patients with the disease. In other words, the more sensitive a test, the fewer false negatives occur and the less likely the disease will be missed. Specificity refers to the ratio of true negatives to the total number of patients without the disease. The more specific a test, the fewer false positives it yields and the more likely a patient is to have the disease when the test is positive. Tests are rarely both highly sensitive and specific for a given disease state. For example, blood tests for elevated liver enzymes are sensitive for active liver inflammation due to heavy alcohol ingestion, but they are not specific, as elevated liver enzymes may occur due to other reasons, such as infection or medications. Finally, the incidence and prevalence of a disease state must be considered. No matter how technically valid, sensitive, or specific a test, its value is wasted when indiscriminately ordered on a large group of patients thought to have a very low incidence or prevalence of the abnormality being tested [3].

ROUTINE SCREENING TESTS

In the outpatient setting, a patient with alcoholism but with an otherwise benign history and physical may require only a baseline of recommended testing. Using the guidelines delineated by the American College of Physicians, laboratory tests would include: a stool for occult blood, a PPD, a Pap smear, a VDRL, and a serum cholesterol.

The above are tests recommended for "minimal preventive measures" and were a synthesis of four major studies in the area of periodic examinations and preventive health care [4]. The test for occult blood in the stool was recommended by all four studies essentially yearly after the age of 45. This should be done at least once in all patients suspected of heavy alcohol intake due to its inflammatory effect on the gastrointestinal system and the increased risk of gastrointestinal bleeding. Testing a stool sample on rectal exam emphasizes the additional information obtained by an examination (evaluating the prostate gland, probing for rectal carcinoma) rather than a collected stool. A tuberculin skin test (the purified protein derivative or PPD) was recommended by only one of the four studies, once every decade. However, since patients suffering from alcoholism have an increased incidence of tuberculosis, they should be tested more frequently and with greater vigilance for the systemic symptoms of tuberculosis. The ideal frequency has not been established. The Pap smear is currently recommended every two years after two consecutive normal exams, from the onset of sexual activity or the age of 20, whichever occurs first. The VDRL was recommended on a screening basis by only one study, to be done every five years. Similarly, the serum cholesterol was recommended by only two studies, to be done every four to five years. The mammogram as a screening procedure has been a topic of controversy and is beyond the scope of this brief discussion. It should be noted that two of the studies recommended yearly mammograms for all females after the age of 50. We also note that several commonly included tests were not mentioned: routine electrocardiogram, chest roentgenogram, urinalysis, or complete blood count.

In summary, for the asymptomatic, otherwise well patient who may have alcoholism, the recommended minimal preventive laboratory tests should include:

1. Stool for occult blood, obtained on rectal exam
2. PPD
3. Pap smear

EVALUATING THE PATIENT FOR DISULFIRAM THERAPY

Disulfiram (Antabuse, Ayerst) has been prescribed for patients needing extra support to maintain abstinence from alcohol. In itself, disulfiram is relatively innocuous. The most common side effects are transient drowsiness, a metallic or garlic taste in the mouth, and impotence. Rarely, an organic brain syndrome or seizure occurs. The real danger is an alcohol-disulfiram reaction, occurring minutes after accidental or purposeful ingestion of alcohol. Depending on the amount of alcohol ingested, the adverse reaction may range from mild nausea, flushing, headache, lightheadedness, and tachycardia, to profound hypotension, loss of consciousness, arrhythmias, convulsions, and death. With these potential reactions in mind, a thorough history and physical examination are of obvious importance. The laboratory evaluation must assess other disease processes which would be dangerously exacerbated by an alcohol-disulfiram reaction. If diabetes mellitus is clinically suspected, a fasting blood sugar should be done. Likewise, thyroid function tests to rule out hypothyroidism and an electrocardiogram (EKG) to screen for myocardial problems should be done. Since disulfiram is primarily metabolized by the liver, baseline liver enzymes should be ordered initially then repeated after three months. A complete blood count, electrolytes, and a urinalysis complete the baseline evaluation, along with the previously mentioned preventive tests in the asymptomatic patient.

In summary, laboratory tests to be considered for the patient about to commence disulfiram therapy include:

1. Tests mentioned for the asymptomatic patient
2. Complete blood count (CBC)
3. Electrolytes (Na and K)

4. Renal function (blood urea nitrogen and creatinine)
5. Liver enzymes (gamma-glutamyl transpeptidase or GGT, serum glutamic-oxalacetic transaminase or SGOT, serum glutamic-pyruvic transaminase or SGPT, alkaline phosphatase)
6. Urinalysis (UA)
7. Fasting blood sugar (if symptomatic or family history is positive)
8. Thyroid function tests (if clinically suspected)
9. Electrocardiogram (for patients over the age of 35, or if there is any history of cardiac symptoms or disease)

Subsequent clinic visits by the patient, which should be at least weekly at the beginning of therapy, will determine the need for any repeat laboratory tests.

EVALUATION OF THE PATIENT WITHDRAWING FROM ALCOHOL

The large majority of individuals withdrawing from alcohol will suffer only minor untoward effects, such as a hangover, nausea, minimal vomiting, palpitations, or even mild tremors. Most of these individuals are able to undergo detoxification on their own, under the watchful eye of a friend or family member, or in a social-setting detoxification program. These individuals may require only the minimal tests, such as a stool for occult blood, or electrolytes and renal function testing if they appear mildly dehydrated. However, if the individual has major withdrawal complications (seizures, delirium tremens, or hallucinosis) or secondary medical complications (such as cardiac dysrrhythmias, alcoholic liver disease, pancreatitis or pneumonia) then extensive testing is required.

SEVERE ALCOHOL WITHDRAWAL SYNDROMES

Seizure is the most common major withdrawal syndrome occur. ing in patients with alcohol withdrawal. The seizures are major motor, generalized rather than focal from the outset, and are usually self-limited to no more than two or three. Rarely (less than 1%) do they proceed to status epilepticus. The question often arises as to how extensive a work-up should be ordered for what clearly appears to be withdrawal seizures. An individual with a clear-cut alcohol withdrawal seizure, who does not go into status epilepticus, and who has been thoroughly evaluated in the past may not need more than a thorough physical examination including a complete neurologic exam, CBS, and electrolytes. Additional abnormal findings or concerns guide the ordering of additional tests. For example, concomitant head trauma might lead to roentgenograms of the skull; a possible aspiration during the seizure calls for a chest x-ray; an abnormal reflex or asymmetry of the neurologic exam might suggest a subdural hematoma requiring a computerized axial tomogram (CAT scan) to rule out this possibility.

The work-up of a patient with first time seizures, even when presumptively due to alcohol withdrawal, should include:

1. All previously mentioned tests, for the asymptomatic patient as well as the pre-disulfiram therapy evaluation
2. Serum calcium, magnesium, and inorganic phosphate
3. Serologic test for syphilis
4. Toxic screen for barbiturates and benzodiazepines and, if indicated, lead, organophosphates, and blood alcohol level
5. Chest x-ray
6. Lumbar puncture (LP) to rule out infection, subarachnoid hemorrhage, and syphilis
7. Electroencephalogram (EEG), which should be done some days after the seizure to look for an epileptic focus. The EEG should then be normal if the seizure was only due to withdrawal [5]
8. Skull x-rays, which might detect skull fracture, abnormal calcifications, or a meningioma
9. Computerized axial tomography of the brain (CAT scan), depending on the clinical situation

A special mention should be made regarding the blood alcohol level. Withdrawal seizures occur even when there is measurable alcohol in the blood since their occurrence has more to do with the relative drop in blood alcohol rather than with the absolute level. The presence of alcohol in the blood does not preclude the diagnosis of alcohol withdrawal seizures.

DELIRIUM TREMENS

Delirium tremens, characterized by confusion, hyperactivity, severe tremulousness, disoriented combativeness, visual and/or auditory hallucinations, vasomotor instability, and fluid and electrolyte imbalance, can be the most severe and life threatening of the withdrawal syndromes. All of the previously mentioned laboratory tests must be taken into consideration in evaluating and treating this medical emergency. However, meticulous attention must be paid to the patient's hydration status in order that hypoglycemia or hypotension do not occur, that serum electrolytes stay within normal concentrations, and that the many nutritional demands of the body are met under this high stress situation. Cardiovascular instability may be worsened by dysrhythmias and by the direct toxic effect of chronic alcohol exposure to the heart [6]. Severe hypokalemia, hypomagnesemia, and hypophosphatemia occur frequently in this clinical setting and must be diagnosed because of the myriad of complications which then ensue [7-10]. Therefore, a checklist of laboratory tests which should be considered are:

1. Blood urea nitrogen (BUN) and creatinine to monitor the fluid status and kidney function
2. Serum sodium, potassium, calcium, magnesium, and inorganic phosphate
3. Blood glucose
4. All the additional tests previously mentioned where clinically relevant.

The replacement of several vitamins in patients with malnutrition, and those with delirium tremens, should be considered without routinely ordering laboratory tests to prove deficiency. Necessary replacement vitamins include thiamine, folate, niacin, pyrodoxine, riboflavin, and ascorbic acid.

HALLUCINOSIS

Isolated hallucinosis occurs less frequently than withdrawal seizures of delirium tremens. When it occurs, consideration must be given to other potential causes of an acute organic brain syndrome, or toxic psychosis. Metabolic disorders, infections (particularly meningitis), and especially other drugs or toxins need to be considered in the differential diagnosis. When an acute brain syndrome occurs in an alcoholic patient with or without hallucinations, impending hepatic coma must be included in the differential. The usual laboratory tests are of no help in establishing this diagnosis, though they may establish the presence and the severity of the liver disease. Blood ammonia, a toxic by-product of the gut usually metabolized by the liver, may increase in the presence of liver failure. While not 100% sensitive (cases of normal blood ammonia have been reported in patients with hepatic failure), "The state of consciousness correlates with blood ammonium content better than with any other biochemical measurement made to date" [11]. The blood ammonia level is not specific to liver failure due to alcoholism and may be elevated in liver failure of any cause.

THE DEBILITATED PATIENT

Some special circumstances may occur in the patient with severe alcoholism that deserve special mention. The debilitated malnourished alcoholic may present with general malnutrition. Several concerns have already been mentioned, such as an extensive list of electrolytes, which require serial evaluation, and several vitamins, which should be replaced presumptively.

Alcoholic ketoacidosis may be missed because the nitroprusside test for detecting plasma ketones is more sensitive for the acetoacetate of diabetic ketoacidosis than the beta-hydroxybutyrate ketoacidosis associated with alcoholism [12]. This can be diagnosed by a combination of a high index of suspicion in this clinical setting of alcoholism, poor nutritional intake, protracted vomiting, and by the simple calculation of the anion gap from the electrolytes. These unmeasured anions may be calculated by taking the plasma sodium concentration and subtracting the sum of the plasma bicarbonate and chloride, the normal range being 4-12 mmol per liter. An elevated anion gap indicates the presence of an unmeasured anion, which in the case of a malnourished, vomiting alcoholic patient, may be beta-hydroxybutyrate. The lab evaluation should include:

1. Calculation of the anion gap
2. Arterial blood gas (arterial pH, pO_2, pCO_2, HCO_3^-)
3. Serum lactate (to rule out lactic acidosis)
4. Blood glucose (to rule out diabetic ketoacidosis)

The debilitated patient risks the development of severe hypophosphatemia when the initial test shows the level of inorganic phosphate to be slightly low or even in the low-normal range. This level often drops precipitously after the patient begins to eat again and needs to be rechecked within two to three days.

LABORATORY SCREENING FOR OCCULT ALCOHOLISM

There is no biologic marker for the disease of alcoholism. Even the blood alcohol level (BAL) is of limited use, since most patients with alcohol dependence will abstain prior to a scheduled clinic visit. When positive, this test does not discriminate the "heavy social drinker" from the "alcohol abuser" or the "alcohol dependent." It may diagnose alcohol tolerance, one of the criteria of alcohol dependence from the Diagnostic and Statistical Manual of Mental Disorders, third edition. [13]. If the BAL is 150 mg or more and the person exhibits no gross signs of inebriation, then he or she is exhibiting tolerance to the substance. However, the blood alcohol level is both insensitive and nonspecific in diagnosing alcoholism.

A number of laboratory tests, when abnormal, may suggest the diagnosis of alcohol abuse or dependence, but all suffer from the same difficulty of being insensitive and nonspecific. The complete blood count may reveal macrocytic anemia, due to the inhibition of folate metabolism by alcohol as well as poor folate intake, or thrombocytopenia and leukopenia due to the toxic effect of alcohol on the bone marrow [14]. Sequential multiple analysis of the blood biochemistry (SMA6, SMA12) may also show elevated liver enzymes, such as the GGT, SGOT, or SGPT. Triglycerides may be elevated due to alcohol's effect on liver lipid metabolism.

Serum urate may be elevated due to alcohol's effect of both increasing uric acid production and decreasing its renal excretion [15]. The BUN is often low when there is poor nutritional intake reflecting a decreased protein metabolism.

If each of the above tests are by themselves insensitive and nonspecific, could chronic alcohol intake cause a unique *profile* among all these tests which is sensitive or specific for alcoholism, even if each of the tests were normal? Ryback and his associates posed this question in a clinical investigation, utilizing 25 parameters in SMA6, SMA12, and CBC. Applying a quadratic multiple discriminant analysis to these biochemical and hematologic values, they were able to identify 100% of medical ward alcoholics as alcoholics (n = 63) and 94% treatment program alcoholics (n = 412), which suggests a high degree of sensitivity in this group of patients as the false negative rate was only 6%. Of the group of nonalcoholic hospitalized controls (n = 40), the profile correctly identified 100% as nonalcoholic, hence being highly specific when applied to this population [16].

Beresford and his associates performed a subsequent study on 104 hospitalized medical and orthopedic patients, 38 of whom met the DSM III criteria for alcohol dependence and 66 of whom did not. Similarly, a computerized linear discriminant analysis program was applied using seven hematologic parameters, 20 biochemical parameters (which included the GGT, not included in the Ryback study), and the anion gap. Unlike previous results, this study only found a profile of three direct measurements (mean cell volume or MCV, serum creatinine, and SGOT) and four logarithmic functions (1g BUN, 1g uric acid, 1g total bilirubin, and 1g lactate dehydrogenase) to be useful in correctly assigning the patients to the alcoholic or the nonalcoholic groups. The test was accurate in diagnosing 79% of the alcoholics and 80% of the nonalcoholics. The sensitivity and specificity were poorer in this population of patients. The GGT, purported by some to be a more sensitive measure of alcoholic liver disease than the other liver enzymes, was not as helpful in this study as the SGOT [17].

More research needs to be done to determine the applicability of this multiple discriminant analysis as a screening test. Certainly, this device is not needed to diagnose the patient already in an alcohol treatment program or suffering from end-stage cirrhosis. It needs to be tested adequately on younger patients, patients of both sexes, and on "heavy" drinkers who do NOT fit the criteria of alcoholism to determine its applicability. Additionally, patients no longer routinely receive all of the above mentioned tests required to establish this "biochemical profile." In this age of burgeoning healthcare costs, none of these tests are considered essential for health screening or maintenance. Its niche may be to test a population which is thought to have a high risk for alcoholism, but is likely to deny drinking, or inaccurately report the amount (e.g., drug abusers). The majority of patients suffering from alcoholism can be diagnosed with a careful history done by an experienced clinician. In fact, Beresford's group also demonstrated the superiority of an interviewing instrument known as the CAGE Questionnaire over the multiple discriminant analysis, both in sensitivity and specificity for the diagnosis of alcoholism [18].

We end this chapter as we began it, with the caveat that laboratory tests have added new dimensions to the diagnosis and treatment of alcoholism and its complications, but they cannot replace the thoughtful care of the physician.

REFERENCES

1. Osler W: The Principles and Practice of Medicine. New York, D. Appleton and Co., 1892.
2. Beresford TP, Low DG, Adduci R, et al: Alcoholism assessment on the orthopedic surgery service. J Bone and Joint Surg 64(5):730, 1982
3. Burke MD: The importance of prevalence in the interpretation of laboratory tests. Internal Medicine for the Specialist 4(4):45, 1983
4. Medical Practice Committee, American College of Physicians, Periodic Health Examination: A guide for designing individualized preventive health care in the asymptomatic patient. Ann Int Med 95(6):729, 1981
5. Adams RD, Victor M: Alcohol and alcoholism. In Principles of Neurology. New York, McGraw-Hill, 1977
6. Knochel JP: Cardiovascular effects of alcohol. Ann Int Med 98(2):849, 1983
7. Rubenstein AE, Wainapel SF: Acute hypokalemic myopathy in alcoholism. Arch Neurol 34:553, 1977
8. Shils ME: Experimental human magnesium depletion. Med 48(1):61, 1969
9. Ryback RS, Eckardt MJ, Pautler CP: Clinical relationships between serum phosphorus and other blood chemistry values in alcoholics. Arch Int Med 140:673, 1980
10. Knochel JP: Hypophosphatemia in the alcoholic. Arch Int Med, 140:613, 1980
11. Davidson CS, Gabuzda GJ, Schiff L: Hepatic coma. In Diseases of the Liver. Philadelphia, J. B. Lippincott Co, 1975
12. Levy LJ, Duga J, Girgis M, et al: Ketoacidosis associated with alcoholism in nondiabetic subjects. Ann Int Med 78:213, 1973
13. American Psychiatric Association, Diagnostic and Statistical Manual of Mental Disorders, 3rd ed, 1980
14. Lieber CS: Alcohol and the hematologic system. In Medical Disorders of Alcoholism. Philadelphia, WB Saunders Co, 1982
15. Korsten MA, Lieber CS, Mendelson JH: Hepatic and gastrointestinal complications of alcoholism. In The Diagnosis and Treatment of Alcoholism. McGraw-Hill, 1979
16. Ryback RS, Eckardt MJ, Pautler CP: Biochemical and hematological correlates of alcoholism. Res Commu in Chemical Pathol and Pharmacol 27(3):533, 1980
17. Beresford TP, Low DG, Hall RCW, etal: A computerized diagnostic biochemical profile for the detection of alcoholism. Psychosomatics 23:713-720, 1982

18. Beresford TP, Low DG: A comparison of the effectiveness of the CAGE Questionnaire, diagnostic algorithm, and biochemical data profile in the screening of alcoholism. In Abstracts of the Proceedings of the Sixth World Congress of the International College of Psychosomatic Medicine, Sept 1981

CHAPTER 9

The Patient with Anorexia Nervosa or Bulimia

WILLIAM L. WEBB

Anorexia nervosa and bulimia are partially understood eating disorders characterized by a relentless pursuit of thinness. Recently, the syndromes have been more clearly defined and demonstrated to be on the increase [1]. The onset and course may be insidious, and the patient, through denial or shame, may not reveal to the physician the true nature of the disorder.

The clinical history is crucial in arriving at the proper diagnosis, and in its absence, the weight loss and abnormalities in test results may be very confusing leading to further fruitless investigation. Laboratory abnormalities appear secondary to starvation, medical complications of malnutrition, or artificial efforts to control weight. Once this is understood, laboratory findings may be very helpful in differentiating anorexia nervosa/bulimia from other medical or psychiatric conditions. Complications derived from self-induced vomiting, laxative abuse, or treatment effects, can be picked up in the laboratory. Sharing these abnormal findings with patients can sometimes assist in overcoming their resistance to treatment. Some test results have raised questions about hypothalamic-pituitary neurotransmitter abnormalities in anorexia/bulimia, but at present, there are no clear-cut biologic abnormalities or specific diagnostic tests identified for the disorders. This chapter will review laboratory abnormalities associated with anorexia nervosa and bulimia with the speculations about hypothalamic dysfunction triggered by these findings.

Patients with a fear of weight have been divided into two syndromes, anorexia nervosa, those who persistently starve themselves, and bulimia, those who binge

---

Handbook of Psychiatric Diagnostic Procedures, vol. 2, edited by R. C. W. Hall and T. P. Beresford. Copyright © 1985 by Spectrum Publications, Inc.

eat and attempt to control weight through the use of self-induced vomiting or purgatives. Although they are designated as separate disorders in the Diagnostic and Statistical Manual III with distinct inclusion criteria, there is considerable overlap [2]. Both have a phobia about weight and telescope a myriad of psychological problems with self-esteem, cognitive functions, and interpersonal relationships into the concrete idea, "All will be solved if I am thin." A number of persistent dieters become binge/vomiters after treatment with tricyclic antidepressants or chlorpromazine. Some bulimics become anorectic and require treatment for weight loss. The two groups share a number of behavioral characteristics that may complicate the diagnostic process. Either through denial or shame, they may not be completely truthful about their eating habits, vomiting, or laxative abuse; the weight loss and laboratory abnormalities may be hard to understand.

There are important differences in the clinical behavioral picture between anorexia nervosa and bulimia. It is important to understand these differences, because these are reflected in specific abnormalities in the associated laboratory findings.

LABORATORY FINDINGS ASSOCIATED WITH MALNUTRITION

Anorexia Nervosa—The Persistent Dieters and the Ravages of Malnutrition: The Clinical Picture

The label of anorexia nervosa is misleading. Most patients do not experience a complete loss of appetite until a late stage of the illness. Fluctuations in appetite seem very much related to the psychological state of the patient. Attempts to stimulate appetite characterized a number of well meant but misdirected treatment attempts [3,4]. The anorectic's behavior can best be understood as a massive struggle to achieve maximum thinness. The inclusion criteria for the diagnosis of anorexia emphasize the intense fear of becoming obese, the feeling of being fat even when emaciated, a 25% weight loss of the original body weight, and a refusal to maintain body weight. It is primarily a disorder of young women. Halmi only diagnosed six males in one study of 94 patients [5]. The dieting behavior usually begins in adolescence. It may be stress related or develop insidiously. Hyperactivity is a prominent characteristic of anorectic patients. They are hyperactive before weight loss, but this becomes more pronounced as emaciation progresses.

Early in the course of the illness, amenorrhea may appear. Amenorrhea may occur before the weight loss is obvious and seems tied to a given percentage of body fat related to body mass. Early onset of amenorrhea may be stress related. The appearance of amenorrhea and other hypoestrogenic changes in vaginal mucosa and secondary sexual characteristics are associated with significant changes in circulating gonadotropins. Jeuniewic et al demonstrated that low resting levels of luteinizing hormone causing the amenorrhea were correlated with percentage fat, body weight, and percentage weight loss [6].

With the progress of weight loss, several other clinical features appear. The patient seems constantly preoccupied with food, food preparation, and a series of behaviors to avoid calories. Food is cut into small pieces, and idiosyncratic food preferences become evident. The patient will blatantly deny her emaciation and react negatively to any change in body contour that suggests weight gain.

When the fat falls below 70 pounds, the picture takes on a more ominous character. The patient shows evidence of increased fatigue and muscle weakness. Medical complications associated with starvation become apparent. Starvation may lead to death. Mortality in anorexia nervosa has been estimated from 4–9%.

Many of the unusual laboratory findings in anorexia are related to malnutrition. Anorexic patients differ from starving patients in a number of significant ways. Most starvation diets are protein deficient, but anorectics usually preserve minimal protein intake and selectively avoid carbohydrates. Although some show vitamin deficiencies, most anorectics do not suffer evidence of vitamin deficiency but may have trace metal deficiencies. These nutritional idiosyncracies are reflected in laboratory findings.

Hematological Findings Clinical symptoms in anorexia secondary to blood changes are rare, but the changes in the blood picture are quite characteristic. Anemia is frequent but usually mild. Values for hemoglobin below 12 grams or hematocrit below 30 percent are rare. Red cells do show evidence of anisocytosis, poikilocytosis, and acathocytosis. There are seldom reticulocytes or other evidence of hemolysis. Serum iron and iron-binding capacity are in the low-normal range. There may be a mild thrombocytopenia, and rarely, patients with petechia are reported. Serum fibrinogen levels are low but not low enough to compromise the patient's clotting mechanism [7].

Commonly, anorectics demonstrate some degree of leukopenia. White blood counts are usually above 2,400 white cells per millimeter [8]. Palmblad reported that polymorpholeukocytes from anorectic patients demonstrate decreased bactericidal activity and adherence to bacteria in viral preparations [9]. Several reports note that the bone marrow is characteristically hypocellular with increased histiocytes and a clear, thick, sticky substance high in hyaluronic acid. All of these changes in marrow and peripheral blood are reversed after refeeding [7].

There has been some controversy about the susceptibility of anorectics to infection. At one time, they were thought to be at risk for bacterial infections, particularly TB. Recently, Bowers reported that anorectics show no differences in infection rates [10]. Immune mechanisms seem to be intact. Palmblad reported some decreased plasma complement, but immune responses in anorectics are quite adequate, and other authors have reported increased circulating globulins that afford protection to viral infections [11].

Blood Chemistry Findings Anorectics may betray a yellowish tint to their skin that can be misconstrued as jaundice by the unsuspecting physician. It directly derives from the elevated blood carotene found in 57% of one study of anorectics [12]. It has not been satisfactorily established why they show elevated carotene levels in the blood. Anorectics do show a preference for foods high in carotene, but it may also be related to some metabolic defect.

Plasma cholesterol is commonly elevated. This seems unrelated to depressed thyroid function or excessive intake of high cholesterol foods during binge eating. The elevated concentrations of cholesterol are the low density lipoprotein cholesterol [13].

Although vitamin deficiencies are rare, there are cases of beri beri reported. Occasional patients show low values of vitamin K or A. Deficiencies of trace metals, especially zinc and copper, are common. Zinc and copper content in the hair of anorectics is usually within normal limits [14]. It has been suggested that some of the taste idiosyncracies observed in anorexia may be related to zinc or copper deficiency. Occasionally, patients with anorexia will suffer hair loss, and at least one etiologic factor may be zinc deficiency. Most of the changes discussed above are clinically quite benign and easily reversed with adequate nutritional intake.

The more serious blood chemistry changes are associated with electrolyte abnormalities. These most commonly occur in those patients who self-induce vomiting.

Endocrine Changes with Malnutrition Berkman, at the Mayo Clinic, believed that "Patients (anorexia nervosa) demonstrated, as a feature of their illness, a reversible insufficiency of the anterior pituitary gland." [15]. He was reporting on patients seen between 1917–1929 and was one of the first to note endocrine changes in patients suffering with anorexia. However, it is oversimplified to see anorexia nervosa as a pituitary deficiency, and a number of more recent findings would refute this and suggest that the problem resides at the hypothalamic level. It is still unclear whether anorexia represents a primary hypothalamic disturbance or whether this is secondary to starvation. In a study of 101 patients from the Mayo Clinic in 1977, 50% of the patients demonstrated elevations of serum corticosteroids and a reversal of the usual diurnal variation in plasma cortisol levels [16]. Walsh et al studied 19 emaciated women with anorexia nervosa [17]. He found that relative to body size, the patients demonstrated mean cortisol production rates pf 0.591 mg/kg/day and 16.4 mg/m^2/day. These findings were significantly elevated compared to those of 0.322 mg/kg/day and 11.4 mg/m^2/day for age and sex match controls. The 24-hour mean plasma cortisol concentration in 18 patients was 10.6 μg/day and was significantly higher than the controls (6.8 μg/dl, p < 0.001).

Anorectic patients during the starvation period demonstrate a failure to suppress serum cortisol with the ingestion of dexamethasone 12 hours previously (DST test). This is another finding demonstrating the hyperactivity of the adrenal cortex in cachetic anorectics and lack of hypothalamic-pituitary responsivity [34].

Thyroid studies support the hypothesis of pituitary dysfunction secondary to hypothalamic–pituitary insufficiency. Circulating levels of T_3 are low with the preservation of low-normal T_4 and TSH concentrations. The low T_3 is thought to result from hepatic dysfunction secondary to cachexia and a diminished deiodination of T_4 to T_3 [18]. T_2, the deiodinated product from T_3 and T_4, is also lowered in anorexia nervosa [19]. Casper and Gold have reported delayed TSH response to the injection of 500 m of thyrotropin-releasing hormone (TRH) [20,21]. The delayed TSH response occurred in 10 patients whose weight had been stabilized. Six patients continued to show this delay after an extended period of weight stabilization suggesting only a partial reversal of hypothalamic-pituitary-thyroid abnormalities with improvement in the illness. Basal metabolism is low when the patients are cachetic and transient elevations of T_3 and T_4 to hyperthyroid levels have been reported during refeeding [22].

Growth hormone is elevated during the malnourished phase of anorexia. The usual perturburation tests utilizing insulin or arginine produce a sluggish or minimal response in growth hormone levels. Gold has reported a delayed response of growth hormone to thyroid-stimulating hormone and cited this as evidence of possible hypothalamic dysfunction in anorexia [21]. Halmi et al showed a lack of growth hormone response to L-dopa both during pretreatment and after weight gain in anorectics [23]. She hypothesized an impairment in dopaminergic regulation in growth hormone at the level of the pituitary cell in anorexia nervosa.

Serum prolactin levels have been reported to be normal in anorexia nervosa [24]. This contradicts a favorite theory of the etiology of anorexia. It had been hypothesized that anorexia resulted from a depletion of central nervous system dopamine. Since dopamine controls the release of prolactin, a depletion of dopamine would ordinarily produce an elevated plasma prolactin level. Treatment of anorectics with bromocriptine, a dopamine agonist, produced a lowering of prolactin level in anorectics and normals but produced no weight gain in anorectics [25]. Beumont reported a paradoxical rise of prolactin to an infusion of gonadotropin-releasing hormone (GNRH) in those anorectics who were gaining weight [26]. This paradoxical response of a pituitary hormone to an inappropriate hypothalamic-releasing factor has also been reported in acromegaly and depression. Beumont suggested that whatever the mechanism is, it points to a dysfunction of neurotransmitter systems in the hypothalamus of patients with anorexia nervosa.

The cardinal symptom of amenorrhea in anorexia nervosa in females is associated with very striking changes in circulating gonadotropins. Katz indicates that the plasma and urinary levels of the two pituitary polypeptides, luteinizing hormone (LH) and follicle stimulating hormone (FSH) are low during the emaciated state of anorexia nervosa [27]. The circadian rhythm of LH is prepubertal, and patients fail to respond to clomiphene citrate with an initial rise of LH as occurs in the normal response. The delayed rise is also absent and continues even after adequate weight is restored. In six women with active anorexia nervosa, Katz demonstrated a normal release of LH in response to the single administration of luteinizing-releasing hormone (LHRH) [27]. Marshall and Kelch were able to reproduce the normal maturational response to gonadotropin-releasing hormone in three amenorrheal women with anorexia with low-dose injections of GNRH over a five-day period [28]. Initially, the patients showed a predominance of FSH secretion followed by increasing secretion of LH. On the fifth day, the LH response exceeded the FSH level, which is the normal response. These studies emphasized that the low level of circulating LH and FSH found in patients with anorexia is secondary to diminished secretion of endogenous gonadotropins releasing hormone by the hypothalamus. Whether this represents a primary vulnerability in the hypothalamus or simply is related to starvation is unclear.

Disturbances of sex hormones in male patients in the acute phase of anorexia nervosa have also been reported, but the number has been lower because of the less frequent occurrence of the disorder in males. Low testosterone and gonadotropins levels appear to be a universal feature during the acute phase of the disorder in males, and serial estimations suggest that the abnormalities do not return to normal after weight gain. McNab and Haughton report a single case in which the patient's low gonadotropins level returned to normal after weight gain, but his testosterone level remained low for several months after his recovery [29].

Cardiovascular Findings Fohlin et al examined the cardiovascular and oxygen transporting systems in 17 female and 11 male patients with anorexia nervosa [30]. Both groups had lost 25% of body weight. The measurements included blood and heart volume, heart rate, blood pressure, oxygen uptake (VO_2), blood lactate (LA), and in six patients cardiac output. Bradycardia and hypotension were apparent at rest in all patients. Blood and heart volume were decreased in proportion to weight loss. When exercised to a given workload, the oxygen capacity was reduced out of proportion to the circulatory dimensions, and maximum heart rate was slow. There was no evidence of myocardial impairment, and circulation flow seemed normal. The reduced oxygen capacity seemed due to the reduced muscle mass. Kalager measured systolic time intervals and cardiac output in 15 patients with anorexia nervosa [31]. He felt that the lengthened preinjection period, which was prolonged in 87% of cases, was indicative of impaired left ventricular contractility. In the later stages of anorexia, patients tire easily, and occasionally, sudden deaths occur. This is most likely related to multiple cardiac problems due to reduced muscle mass and electrolyte imbalances.

Limb circulation studies, conducted by Freyshuss et al demonstrate a heat conserving selective peripheral vascular constriction in the six anorectic females they studied [32]. Skin temperature was lower in the knees and toes, and the calf peripheral blood flow was 50–60% lower in the anorectic group. Luck and Wakeling have suggested that the preference of anorectic patients for warmer temperatures is related to increased cutaneous reactivity and vasospasm in anorexia nervosa [33]. They hypothesize that this is related to a displacement of the set point for behavioral thermoregulation probably located in the hypothalamus.

Gastrointestinal Findings Anorectic patients frequently complain of abdominal discomfort and bloating particularly during the refeeding process in early treatment. Some actually demonstrate abdominal swelling which is upsetting to the patient who misinterprets it as precipitous weight gain. Holt et al measured the gastric emptying time in ten female anorectics employing a test meal and a computer analysis of successive abdominal scans [34]. Gastric emptying time for both liquid and solid contents of the test meals was significantly slower for the anorectic group than the healthy controls. Being aware of the delayed emptying time in anorectic patients, some clinicians have employed metoclopramide, a properistaltic agent to relieve the gastric discomfort experienced by anorexia patients when eating [35].

Hepatic and pancreatic dysfunction have been reported secondary to malnutrition. Several reports have noted symptoms of abdominal pain associated with elevated serum amylase levels. It is hypothesized that the pancreatitis is secondary to malnutrition, but several authors have speculated that it may be etiologically related to anorexia nervosa [36].

Elevations in the liver enzymes SGOT and SGPT have been reported in anorectic patients during the cachetic phase [31]. Since loss of appetite is associated with hepatic dysfunction, this too might contribute to the diminished appetite seen in the later stages of anorexia. The liver enzymes returned to normal following adequate refeeding.

Renal Findings Although edema and decreased urinary concentrating capacity are common findings in emaciated anorectic patients, their etiology has not been clear, and they were not thought to be secondary to renal dysfunction. Aperia et al studied eight anorectic females, ages 12-18 years, with a variety of renal function determinations including glomerular filtration rate, clearance of PAH, and urinary concentrating capacity [37]. The test revealed a concentrating defect in anorexia nervosa that was primarily of renal origin. The concentrating capacity was not normalized by the administration of vasopressin. This suggests that the edema that occurs in anorexia may be related to a renal defect in fluid reabsorption.

Central Nervous System Transmitter Changes The central nervous system transmitters norepinephrine and dopamine are lowered in the acute phase of primary anorexia nervosa. Halmi documented this by demonstrating that the urinary MHPG (3-methoxy-4 hydroxyphenylglycol) is diminished during cachexia and restored to normal by weight gain [38]. Gerner and Gwertsman have shown that the failure of dexamethasone to suppress the diurnal variation of plasma cortisol (a positive DST test) is correlated with lowered urinary MHPG in anorexia nervosa [39]. Halmi had suggested that the lowered catecholamines in the emaciated anorectic might be correlated with depressive affect [38], but Abraham et al demonstrated in seven anorectic patients that the lowered urinary MHPG is correlated with weight only and unrelated to the patient's affective state [40].

Conflicting reports on the activity of the cerebrospinal fluid peptides during anorexia are confusing and have brought into question a therapeutic approach that employed naloxone in the treatment of anorexia nervosa. Kaye et al reported higher levels of cerebral spinal fluid opioid activity determined by radioreceptor assay in patients with anorexia nervosa [41]. Patients with chronic anorexia nervosa without weight loss demonstrated normal levels of cerebrospinal fluid opioid activity. Gerner measured cerebrospinal fluid endorphins in 75 medication-free-subjects including 25 with active anorexia nervosa [42]. He was not able to demonstrate any differences in the beta-endorphin concentrations in anorectic patients as compared to normals utilizing an immunoreactivity test. Animal data on appetite regulation suggests that opioid agonists stimulate eating and antagonists diminish eating. Opioid antagonists may well have a role in the therapy of anorexia nervosa, but the results of treatment of anorexia nervosa with naloxone, an opiate antagonist, are at best unclear.

LABORATORY FINDINGS ASSOCIATED WITH PATHOLOGICAL ATTEMPTS TO CONTROL WEIGHT, TREATMENT ATTEMPTS, OR MEDICAL COMPLICATIONS

Bulimia—The Gorgers and Vomiters: The Clinical Picture

Since the disorder of bulimia is characterized by many pathologic attempts to control weight, the clinical picture is presented here. It should be remembered that even though bulimia is given a separate diagnostic identity in the Diagnostic Statistical Manual III with specific inclusion criteria, it is difficult to know how much overlap there is with primary anorexia nervosa (the dieters). There are clearly many areas of overlap as previously pointed out.

Recently, certain distinctions in behavior and character have been recorded for the two groups. Binge-eating usually makes its appearance in late adolescence, whereas anorexia nervosa commonly appears in early adolescence. Patients with anorexia are characterized as demonstrating greater rigidity, social immaturity, and obsessive traits, whereas bulimics show characterologic problems and poor impulse control. Binge-eaters demonstrate more sexual acting out, kleptomania, and alcohol or substance abuse.

Binge-eating is characterized by the rapid consumption of large amounts of food in a discrete period of time, usually less than two hours. Associated behaviors include consumption of high-caloric, easily ingested food, inconspicuous eating during a binge, termination of binges by abdominal distention, sleep, social interruption, or self-induced vomiting. There are repeated attempts to lose weight by severely restrictive diets with frequent weight fluctuations. Patients are aware that the eating pattern is abnormal and are afraid they cannot stop eating voluntarily. Binges are followed by depressed mood and self-depreciating thoughts. From a clinical standpoint, the two most ominous aspects of bulimia are the suicidal impulses associated with binging and the medical complications associated with self-induced vomiting and laxative abuse. Anorectics die from complications of starvation, and bulimics die from suicide and the complications associated with vomiting or laxative abuse.

LABORATORY FINDINGS

Blood Chemistry Findings

The most serious consequence of repeated self-induced vomiting is hypokalemia. Potassium levels as low as 2.6 mE/l have been reported in 6% of vomiters [44]. To a lesser extent, the plasma sodium and chloride may be reduced resulting in a hypochloric alkalosis. Serum calcium and albumin may also be lowered in patients with significant vomiting.

Hypokalemia may develop rapidly or slowly with an insidious onset of symptoms. Common symptoms of hypokalemia include muscle weakness, cardiac arrythmias, outright paralysis, and tetany. The cardiac abnormalities may occasionally result in sudden death. Prolonged hypokalemia exerts a malignant influence on renal function. Initially there is an increase in plasma renin and an increased secretion of aldosterone. Prolonged hypokalemia can result in renal tubular vacuolization and ultimately renal failure.

Patients with hypokalemia should have serial EKGs, plasma potassium levels, and urinary potassium levels until potassium concentrations are returned to normal with oral and intravenous potassium supplements.

EKG Findings

Electrocardiographic findings in anorexia are quite common. Aberrant EKG findings have been reported as high as 69% among patients with anorexia nervosa. These changes included sinus bradycardia, low-voltage T-wave inversions, AV block, and ST wave depression. During exercise, one out of 11 patients showed bursts of ventricular tachycardia, and several patients showed prolonged QT intervals [43].

Some patients assist their vomiting with ipecac which may produce serious myocardial effects including ventricular tachycardia and myocardial myopathy. Most of the serious EKG findings are related to hypokalemia [44].

Gastrointestinal Complications

Abuse of laxatives may produce diarrhea that is hard to discriminate from chronic gastrointestinal disease. This is complicated by the frequent association of anorexia nervosa with Crohn's disease. A small bowel series, barium enema, and sigmoidoscopic examination will rule out chronic bowel disease.

Forced feeding and vomiting combined with delayed gastric emptying may occasionally produce serious upper GI complications. There are several reports of gastric obstruction and perforation resulting from compression of the duodenum by the superior mesenteric artery [45,46]. Self-induced vomiting may aggravate episodes of pancreatitis occurring in anorexia nervosa.

Pulmonary Complications

Pulmonary complications are rare in anorexia and are likely to occur in patients who self-induce vomiting. Clinical examination and chest x-ray may reveal evidence of pneumomediastinum and subcutaneous emphysema [47]. Apparently, starvation weakens the lining of the alveoli, and the added stress of vomiting may produce mediastinal or subcutaneous air collections.

Oral-Pharyngeal Complications

Repeated vomiting places severe stress on the enamel and dentin of the teeth. The repeated assault of vomit high in acid content produces poor dental hygiene and numerous caries. Repeated vomiting also produces enlargement of the salivary glands giving the patient a chipmunk-like appearance. Acute parotitis is rare and biopsy of the glands shows evidence of chronic inflammatory reaction and lymphocytic infiltration. Except for the unsightly appearance, there are no other complications associated with salivary gland enlargement [48].

Ophthamologic Complications

Archer reports on three anorectic patients with chronic vomiting who presented with sublenticular cataracts identified on slit-light examination [49]. Cataracts are commonly associated with severe constitutional and metabolic disturbances. He hypothesized that the hypokalemia and hypomagnesemia associated with weight control efforts may be etiologic in cataract formation.

Neurological Complications—Electroencephalographic Findings
and CAT Scan Findings

Seizures in anorexia nervosa are common. It was estimated in one study that seizure activity occurred in 9% of patients [50]. Commonly, they are due to metabolic changes secondary to electrolyte deficiencies, decreased blood sugar, or alcohol or drug excess. The findings on EEG reflect these changes. Crisp, in a systematic study of the EEG in anorexia nervosa in a series of 32 patients, reported that 59% had abnormal EEG background activity, 31% had unstable response to hyperventilation, and 12.5% displayed an epileptiform paroxysmal dysrhythmias [51]. The majority of these findings were attributed to reversible secondary manifestations of self-starvation, electrolyte imbalance, metabolic alkalosis, and relative hypoglycemia. Nell et al in a report of 36 patients with the diagnosis of primary anorexia nervosa who underwent all-night sleep EEGs showed significant decreases in phasic REM sleep parameters [52]. REM activity and REM density were found to be lower in those patients demonstrating an abnormal waking EEG. The patients exhibiting bulimia and vomiting, those abusing laxatives and diuretics, showed the greatest degree of EEG abnormality.

Several studies have recently reported reversible ventricular dilatation in anorexia identified by computerized axial tomography (CAT scan) [53]. Patients with these abnormal scans showed either evidence of cortical atrophy or ventricular dilatation. Evidence of cerebral atrophy associated with anorexia nervosa seems particularly prevalent in male anorectics. Apparently, the signs of atrophy are reversible with refeeding.

Laboratory of Determinations in the Different Diagnosis of Anorexia
Nervosa from Other Psychiatric and Medical Conditions

Anorexia and weight loss are common symptoms in a variety of psychiatric and medical syndromes. Differentiating anorexia nervosa from other psychiatric syndromes is largely a clinical process with an emphasis on good clinical history. The most difficult differential diagnosis is distinguishing anorexia nervosa from primary affective disorder. Bulimic patients are particularly prone to depression and may manifest sleeping disturbances, lowered energy level, and subjective depressive feelings. There is an increased prevalence of depressive illness in the family histories of eating disorder patients. It has been mentioned that catecholamines are low in the cachetic stage of anorexia, and the dexamethasone suppression test is likely to be positive. This has led some authors to speculate that anorexia may be an example of an atypical depressive disorder. The depression commonly seen with eating disorders seems more reactive to the patient's phobia about gaining weight. Anorectics get depressed when they feel they have gained too much, and bulimics are often suicidally depressed after a binge is concluded. The catecholamines, urinary MHPG, and positive dexamethasone suppression test return to normal after the patient's weight is restored.

Occasionally, anorexia presents as a symptom of schizophrenia. MMPI data on anorexia patients resembles the profile produced by schizophrenic patients. Many patients with anorexia demonstrate characteristics of a borderline personality disorder, but it is unusual for patients with anorexia to present with symptoms of a thought disorder. Those patients that have a combination of schizophrenia and anorexia are often older and show clear-cut evidence of the cardinal symptoms of schizophrenia.

Sometimes, patients with conversion disorders or Briquet's syndrome (somatization disorder) will demonstrate loss of appetite or vomiting as a feature of the clinical picture. A careful history will usually demonstrate that the symptoms are clearly stress related and are associated with other tell-tale symptoms of somatiform disorder. Usually, the MMPI will show the typical conversion triad with elevations on the HY, HS, and D Scales. This is not usually the profile seen in anorexia nervosa, and patients with somatization disorders are not weight phobic.

A variety of chronic medical illnesses can present with anorexia and weight loss. This includes endocrinopathies (hyper and hypothyroidism), malignancies (leukemias, lymphomas, solid tumors), cystic fibrosis, sickle cell disease, chronic pyelonephritis, subacute bacterial endocarditis, juvenile rheumatoid arthritis, and systemic lupus erythematosis. All of these illnesses have characteristic clinical histories which are significantly different from anorexia nervosa and bulimia.

Drug and environmental toxins may present with weight loss and anorexia. Children treated with methylphenidate for hyperactivity may demonstrate weight loss. Amphetamine abuse and heroin addiction are accompanied by weight loss. Exposure to ammonia and other environmental toxins may produce symptoms of lassitude, cachexia, and loss of weight. Careful clinical history can rule out drugs and environmental toxins. Doering has suggested a series of standard laboratory tests that can act as a screen for differential diagnosis of anorexia nervosa from other medical illnesses and for identifying those medical illnesses commonly associated with anorexia nervosa [54].

Standard Tests for Differential Diagnosis of Anorexia Nervosa from Other Medical Illnesses

1. Hemoglobin level, white blood count, differential, hematocrit.
2. Sedimentation rate.
3. Quantitative stool fat level.
4. SMA-18 or equivalent.
5. Urinalysis.
6. Purified protein derivative (PPD) tuberculin test with chest x-ray.

7. Triiodothyronine (T_3) plus total thyroxin concentration (T_4), or free thyroxin index.
8. Morning and evening plasma cortisol, luteinizing hormone (LH), follicle-stimulating hormone (FSH), and prolactin assay.
9. Head CAT scan and lateral skull x-rays.
10. Complete gastrointestinal series including small bowel study.
11. Pelvic examination.
12. Electrocardiogram.

A brief inspection of these screening tests will demonstrate that they are designed to rule out chronic medical conditions of endocrine, infectious, or malignant origin. It is worth emphasizing that certain rare illnesses may stimulate anorexia nervosa. Several reports of craniopharyngiomas or malignant tumors invading the hypothalamic area have emphasized the similarity of symptoms to anorexia nervosa. Usually, there have been other symptoms of visual disturbance or headache. A computerized axial tomograph is diagnostic.

Anorexia nervosa is associated on a greater-than-chance basis with Turner's syndrome and Crohn's disease. The diagnostic features of the former are obvious, but it may be difficult to differentiate the latter from the diarrhea or abdominal complaints associated with laxative abuse and anorexia. A gastrointestinal series with small bowel study is diagnostic.

SUMMARY AND CONCLUSIONS

Anorexia nervosa and bulimia influence changes in many body systems. The changes are reflected in laboratory findings, the electrocardiogram, tests of endocrine function, and radiologic findings. An awareness of these test abnormalities and a firm grasp on the clinical picture enables the physician to differentiate anorexia/bulimia from other medical and psychiatric conditions. Endocrinopathies show characteristic changes while the hypothalamic-pituitary axis abnormalities seen in anorexia resolve when the patient is adequately nourished. Symptoms of depression and urinary MHPG secretion return to normal in the anorexic with adequate nutrition. The dexamethasone suppression test is abnormal in anorexia but returns to normal when the patient is adequately nourished.

Equally important is the identification of the occasional medical illness that simulates anorexia nervosa. The rare case of achalasia with anorexia and vomiting can be identified by barium swallow and specialized tests of esophageal function. The direct invasion of the hypothalamic-limbic system by malignancy or infection will demonstrate characteristic changes in the cerebrospinal fluid, sedimentation rate, and computerized axial tomography. A variety of chronic medical diseases can present with anorexia and emaciation as a major diagnostic feature. Endocrinopathies, cystic fibrosis, chronic pyelonephritis, subacute bacterial endocarditis, rheumatoid arthritis, and systemic lupus erythematosis show characteristic laboratory changes. Anorexia may be associated with certain diseases on a greater-than-chance basis. Patients with anorexia may also demonstrate hypothyroidism, hyperthyroidism, Turner's syndrome, and Crohn's disease.

Laboratory findings become of paramount importance in following the course of anorexia and bulimia. Hypokalemia can result in sudden death from arrhythmia or produce irreversible renal damage. Frequent checks of potassium blood levels and electrocardiograms can alert the physician to the necessity of hospitalization. Understanding the impact of starvation, pathological attempts to control weight, and associated medical complications on the laboratory profile can greatly strenthen the physician's hand in the management of these difficult eating disorders.

REFERENCES

1. Kendell RE, Hall DJ, Hailey A, et al: The epidemiology of anorexia nervosa. Psychol Med 3:200-203, 1973
2. American Psychiatric Association: Diagnostic and statistical manual of mental disorders. (3rd ed), Washington DC, APA, 1980
3. Dally P, Sargant W: Treatment and outcome of anorexia nervosa, Br Med J 2: 793-795, 1966
4. Tolstrup K: The treatment of anorexia nervosa in childhood and adolescence. J Child Psychol Psych 16:75-78, 1975
5. Halmi K: Anorexia nervosa. In H Kaplan, A Freedman, B Saddock (eds): Comprehensive Textbook of Psychiatry, Vol 2, Baltimore, Williams & Wilkins, 1980 pp. 1882-1890
6. Jeuniewic N, Brown GM, Garfinkel PE, et al: Hypothalamic function as related to body weight and body fat in anorexia nervosa. Psychosom Med 40:187-198, 1978
7. Myers TJ, Perkerson MD, Witter BA, et al: Hematologic findings in anorexia nervosa. Conn Med 45:14-17, 1981
8. Rieger W, Brady JP, Weisberg E, et al: Hematologic changes in anorexia nervosa. Am J Psych 135:984-985, 1978
9. Palmblad J: Anorexia nervosa and polymorphonuclear granulocyte reactions. Scand J Haematol 19:334-342, 1977
10. Bowers TK, Eckert E: Leukopenia in anorexia nervosa. Arch Int Med 138: 1520-1523, 1978
11. Palmblad J, Fohlin L, Norberg R, et al: Plasma levels of complement factors 3 and 4, orosomucoid and opsonic functions in anorexia nervosa. Acta Paediatr Scand 68:617-618, 1979
12. Silverman JA: Anorexia nervosa: Clinical observations in a successful treatment plan. J Pediatr 84:68-73, 1974
13. Mordasini R, Klose G, Greten H, et al: Secondary type II hyper lipoproteinemia in patients with anorexia nervosa. Metabolism 27:71-79, 1978
14. Casper RC' Kirschner B, Sandstead HH, et al: An evaluation of trace metals, vitamins and taste function in anorexia nervosa. Am J Clin Nutr 33:1801-1808, 1980

15. Beckman JM: Anorexia nervosa; Anorexia. Inanition and low basal metabolic rate. Am J Med Sci 180:422–424, 1930
16. Hurd II HP, Palumbo PJ, Gharib H, et al: Hypothalamic-endocrine dysfunction in anorexia nervosa. Mayo Clin Proc 52:712–716, 1977
17. Walsh BT, Katz JL, Levin J, et al: Adrenal activity in anorexia nervosa. Psychosom Med 40:499–506, 1978
18. Croxson MS: Low serum triiodo thyronine (T_3) and hypothyroidism in anorexia nervosa. J Clin Endocrinol Metab 44:167–174, 1977
19. Burger A, Sakoloff C: Serum 3,3'-L-diiodothyronine, a direct radioimmunoassay in human serum: Method and clinical rejects. J Clin Endocrinol Metab 45:1:384–391, 1977
20. Casper R: Delayed TSH release in anorexia nervosa following injection of thyrotropin-releasing hormone (TRH). Psychoneuroendocrinol 7:1:59–68, 1982
21. Gold MS: Thyroid stimulating hormone and growth hormone responses to thyrotropin-releasing hormone in anorexia nervosa. Int Psych Med 10:1:51–55, 1980–1981
22. Moore R, Mills I: Serum T_3 and T_4 levels in patients with anorexia nervosa showing transient hyperthyroidism during weight gain. Clin Endocrinol 10:443–449, 1979
23. Halmi K, Sherman B: Dopaminergic and serotonergic regulation of growth hormone secretion in anorexia nervosa. Psychopharmacol Bull 13:1:63–65, 1977
24. Giusti M, Mazzocchi G, Mortara R, et al: Prolactin secretion in anorexia nervosa. Horm Metab Res 13:585–586, 1981
25. Harrower AD, Yap PL, Nairn IM, et al: Growth hormone, insulin, and prolactin secretion in anorexia nervosa and obesity during bromocriptine treatment. Br Med J 2:156–159, 1977
26. Beumont PJ: Paradoxical prolactin response to gonadotropin releasing hormone during weight gain in patients with anorexia nervosa. J Clin Endocrinol Metab 51:6:1282–1285, 1980
27. Katz JL, Boyar RM, Roffwarg H, et al: LHRH responsiveness in anorexia nervosa intactness despite prepubertal circadian LH pattern. Psychosom Med 39:4:241–250, 1977
28. Marshall JC, Kelch RP: Low-dose pulsatile gonadotropin-releasing hormone in anorexia nervosa: A model of human pubertal development. J Clin Endocrinol Metab 49:5:712–718, 1979
29. McNab D, Hawton K: Disturbances of sex hormones in anorexia nervosa in the male. Postgrad Med J 57:254–256, 1981
30. Rohlin L, Freyschuss U, Bjarke B, et al: Function and dimensions of the circulatory system in anorexia nervosa. Acta Paediatr Scand 67:11–16, 1978
31. Kalager T, Brubakk O, Bassoe HH, et al: Cardiac performance in patients with anorexia nervosa. Cardiol 63:1–4, 1978
32. Freyschuss U, Fohlin L, Thoren C, et al: Limb circulation in anorexia nervosa. Acta Paediatr Scand 67:225–228, 1978
33. Luck P, Wakeling A: Set point displacement for behavioral thermoregulation in anorexia nervosa. Clin Sci 62:677–682, 1982
34. Holt S, Ford MJ, Grant S, et al: Abnormal gastric emptying in primary anorexia nervosa. Br J Psych 139:550–552, 1981

196   WEBB

35. Saleh J, Lebwohl P: Metoclopramide-induced gastric emptying in patients with anorexia nervosa. Am J Gastroenterol 74:127-132, 1980
26. Nordgen L, Von Scheele C: Hepatic and pancreatic dysfunction in anorexia nervosa. Biol Psych 12:5, 1977
37. Aperia A, Broberger O, Fohlin L, et al: Renal functions in anorexia nervosa. Acta Paediatr Scand 67:219-224, 1978
38. Halmi K, Dekirmenjian H, Davis JM, et al: Catecholamine metabolism in anorexia nervosa. Arch Gen Psych 35:458-460, 1978
39. Gerner RH, Gwertsman HE: Abnormalities of dexamethasone suppression test and urinary MHPG in anorexia nervosa. Am J Psych 138:650-653
40. Abraham SF, Beaumont PJ, Cobbin DM, et al: Catecholamine metabolism and body weight in anorexia nervosa. Br J Psych 138:244-247, 1981
41. Kaye W, Pickar D, Naber D, et al: Cerebrospinal fluid opiod activity in anorexia nervosa. Am J Psych 139:643-645, 1982
42. Gerner R, Sharp B: CSF bendorphin—immuno reactivity in normal, schizophrenic, depressed manic and anorexic subjects. Brain Res 237:244-247, 1982
43. Thurston J, Marks P: Electrocardiographic abnormalities in patients with anorexia nervosa. Br Heart J 35:719-723, 1974
44. Garfinkle PE, Garner D: Anorexia Nervosa: A Multidimensional Perspective. New York, Brunner/Mazel, 1982
45. Saul SH, Dekker A, Watson CG, et al: Acute gastric dilatation with infarction and perforation. Report of fatal outcome in patient with anorexia nervosa. Gut 22:978-983, 1981
46. Pentlow BD, Dent RG: Acute vascular compression of duodenum in anorexia nervosa. Br J Surg 68:665-666, 1981
47. Altmeyer RB, Morgan EJ: Spontaneous pneumodiastinum as a complication of anorexia nervosa. W Va Med J 77:189-190, 1981
48. Walsh BT, Croft CB, Katz JL, et al: Anorexia nervosa and salivary gland enlargement. Int J Psych Med 11:255-260, 1981-1982
49. Archer AG: Cataract formation in anorexia nervosa. Br Med J. 280:274, 1981
50. Dally P: Anorexia Nervosa. London, William Heinemann, 1969
51. Crisp AH, Fenton GW, Scotton L, et al: A controlled study of the EEG in anorexia nervosa. Br J Psych 114:1149-1160, 1968
52. Neil JF, Merikangas JR, Foster FG, et al: Waking and all night sleep EEG'S in anorexia nervosa. Clin Electroencephalogr 11:9-15, 1980
53. Nussbaum M, Shenker IR, Marc J, et al: Cerebral atrophy in anorexia nervosa. J. Pediatr 96:867-869, 1980
54. Doering EJ: The role of the primary care physician in the diagnosis and management of anorexia nervosa. In M Gross (ed): Anorexia Nervosa: A Comprehensive Approach, Lexington MA, Gillmore Press, 1982

CHAPTER 10

The Provisional Diagnosis of Dementia: Three Phases of Evaluation

MICHAEL K. POPKIN and THOMAS B. MACKENZIE

The term dementia is derived from the Latin "dement" which means literally to be out of one's mind. Within psychiatry dementia is considered to be an organic mental disorder, the essential feature of which is a loss of intellectual abilities of sufficient severity to interfere with social or occupational function.

Diagnostic criteria for dementia are specified in the Diagnostic and Statistical Manual, third edition, of the American Psychiatric Association. They include a critical loss of intellectual ability, memory impairment, and at least *one* of the following: impaired abstract thinking, impaired judgement, disturbance of higher cortical function, or personality change. Clouding of consciousness, as seen in delirium and intoxication, is not permitted.

This chapter will discuss the evaluation of the demented patient with special attention to use of diagnostic procedures. Our approach to this task will emphasize that evaluation is best viewed as a phasic process, consisting of three sequential components. They are: (1) validation of the provisional diagnosis, (2) identification of an etiology, and (3) diagnostic persistence in the face of uncertainty.

Handbook of Psychiatric Diagnostic Procedures, vol. 2, edited by R. C. W. Hall and T. P. Beresford. Copyright © 1985 by Spectrum Publications, Inc.

PRIMARY PHASE OF EVALUATION: VALIDATION

Dementia is a clinical diagnosis. Of all the organic mental disorders set forth in DSM-III, it is the only one that can be diagnosed in the absence of evidence for a specific etiology. The manual states that the organic factor can be presumed "if conditions other than organic mental disorders have been reasonably excluded and if the behavioral change represents cognitive impairment in a variety of areas."

Evidence to satisfy diagnostic criteria for dementia is derived from a skillful clinical interview, a reliable corroborative history, a review of systems, a thorough physical exam, and a knowledgeable laboratory workup. Insofar as possible the initial interview should precisely quantitate the patient's cognitive status. Particular attention should be paid to memory, language, and thought. Resistance to formal testing on the part of the patient may force the clinician to integrate the cognitive exam in the conversational moments of the interview. Since the diagnosis of dementia is often revealed by changes in function over time, and since the patient cannot provide such a history, a corroborative history is crucial. The corroborative historian needs to be an unbiased observer with a detailed knowledge of the patient's function. Additional medical and psychiatric problems should be sought in a careful review of systems. If cognitive deficits are evident or suspected, a thorough medical exam to detect undiagnosed medical conditions is indicated. This may be performed by the initial examiner or a colleague in neurology, internal medicine, or primary care. What is included in the initial, or first line, laboratory work-up depends upon several factors. Medical complaints on review of systems or positive findings on physical exam may dictate certain laboratory procedures. Certain tests may have been done recently and be available on request. Finally, each physician and medical community will have a standard battery of tests and studies routinely drawn on all patients with medical complaints. The extent of this battery is variable. This usually includes a complete hemogram, a urinalysis, an electrocardiogram (if not done in the last year), blood urea nitrogen, sodium, chloride, potassium, bicarbonate, liver function studies and a chest x-ray. Though such batteries may assist in identification of concurrent medical illness, data presented in the subsequent section do not suggest such studies are useful in determining the etiology of dementia.

The differential diagnosis of an apparent loss of intellectual abilities includes depression and delirium as well as dementia. Distinguishing dementia from these entities can be extremely difficult and may force the diagnostician to consider both possibilities simultaneously.

In contrast to dementia, depression, sometimes called pseudodementia when it imitates dementia, usually begins more discretely and progresses more rapidly. There may be a history of previous depressive illness and performance on cognitive testing tends to be marked by poor motivation and variable performance. The disturbance in mood characteristic of depression is usually more pervasive and less responsive to distraction. Despite these differences in clinical presentation, measurements of mood or cognition which definitively distinguish depression from dementia or quantitate their relative contribution to intellectual impairment are unavailable [1]. Further, the ability of laboratory measures, such as the dexamethasone test, to differentiate dementia from depression is unresolved [2]. For that reason many authorities would recommend a trial of antidepressants if the question of depression or dementia cannot be resolved.

According to DSM-III, delirium is distinguished from dementia by the presence of "clouding of consciousness" and an unstable course marked by an abrupt onset and fluctuating symptomatology. The manual suggests that when there is uncertainty as to whether the symptoms of a given individual are those of delirium or dementia, it is wise to make a provisional diagnosis of delirium. Such an approach directs that the common etiologies of delirium be sought acutely and that further investigation be undertaken if these are unrevealing. Thus, if a patient's clinical presentation includes evidence of clouding of consciousness such as difficulty sustaining attention to external and internal stimuli, sensory misperception, a disordered stream of thought, disturbances in sleep-wakefulness, or psychomotor disturbances, a search for causes of delirium should be initiated.

A systematic search for the cause of a delirium is complicated by the virtually unlimited number of entities known to cause the disorder. Lipowski points out that the search for an etiology can be rendered more focused if specific attention is paid to pre-existing illnesses, medication and drug history, potentially harmful occupational exposure, and occurrence of head trauma [3]. If an obvious cause is not revealed, he recommends a specific sequence of laboratory investigations.

If the presence of intellectual deficits, memory impairment, and of impaired abstract thinking, impaired judgement, disturbance of higher cortical function or personality change is confirmed and delirium and depression can be confidently excluded, the diagnostician should undertake a search for a reversible etiology.

THE SECONDARY PHASE OF EVALUATION: ATTEMPT TO IDENTIFY AN ETIOLOGY

Once the provisional diagnosis of dementia is given credence by the steps enumerated above, the clinican's focus must be directed to the question of etiology. If the primary phase identifies a probable cause for the dementia, this should be pursued in advance of the secondary phase outlined below. In the absence of a recognized etiology, the foremost consideration is the identification of "potentially reversible" dementiform processes. Other objectives include minimizing the deficits incurred by irreversible processes, clarifying the genetic implications of dementia for a patient's progeny and extended family, and in rare instances, identifying the communicability of the dementing process. What must the clinician appreciate as regards the etiologies of dementia? What should guide his/her investigations and efforts, his/her use of the laboratory, to identify the specific etiology? To address these questions, we have reviewed a series of studies conducted in the preceding decade. They afford data-based answers to the questions at hand.

Table 1 presents data compiled from 7 major investigations conducted in the years 1972-1982 [4-10]. The authors of these studies, numbering both psychiatrists and neurologists, examined subjects given provisional (or final) diagnoses of dementia (e.g., organic mental disorder, dementia if viewed in the context of DSM-III). They sought to establish specific etiologies for the clinical presentations. Of 659 subjects in the 7 studies, 568 (86%) had the presumed diagnosis of dementia confirmed. In the five studies of truly provisional diagnoses [4,5,6,7,10] dementia was confirmed in 82% of cases (427 of 518 patients).

In reviewing the data from the 7 studies, it should be underscored that the methods by which the specific etiologies were established are not belabored by any of the investigators. Rather, they have for the most part indicated in a phrase or two the diagnostic studies addressing particular problems. Thus, we can offer no assurance that equally rigorous or even highly similar criteria were uniformly applied. This limitation must be recalled in terms of the section that follows, the one dealing with clinical guidelines derived from the data. In addition, in the decade spanning the 7 studies, investigative techniques and procedures have evolved rapidly. This too complicates the question of what suffices to establish the etiology of a dementing process. Current tests and criteria have been and may be outmoded overnight. As discussed by Griner and Glaser [11], the proliferation of diagnostic measures has outstripped the capacity of many clinicians to keep abreast.

Table 2 shows primary psychiatric diagnoses other than dementia resulting from the evaluations in four studies [4,5,7,10]. (The other studies did not present this data or were restricted to confirmed, final diagnoses of dementia.) Though the data vary noticeably, 18% of patients (86 of 466) received a primary psychiatric diagnosis other than dementia. In half these cases, depression was the diagnosis. Remaining diagnoses included schizophrenia and a cadre of organic mental disorders (particularly delirium).

Coupled with the finding that 15-20% of provisional diagnoses of dementia are not confirmed, there are follow-up studies, such as that of Ron, Toone, Garralda, and Lishman [12], which have demonstrated that as many as *30%* of original diagnoses of dementia cannot be supported on re-examination several years later. Ron anad colleagues concluded that unappreciated affective disorders with concomitant cognitive dysfunction chiefly explained the outcomes they observed. Hence, the clinician must expect that *at least 20%, if not 40%* of patients presenting with an apparent dementiform process *do not have dementia*. This alone should prompt careful examination and a vigorous approach by the clinician faced with a provisional diagnosis of dementia.

Table 1. Evaluations for Provisional Diagnosis of Dementia

	Number in original sample	Confirmed dementia	Alzheimer's type (diagnosis by exclusion)	Specific etiology established (diagnosis by inclusion)
Marsden, Harrison [4]	106	86 (81%)	48/86 (56%)	38/86 (44%)
Freeman [5]	60	59 (98%)	26/59 (44%)	33/59 (56%)
Victoratos et al. [6]	52	49 (94%)	30/49 (61%)	19/49 (39%)
Smith, Kiloh [7]	200	164 (82%)	84/164 (51%)	80/164 (49%)
Rabins [8]	41	41 (100%)	29/41 (71%)	12/41 (29%)
Delaney [9]	100	100 (100%)	49/100 (49%)	51/100 (51%)
Maletta et al. [10]	100	69 (69%)	43/69 (62%)	26/69 (38%)
Total	659	568 (86%)	309/568 (54%)	259/568 (46%)

Table 2. Primary Psychiatric Diagnoses (Other than Dementia) Resulting from Evaluations

	Marsden, Harrison [4] 106	Freeman [5] 60	Smith, Kiloh [7] 200	Maletta et al [10] 100	Totals 466	%
Depression	8	1*	10	24	43	(9)
Mania	1	—	2	—	3	(1)
Hysteria	1	—	—	—	1	(<1)
Schizophrenia	0	—	7	4	11	(2)
Other OMD	—	—	16	—	16	(3)
Other	7	—	—	1	8	(2)
Uncertain	3	—	1	—	4	(1)
	20 (19%)	1 (2%)	36 (18%)	29 (29%)	86	(18)

*"Many depressed but only 1 responded to TCA"

Table 1 also indicates that in 54% of the confirmed dementias, a specific etiology was established by the evaluations. In these cases, the diagnosis was made according to criteria of inclusion. In the remaining 46% of cases, a diagnosis of dementia of the Alzheimer's type (DAT) was made. These diagnoses were made by exclusion. None of the authors report postmortem findings. For the etiologies established by criteria of inclusion, rates ranged from 44-71% in the 7 studies. For DAT, the range was 29-56%. These results suggest a slightly lower prevalence of DAT than commonly cited [13]. This of course does not address the question of DAT found at autopsy to accompany other etiologies of dementia [14].

As noted at the outset of this section, the clinician's first responsibility in the work-up of the patient with a provisional diagnosis of dementia is to identify potentially reversible etiologic processes. As Tables 3 and 4 make apparent, only a small fraction of confirmed dementias were categorized as "potentially reversible" after careful evaluation with respect to etiology. Of 499 confirmed cases in 6 studies [4-9] examining reversibility of the dementias, only 77 (15%) were assigned by the investigators to "potentially reversible" groupings. The percentage of "reversible" dementias ranged from 8-29 in the six studies. Restricting the focus to non Alzheimer's cases (Table 4), 33% of patients were identified as having "potentially reversible" etiologies for their clinical presentations. This rate ranged from 16-52% in the individual 6 studies.

These data are clear. The clinician confronting the patient with a provisional diagnosis of dementia must appreciate that the likelihood of identifying a potentially reversible etiology is small (e.g., less than one in seven on the average!). Yet, were the chances even 1 in 20 or less, there could be little doubt that the obligation to be most circumspect would remain. As we shall consider subsequently, cost-effectiveness factors do come to play; and there is a difference between potential and actual reversibility; nevertheless, to miss a potentially reversible etiology of dementia borders on negligence. We are particularly concerned lest clinicians encountering dementia presume it represents DAT (which is, of course, the statistical probability) and forego even the most rudimentary assessment. At the risk of redundancy, DAT is as yet a diagnosis of exclusion—to be made only when all other specific causes of dementia have been addressed and ruled out.

The conditions known to be etiologically associated with dementia are myriad. These have been reviewed in detail by Wells [15-17] and others [18-20]. For in depth considerations, the reader is referred to those reviews. We shall confine attention to the picture emerging from the six previously identified studies. These offer some surprising perspectives as regards etiologies of "potentially reversible" dementias. Though each of the studies explores the issue of reversibility, none has offered explicit criteria for or definitions of the term. Full resolution and/or restitution of functions [17] seem in our view central to the matter of reversibility.

Table 5 provides a delineation of the etiologies assigned to the 77 cases of "potentially reversible" dementia in the series of 6 studies. Eleven specific medical

Table 3. Reversibility of All Confirmed Dementias: Those with Specific Etiology Established and Those of the Alzheimer's Type

Study	Confirmed cases	Number irreversible	(%)	Number potentially reversible	(%)
Marsden, Harrison [4]	86	71	(83)	15	(17)
Freeman [5]	59	42	(71)	17	(29)
Victoratos et al [6]	49	44	(88)	5	(12)
Smith, Kiloh [7]	164	151	(92)	13	(8)
Rabins [8]	41	37	(90)	4	(10)
Delaney [9]	100	77	(77)	23	(23)
Total	499	422	(85)	77	(15)

Table 4. Reversibility of Confirmed Dementias Other than Alzheimer's Type

Study	Confirmed cases	Number irreversible	(%)	Number potentially reversible	(%)
Marsden, Harrison [4]	38	23	(61)	15	(39)
Freeman [5]	33	16	(48)	17	(52)
Victoratos et al [6]	19	14	(74)	5	(26)
Smith, Kiloh [7]	80	67	(84)	13	(16)
Rabins [8]	12	8	(67)	4	(33)
Delaney [9]	51	28	(55)	23	(45)
Total	233	156	(67)	77	(33)

Table 5. Etiologies Assigned to the "Potentially Reversible" Dementias and Their Actual Clinical Outcomes

Studies:	Marsden Harrison [4] (n=86)	Freeman [5] (n = 59)	Victoratos* et al [6] (n=49)	Smith, Kiloh [7] (n=164)	Rabins* [8] (n=41)	Delaney [9] (n=100)	Total N	Total Pct	Cumulative (%)	No change N	No change Pct	Partially improved N	Partially improved Pct
NPH	5	7	1	8	1	2	24	31	31	12	55	6	27
Tumor/cyst	8	0	0	3	0	5	16	21	52	8	50	5	31
Drug toxicity	2	5	0	0	0	2	9	12	64	0	0	0	0
Subdural hematoma	0	2	1	0	1	3	7	9	73	0	0	5	100
Hypothyroidism	0	1	0	2	1	0	4	5	78	0	0	1	33
ETOH	0	0	1	0	0	3	4	5	83	0	0	0	0
Paresis	0	1	1	0	0	1	3	4	87	1	50	1	50
Hyperthyroidism	0	0	0	0	1	1	2	3	90	0	0	0	0
Hepatic encephalopathy	0	1	0	0	0	1	2	3	93	0	0	0	0
Fungus	0	0	0	0	0	2	2	3	96	0	0	2	100
Lead	0	0	0	0	0	1	1	0.2	96	0	0	0	0
Other	0	0	1	0	0	2	3	4	100	0	0	2	100
Total	15	17	5	13	4	23	77	-	–	21	27	22	29

*Outcomes not reported by authors

disorders giving rise to presentations of dementia are identified. Of note, 5 of these disorders accounted for >80% of the reversible dementias. These 5 were: normal pressure hydrocephalus (31%); tumors/cysts of the CNS (21%); drug toxicity (12%); subdural hematoma (9%); and thyroid dysfunction (8%). No other single condition, save alcoholic encephalopathy, accounted for as much as 5% of the reversible dementias.

Normal pressure hydrocephalus (NPH) was the most frequent etiology assigned to cases, accounting for almost a third of all reversible dementias. Since Adams, Fisher, Hakim et al [21] offered their theory of the pathogenesis of NPH, this disorder has commanded increasing clinical attention. Though attempts to predict response to surgical shunting have been largely unsatisfactory, there is indication that patients with the classical triad of dementia, gait disorder and incontinence may respond more favorably [22]. Yet, as shown in the "outcomes" portion of Table 5, more than half of the cases of NPH identified by the investigators failed to respond to shunting. A partial improvement was reported in one-quarter of cases and apparent resolution in the remaining 18%. These figures are striking. They underscore the disparity between the concept of "potentially reversible" dementia and actual reversibility. Of the 77 cases comprising the "reversible" dementias, 27% were unchanged after identification and 29% were suggested to have improved partially. Presumptively the remaining 44% proved fully reversible in fact as well as theory. Thus, the data from the studies indicate that perhaps as few as 7% (e.g., 15% X .44) of clinical pictures of confirmed potentially reversible dementias were actually reversed—restitution achieved. The clinician must confront his/her own values and philosophy at this juncture. Diagnostic procedures are not without cost and/or sequelae.

Tempering these facts are the recent findings of Freeman and Rudd [23] corroborating prior work of Fox et al [24]. These workers found that patients with lesser degrees of atrophy on cranial computed tomographic scanning (CT) had greater likelihood of having a "treatable disorder." Wells [25] has likewise suggested that a normal CT scan in the setting of the clinical features of dementia intimates a reversible process. Though data emerging from the 6 studies threaten the myth of "potential reversibility," it may be that *timing* is the critical variable. If recognition of the dementia awaits the development of frank or florid clinical features (versus the earlier, more subtle changes), then outcomes may be as untoward as the figures in Table 5 indicate. Conversely, earlier intercessions may lead to more favorable outcomes. Such a principal would hardly be unique to the realm of dementia.

CNS tumors and cysts accounted for 21% of the "potentially reversible" dementias. These included the following: a meningioma, cysts of the septum pellucidum, and the sylvian fissure, an acoustic neuroma, 4 gliomas, 5 metastases, and 3 primary brain tumors, type not specified [9]. The latter 12 cases, all malignant tumors, do not in retrospect convey a great sense of potential reversibility. Yet, when initially recognized as intracranial mass lesions on CT scan, it was not improbable that the dementias which they evoked might have been resolved. As with NPH, actual reversibility was limited to less than 20% of the cases in the category.

Drug toxicity and subdural hematomas together accounted for another 21% of the assigned etiologies. The studies, however, provide little detail as regards these 2 entities. Restitution was the rule with drug intoxication; it was unlikely with the subdurals. Completing the 5 most common disorders was thyroid dysfunction. Hypothyroidism or hyperthyroidism were diagnosed in a total of 8% of the cases. The former condition was twice as prevalent as the latter; reversibility was reported in all the thyroid-induced disturbances. Alcoholic dementia was included by some of the authors, though as Marsden and Harrison [4] noted, "dementia in alcoholics is not a clearly defined entity." More to the point, its reversibility is not well classified. Thus, the appearance of alcoholic dementia (like CNS tumors) in both Tables 5 and 6, reversible and irreversible etiologies. Completing the major disorders of Table 5 is paresis (3 cases, 4%). In summary, *7 medical disorders* were responsible for >90% of the dementias regarded as potentially reversible.

Before moving to the implications of the findings reviewed above, we briefly turn to Table 6. Wells has recently contended [26] that the preoccupation with treatable or reversible dementias may have contributed to the pattern of "writing off" those patients with irreversible dementing disorders. Given the small numbers/ percentages of actual reversible dementias, this concern appears well grounded. Table 6 reviews etiologies assigned by the various studies to irreversible dementias, which accounted for 86% of confirmed cases. Three conditions, DAT, multi-infarct dementia, and alcoholic dementia, account for upwards of 90% of these cases.

Guidelines Emerging from the Studies

The evaluation of the demented patient has been the subject of much writing and opinion. Many authors have proposed specific approaches involving large batteries of laboratory screens [27,28]; others such as Benson [20] have decried such approaches. It is our contention that few have addressed the more critical questions confronting the clinician, to wit, the appropriate sequencing of studies, the proper balance of history, clinical exam and laboratory tests, and the issues of cost-effectiveness, invasiveness, and yield of testing. Though the studies reviewed in the preceding section are not in any sense definitive, they do offer a data base upon which clinical actions might reasonably be predicated, when integrated with the principals enumerated in the opening section of the chapter.

Once initial screening in all its facets has been effected (clinical exam, first-line laboratory studies, and corroborative history) and the provisional diagnosis of dementia set forth, the data of Table 5 argues that *4* tests currently will suffice to identify 90% of the potentially reversible etiologies of dementing processes.

Table 6. Etiology Assigned to Irreversible Dementias

	Marsden, Harrison [4]	Freeman [5]	Victoratos et al [6]	Smith Kiloh [7]	Rabins [8]	Delaney [9]	Total	Percent of dementias other than Alzheimer's type	Percent of all types of dementia
Alzheimer's	48	26	30	84	29	49	266	—	62%
Multi-infarct	8	5	5	22	8	22	70	43%	16%
Alcoholic	6	4	0	30	0	0	40	25%	9%
Huntington's	3	4	0	5	0	1	13	8%	3%
Tumor	5	1	4	0	0	0	10	6%	2%
Trauma	1	1	1	5	0	0	8	5%	2%
Parkinson's	0	0	1	0	0	4	5	3%	1%
Creutzfeld–Jacob	3	0	1	0	0	0	4	2%	1%
Encephalitis	1	1	0	1	0	0	3	2%	1%
Kuf's: Progressive supranuclear palsy	0	0	1	1	0	1	3	2%	1%
Carbon monoxide encephalopathy	0	0	1	1	0	0	2	1%	<1%
Epilepsy	0	0	0	2	0	0	2	1%	<1%
Subarachnoid hemorrhage	1	0	0	0	0	0	1	1%	<1%

These tests are the CT scan, a full drug screen, thyroid functions (T_4RIA, T_3UP, and TSH) and an RPR. This battery, abbreviated in comparison to many others, is unique in attention to drug screening, and its omission of certain measures, such as B_{12} and folate, currently costs a total of $645 to perform in our hospital. ($108 for the lab studies and $537 for the CT scan with and without contrast.) In the specific case of NPH, it may of course be important following CT evidence of ventricular dilatation to proceed to isotope cisternography. The clinician's acumen and specific features of the case may dictate additional measures, but again the 4 tests should afford the clinician a sound, productive approach. Note that none of the steps are particularly invasive, nor costly—save the CT scan. Table 5 speaks to their yield. Nonetheless, caution is in order, for example, "abnormalities demonstrated by CT scanning do not establish a diagnosis of dementia" [25].

THE TERTIARY PHASE OF EVALUATION: PERSISTENCE AND UNCERTAINTY

In the preceding sections, we have examined initial clinical and laboratory screening and then proposed a specific set of four measures (CT scan, drug screen, TFTs, and RPR) to be implemented routinely when the provisional diagnosis of dementia has been made. As noted, this currently will identify approximately 90% of the potentially reversible etiologies for dementiform presentations. But this leaves unaddressed two major issues, one more readily resolved than the other. First, how vigorous should the clinician be in the pursuit of the remaining 10% of potentially reversible etiologies? We propose that additional laboratory studies should proceed only from a combination of the physician's clinical acumen and appreciation of pertinent individual history. For example, stigmata of an endocrinopathy, history of specific industrial exposure, recognition of subtle, disordered movements or macrocytosis in the CBC, each would justify additional laboratory testing, many times in advance of our secondary phase. We reserve "exhaustive" testing for those few cases with decidedly atypical clinical courses, as eg, the onset of a fulminant dementing process in a previously healthy individual. In closing this area, it seems important to note that we generally have not found the EEG or psychometric testing to be routinely useful in the secondary phase of diagnostic evaluation of the demented patient. Rather, the latter provides a baseline reference for subsequent evaluations and documenting the progression of the patient's clinical course.

A second and more problematic issue is the clinician's pursuit of a definitive diagnosis in those cases with negative findings in the second phase and therefore apparently holding little hope for improvement or palliation. Three factors guide us in the further evaluation of these "irreversible" cases. First, there are genetic implications, especially when a familial pattern of disorder has been previously recognized. Correctly identifying Huntington's chorea has considerable merit for the patient's family; it would be a disservice to accept a diagnosis of DAT in such a case. Second, as noted above, definitive diagnosis seems especially critical in catastrophic presentations as exemplified by herpes simplex encephalitis in a young person. (However, it is beyond our thrust in this chapter to explore criteria for brain biopsy.) In turn, these factors lead to a third consideration: the importance of patient and family alike *knowing* what is happening. Not only does such knowledge prove in our experience constructive in reducing the burden of uncertainty, but we have found a greater tolerance for etiologies established in a medical or biologic sense. There seems in many family members reduced anger and greater capacity for empathy when it is appreciated that the erratic, unpredictable grandmother has encephalomalacia, not merely a passive-aggressive personality disorder.

In the third line of evaluation, as before, a balance is to be struck between cost-effectiveness, invasiveness, and likely yield. As yet, quantitative studies addressing these parameters are lacking. Undoubtedly the advent of techniques such as positron emission tomography and nuclear magnetic resonance will make third line evaluation increasingly feasible for the majority of patients. In turn, this enhanced diagnostic precision will facilitate earlier and more palliative interventions for the patient and family together with an improved recognition and refinements of the large heterogeneous group of disorders currently constituting the dementias.

COMMENT

Should the sequence characterized in the preceding sections be applied without exception? When might it be reasonable to abandon this three phase approach? These are difficult clinical decisions, though they may appear straightforward in the abstract. For example, what can be advised when the steps of phase 1 identify a seemingly obvious etiology for the confirmed dementia? Two considerations seem paramount in this situation. First, if the probable etiology is one routinely diagnosed by exclusion, such as multiinfarct dementia in a patient with a preceding history of hypertension and a stepwise course, proceeding with the second phase of evaluation is very appropriate. Second, even when the etiology is presumed to be a function of known trauma, toxic exposure or the like, we would be inclined to persist with the studies outlined in the second phase of our approach. Such a course of action seems prudent on several counts. There must be concern for concurrent dementing processes (though little data presently exists on this question); and as noted previously, the proposed studies are neither prohibitive in their cost nor especially invasive.

We thus argue for effecting the studies in nearly all situations with a confirmed or validated diagnosis of dementia. The only exceptions would be cases in which medical intervention results in prompt and full resolution of the dementia.

Restitution should obviate the need for further diagnostic measures. However, in such instances, an even more bothersome question is introduced. How long should the physician or consultant be willing to wait to determine full recovery has been achieved? As time is frequently critical to reversibility, this is not an academic issue. Again, the low cost, minimal invasiveness and clear yield of the four studies argue for their inclusion. Only in rare instances should the combination of clinical history and clinical course take precedence over the potential gains of the diagnostic steps of the second phase (e.g., CT scan, TFTs, drug screen, and RPR).

Our approach emphasizes successive phases of evaluation and offers a rationale for their sequencing. It is data based and acknowledges clinical realities, calling the physician's attention to critical issues of timing and the tendency to premature closure when confronted with the provisional diagnosis of dementia.

REFERENCES

1. McAllister TW: Cognitive functioning in the affective disorders. Compr Psych 22:572-586, 1981
2. Raskind M, Peskind E, Rivard MF, et al: Dexamethasone suppression test and cortisol circadian rhythm in primary degenerative dementia. Am J Psych 139: 1468-1471, 1982
3. Lipowski ZJ: Delirium. Springfield, IL, Charles C Thomas, 1980
4. Marsden CD, Harrison MJG: Outcome of investigation of patients with pre-senile dementia. Br Med J 2:249-252, 1972
5. Freeman FR: Evaluation of patients with progressive intellectual deterioration. Arch Neurol 33:658-659, 1976
6. Victoratos GC, Lenman JAR, Herzeberg L: Neurological investigation of dementia. Br J Psych 130:131-133, 1977
7. Smith JS, Kiloh LG: The investigation of dementia: Results in 200 consecutive admissions. Lancet 1:824-827, 1981
8. Rabins PV: The prevalence of reversible dementia in a psychiatric hospital. Hosp Comm Psych 32:490-492, 1981
9. Delaney P: Dementia: The search for treatable causes. South Med J 75:707-709, 1982
10. Maletta GJ, Pirozzolo FJ, Thompson G, et al: Organic mental disorders in a geriatric outpatient population. Am J Psych 139:521-523, 1982
11. Griner PF, Glaser RJ: Misuse of laboratory tests and diagnostic procedures. N Engl J Med 307:1336-1339, 1982
12. Ron MA, Toone BK, Garralda ME, et al: Diagnostic accuracy in presenile dementia. Br J Psych 134:161-168, 1979
13. Butler RN: Charting the conquest of senility. Bull NY Acad Med 4:362-381, 1982
14. Tomlinson BE, Blessed G, Roth M: Observations on the brains of demented old people. J Neurol Sci 11:205, 1970
15. Wells CE: Diagnostic evaluation and treatment in dementia. In CE Wells (ed): Dementia, 2nd ed. Philadelphia, FA Davis, 1977
16. Wells CE: Chronic brain disease: An overview. Am J Psych 131:1-12, 1978

17. Wells CE, Duncan GW. Neurology for Psychiatrists. Philadelphia, FA Davis, 1980

18. Haase GR: Diseases presenting as dementia. In CE Wells (ed): Dementia. Philadelphia, FA Davis, 1977

19. Seltzer B, Sherwin J: "Organic brain syndromes": An empirical study and critical review. Am J Psych 135:13–21, 1978

20. Benson DF: Psychiatric Aspects of Neurological Disease, Vol 2. New York, Grune & Stratton, 1982

21. Adams D, Fisher CM, Hakim S, et al: Symptomatic occult hydrocephalus with normal cerebrospinal fluid pressure. N Engl J Med 273:117, 1965

22. Frank E, Tew JM: Normal pressure hydrocephalus: clinical symptoms, diagnoses, pathophysiology and treatment. Heart and Lung 11:321-326, 1982

23. Freeman FR, Rudd SM: Clinical features that predict potentially reversible progressive intellectual deterioration. J Am Geriatr Soc 7:449–451, 1982

24. Fox JH, Topel JL, Huckman MS: Use of computerized tomography in senile dementia. J Neurol Neurosurg Psych 38:948–953, 1975

25. Wells CE: Chronic brain disease: An update on alcoholism, Parkinson's disease, and dementia. Hosp Comm Psych 33:111–126, 1982

26. Wells CE: Differential diagnosis of dementia. Presented at the Clinical Issues in Geriatric Psychiatry Sumposium of the Meeting of the Academy of Psychosomatic Medicine, Chicago, Nov 20, 1982

27. Lippmann S: Workup and diagnosis of dementia. Resident and Staff Physician, January 1982, pp 50–57

28. Soudemire A, Thompson TL: Recognizing and treating dementia. Geriatr. 36:112–120, 1981

CHAPTER 11

The Comprehensive Evaluation of Cocaine and Opiate Abusers

MARK S. GOLD and
TODD W. ESTROFF

The evaluation and initial treatment of cocaine or narcotic drug-using patients is a complex, demanding and sometimes confusing process. To be complete the physician must coordinate and integrate many diverse aspects of drug abuse, medical and psychiatric specialization. All of this must be done in an atmosphere which protects the patient from himself, from drug-related death, and from the illnesses acquired along with a drug dependence. A thoroughly structured multidisciplinary approach to each patient helps ensure that no aspect of care is overlooked or not treated. Below we will review this structured approach in order of priority which falls under the heading of critical general procedures.

GENERAL PROCEDURES

Control of Patient's Environment

The process begins when the patient is admitted to the hospital and transported to a locked evaluation unit where the patient and his belongings are thoroughly searched for abusable drugs.

Handbook of Psychiatric Diagnostic Procedures, vol. 2, edited by R. C. W. Hall and T. P. Beresford. Copyright © 1985 by Spectrum Publications, Inc.

These procedures effectively control the patients environment so that drug identification, stabilization and initial treatment can begin (Figure 1). This environmental control restricts access to drugs, removes enviromental reinforcers, prevents drugs from entering the hospital, permits observation for symptoms of severe overdose or withdrawal, and permits instantaneous emergency care when such reactions occur. In many cases it will reduce drug craving to the point where it enables the patient to stay in treatment. Addicts should, at the least, have no drug access while in the hospital. Environmental controls are necessary to keep the hospital drug-free. These controls include limiting visitors to immediate family, inspecting all packages, keeping the wards physically separate, locking the entire hospital at night, and comprehensive testing of random supervised urines.

Within one half hour of admission a psychiatrist with substance abuse expertise interviews and examines the patient.

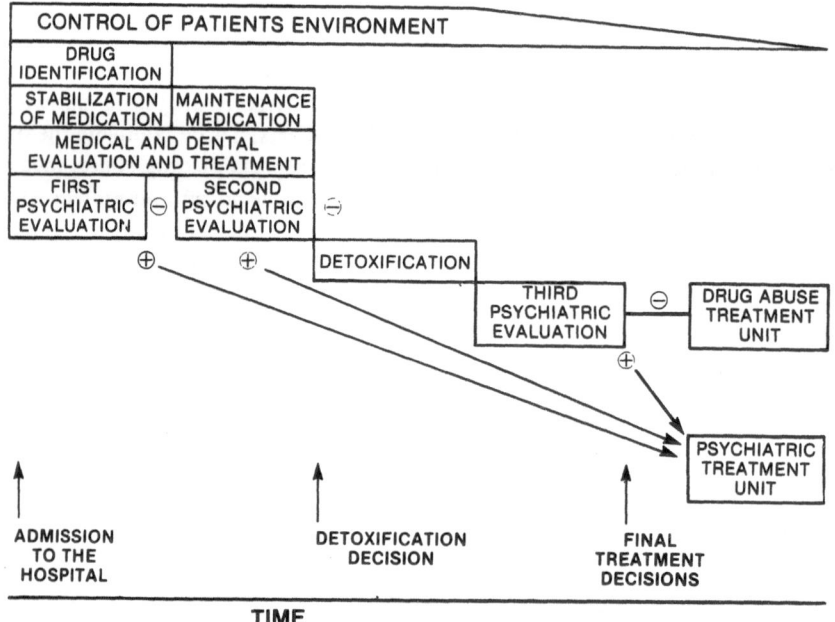

Figure 1. Steps in the control of an addict's environment from admission to the hospital through treatment.

The Interview

The psychiatrist focuses initial interview questions in an attempt to determine which drugs are abused, the magnitude of the habit, and the time of the last dose. This information is unreliable or incomplete in many cases, since some patients minimize or deny the extent of their drug abuse while others exaggerate it.

Medical questions center on past medical history and possible symptoms of bacterial endocarditis, tuberculosis, hepatitis, cellulitis, nutritional and vitamin deficiency, and other medical complications of drug abuse. The answers may help the physician plan for extensive examination and determine which initial laboratory and diagnostic testing are necessary. A preliminary psychiatric assessment is then performed to assess the patients potential for manifesting a major psychiatric disorder during or after detoxification. This assessment is not considered definitive since drug abusing patients can have dramatic changes in their symptoms as stabilization and detoxification proceed [1-5]. This psychiatric evaluation must be repeated at least two other times before arriving at a definitive psychiatric opinion of the patient's underlying psychopathology

The final line of questioning explores the external forces which have brought the patient into the hospital such as pressures from job, family, debts, or legal problems. Many times this information is extremely useful in preventing a patient from prematurely leaving the hospital and relapsing. The leverage provided at a predischarge meeting with the patient's employer telling him that he will definitely lose his job, can be an extremely positive factor if properly utilized. Similarly a confrontation which results in the realization that he will lose his wife or go directly to jail if he leaves the hospital against medical advice or drops out of outpatient treatment can help clarify reality. Additionally these confrontations can be a powerful motivator for continued treatment. Finally, since loss of control and continued use in the face of obvious negative consequences is the definition of an addiction, it is important to have full grasp of the consequences at all times when interacting with the patient.

Physical Examination

The physical examination is first directed toward uncovering impending medical emergencies which might necessitate transfer to a medical floor or hospital. This is important since many patients are so fearful of uncontrolled withdrawal that they may take potentially lethal doses of drugs and alcohol in preparation for admission to the hospital. Even patients who were using only one compound for months or years may mix and take all of their available inventory on the night or day before admission.

Signs of less serious medical problems such as abscesses, cellulitis, hepatitis, endocarditis, arrhythmias and vascular lesions are actively sought during a thorough physical examination and are worked up and treated.

Laboratory Testing

Mistrust of the patients' own reports of the drugs and amount of drugs being abused leads to heavy reliance on objective laboratory testing. In this way the physician does not get angry at the patient for exaggerating, minimizing, and forgetting. As soon as the interview and physical are finished, blood and supervised urines samples are collected and sent for independent identification and quantification of the drugs of abuse. It is essential that all subsequent urine collections be supervised first void urines and that specific gravity is also measured to confirm that the sample is undiluted urine.

If these procedures are followed, complete, comprehensive, and accurate analysis of urine and blood is usually back on the chart within 12 hours of collection. Sensitive antibody-based urinanalysis will detect the vast majority of drugs of abuse which are present in urine at the time that the sample is obtained. Semiquantitative antibody-based urine testing and gas chromatography mass spectroscopic (GC/MS) testing of blood are many times more sensitive and specific than thin layer chromatography (TLC) or urine drug screens. TLC testing is not advisable since it cannot detect several important drugs of abuse at all and several others are detectable only in very high concentrations. TLC is vulnerable to misleading false positives and negatives also [6]. Specific antibody-based urine testing is more desirable than quantitative blood levels, as urine testing can remain positive long after the active drug has left the blood and brain [7]. While blood testing is the most expensive, it is often the preferred sample since drug blood concentrations correlate directly with behavioral effects. Quantitative capillary gas chromatography and GC/MS analysis can be used to detect and quantify drugs in serum that are not easily detected in urine [6,8].

The laboratory is also used to detect drugs which have entered the hospital despite the best preventive measures. In this way the staff can maintain the rules and vigilance but help treat the patient rather than function as a collective warden. Once drugs arrive in the hospital they are eventually taken by drug-abusing patients and are excreted in their urine. Ordering weekly first void random *supervised* comprehensive urines on each drug abusing inpatient and spot urines when unexplained behavioral or motivational changes occur are effective in reducing drug use, as long as the patients learn to believe the credibility of the urine/blood collection/testing procedures.

The initial treatment of the drug abusing patient is adjusted according to these drug testing results. Routine lab work including SMA and CBC is performed along with comprehensive hepatitis antigen and antibody screening. Additional testing is ordered as indicated but should be vigorous enough to establish the presence of common diseases described below.

Stabilization

Regardless of how fast laboratory data becomes available, it is often necessary to provide some medication to stabilize the patient while awaiting the lab results. This dilemma is best resolved by looking at the least risk position. The overdose and withdrawal dangers of each drug are carefully weighed against each other and the least dangerous course is chosen. Opiate overdose can be lethal, whereas withdrawal is uncomfortable but not medically dangerous [9]. Alcohol overdose can also be lethal but it is uncommon [10], whereas withdrawal is potentially one of the most dangerous medical emergencies possible if the patient should develop delirium tremens (DTs) [11]. Cocaine in high doses can cause seizures, hypertension, hyperpyrexia, and sudden death [12-15], whereas withdrawal can produce irritability, negativism, depression, hypersomnia, and psychomotor retardation but is not medically dangerous [16].

Sedative hypnotic overdose is usually much safer; with death, especially using benzodiazepines, being rare [17]. Withdrawal can produce seizures and status epilepticus [18]. Since it is much more dangerous to permit untreated alcohol or sedative-hypnotic withdrawal than to accidentally overmedicate, these drug problems are treated aggressively whereas opiate withdrawal tends to be under treated. Unless patients are showing definite *signs* of opiate withdrawal additional methadone is not given.

Sedative-hypnotic abuse is treated with diazepam usually 10 mg every hour on a PRN schedule. Possible alcohol withdrawal is medicated with chlorodiazepoxide 25 mg every 2-4 hours on a PRN schedule, but if actual withdrawal or impending DT's is suspected a standing dose of 100-200 mg is given in divided doses during 24 hours. The most difficult sedative-hypnotic withdrawals to treat are from glutethimide and ethchlorvynol. This detoxification is done using the agent itself instead of switching to valium. For opiate withdrawal, small doses (eg., 5 mg) of methadone are given every 2-4 hours on a PRN-induced assessment of need basis, unless the actual dosage can be confirmed from the patients methadone maintenance program. The dosage of methadone needed to stabilize most patients is between 20-60 mg with 40 mg/day being the most common. In summary, patients should have all of their complaints evaluated but not necessarily treated. Placebos should never be used or considered a viable treatment option in this setting. Patients should be evaluated, stabilized, re-evaluated, and *then* detoxified.

This system described here could not operate effectively without highly skilled psychiatrist and staff nurses who have been trained in emergency medical/surgical settings necessary to assess and respond to numerous medical problems and alcohol, sedative-hypnotic, and opiate withdrawal. In addition, the staff must be comfortable with the difficult situation of the dependent addicted and polyaddicted patient. The staff must be flexible and pragmatic as actual treatment is frequently modified according to the results of interviews, assessment, and the urine and blood identification and quantification of drugs of abuse.

Behavioral outbursts and fluctuating mental states during this period are treated symptomatically and then are re-examined as possible signs of new drug use, undiagnosed drug dependence or inadequate coverage of the tolerant drugs of abuse. Finally any dramatic changes in motivation for treatment should be scrutinized as possible signs of in hospital drug abuse or attempts to prevent their spouse or employer from being involved in their treatment. The maintenance phase begins when the patient has been comfortably stabilized on PRN medication for several days and he is then given all medication as a standing dose without PRN medication.

Along with these general issues and procedures, specific drug-related diseases must be evaluated, diagnosed, and treated.

COCAINE OR NARCOTIC-RELATED MEDICAL
AND DENTAL COMPLICATIONS

The medical and dental complications of drug abuse are multiple and protean [19-28]. Most are not due to the drugs themselves [20-23] but are secondary to adulterated [20-26,29-33], unsterile drugs [21], lack of sterile techniques, [20,21], sharing of dirty needles with carriers of various infectious diseases [20-23], unusual routes of administration [20,21,30-46] and the addict's particular lifestyle [20,21].

Dental

The most common problem which emerges during detoxification is dental pain. These problems are usually present before admission but are masked by the analgesia of the drugs of abuse. As detoxification proceeds the analgesia is lost and the patient suddenly becomes aware of the pain [28,47-49]. Major dental problems are often diagnosed and require treatment.

Many times the problem is so far advanced that extraction is necessary or the patient develops acute ulcerative gingivitis (trench mouth) [28].

Infections

The addict is prone to develop a wide variety of infections including cellulitis, [20-23], abscesses, [25,26,50,51], endocarditis, [20,21,52-56], pneumonia, tetanus, malaria, [20-22], tuberculosis [57], osteomyelitis, [21,22,58], septic arthritis, [59,60], hepatitis [20-22,61-74], endophthalmitis, [75,76], and veneral diseases [21].

Bacterial infections when they occur tend to be a polymicrobial mixture of aerobic and anaerobic organisms [50,51,56]. When only one organism is involved the offending organism is often unusual or atypical [20,22,52,75].

Hepatitis

Hepatitis in IV addicts occurs commonly and early. It is most often acquired by sharing a needle with another addict who has an acute or chronic viremia. Hepatitis B is most easily acquired and transmitted since it can be passed on in only 0.00004 ml of blood [21,63].

Cocaine and/or heroin addicts, without regard to social class, show increased rates of hepatitis A, [67], non-A/non-B hepatitis [66,73], cytomegalovirus hepatitis, [66], Epstein-Barr virus hepatitis [66], Delta Agent hepatitis [74], chronic active and chronic persistent hepatitis [64,71,72], and superimposed alcoholic hepatitis [20].

Pulmonary

The pulmonary diseases which can occur include pulmonary edema, [20-22], pneumonia secondary to septic emboli or aspiration, [20-22], interstitial pneumonitis, foreign body granulomas and pulmonary hypertension secondary to drug contaminants that are injected IV, snorted, or smoked [30-33,35,77].

Neurology

Neurologic diseases caused by drug abuse include cerebral vascular accidents secondary to hypotensive or hypertensive crisis [78-81] or arterial emboli, [41,82-85], seizures [86], cerebellar ataxia [87,88], peripheral neuropathy [89,90], encephalopathy [91], spongiform leukencophalopathy [36], brain abscesses, and meningitis. Discrete neuropsychologic testing deficits are common in parenteral addicts.

Ophthalmologic

Ophthalmologic problems can result from small particles and bacteria contaminating injected drugs which find their way into the arterial circulation and lodge in retinal arteries [92-96] causing a visual display (talc flash), infection, macular ischemia, [93], neovascularization [94], and foreign body granulomas [95] of the retina.

Renal

Renal disease in addicts often results when antigen-antibody complexes are deposited in the kidney during a variety of infections which include hepatitis B [97-101] and endocarditis [97,102,103]. This may cause a nephrotic syndrome with massive proteinuria [104-109]. Rhabdomyolysis with myoglobinuria [110,111] and polyarteritis nodosa secondary to methamphetamine [112-116] or hepatitis B [116-123] have caused acute and chronic renal failure. Obstructive uropathy secondary to a fungus ball [97] and increased numbers of positive urine cytologies have been reported in opiate abusers [124].

Cardiovascular

Endocarditis and mycotic aneurysms [125] are the major cardiovascular complications of drug abuse. Less common is cocaine induced recurrent angina pectoris, myocardial infarction, hypertension, tachycardia, ventricular arrhythmias, and sudden death [12-14,126].

A necrotizing angiitis indistinguishable from polyarteritis nodosa has been found in IV amphetamine and hepatitis B antigenemic addicts [112-123,127, 128].

Endocrine

Opiate-induced hypoadrenalism has been reported as far back as 1958 [129]. Both ACTH and β-endorphin originate from the same precursor molecule so it is not surprising that chronic opiate administration could block both β endorphin and ACTH production on the basis of exogenous positive feedback inhibition. Lack of ACTH response to naloxone [130] and blunted cortisol response to ACTH in methadone patients [131] are findings consistent with opiate-induced hypoadrenalism.

Increased and decreased testosterone levels have been reported in male opiate addicts but the studies were not controlled for concurrent marijuana (MJ/THC) use [132-134]. Chronic use of narcotics or cocaine can and do produce reduced sexual interest and performance. MJ may have its primary anti-sexual axis effects on pulsatile pituitary LH release. In any case, marijuana and THC are well known to decrease human serum testosterone [135] and sperm motility [136] in males. Opiates and alcohol are more specific and potent testicular poisons.

Toxins and Heavy Metals

Little data exists on environmental toxins or heavy metal disorders in addicts. Since drugs of abuse can be contaminated with anything and such toxin-related disorders are well known to present with psychiatric or organic brain syndrome symptomatology, [137-140] screening for such disorders as a frequent procedure at Fair Oaks Hospital. Behavioral symptoms cannot be explained solely on the basis of the drugs of abuse.

Vitamin and Amino Acid Deficiencies

Many of these abnormalities occur with remarkable frequency in drug addicts since they do not eat regularly or eat a nutritionally adequate diet. Monkeys in bar press paradigms consistently prefer cocaine to food and clinical experience suggests this occurs in human drug users. Some deficiencies may be specific to a certain drug such as cocaine and tyrosine deficiency. Essential amino acid deficiencies (eg., tryptophan, tyrosine) as well as folate, B_6, B_{12} and other B vitamin deficiencies usually occur in chronic drug users without anemia. These deficiencies may contribute to withdrawal complaints and psychopathology.

Drug Effects on the Fetus and Newborn

Valium, barbiturates, and alcohol can produce gross deformity of the newborn [141-142]. These drugs and opiates produce acute and chronic withdrawal after birth [143-145]. Opiates are not teratogenic but many produce behavioral symptoms similar to attention deficit disorder with hyperactivity later in life [143-147]. Amphetamines produce greater early delivery, higher rates of hospitalization, and higher infant mortality [148].

Due to the frequency of drug use by pregnant woman, the field of behavorial teratology is now able to study the long term behavioral effects of maternal drug abuse on children exposed *in utero.*

Severe Acquired Immune Deficiency Syndrome (AIDS)

AIDS, a disease once thought to be exclusively of homosexual men has now been found in IV drug users, Haitians, hemophiliacs, and most recently, in their children [149]. It can present with a variety of unusual infectious diseases that are normally eliminated by cell-mediated immunity in healthy individuals. These diseases include *Pneumocystis carinii* pneumonia, disseminated herpes simplex, cytomegalovirus infections, CNS toxoplasmosis, cryptococcal meningitis, invasive gastrointestinal candida and a variety of typical and atypical disseminated mycobacterial infections. Noninfectious presentations include Kaposi's sarcoma as well as persistent, generalized lymphoadenopathy and diffuse undifferentiated non-Hodgkin's lymphoma.

Decreased amounts of helper T cell [149] and increased suppressor T cell counts result in inverted helper/supressor T cell ratios and this has been postulated to account for the decreased cellular immunity found in AIDS victims

[149,150]. These infections and tumors are thought to be eventually fatal to 65% or more of AIDS cases [149].

TREATMENT

If any of the previously described medical and dental problems are found, they are treated as rapidly and as definitively as possible. Only after the addict has been stabilized on maintenance medication, medical disorders found and treated, and the preliminary psychiatric evaluation finished, is the decision made to proceed with detoxification.

DETOXIFICATION

Detoxification in this type of controlled hospital environment is usually straightforward and uncomplicated. Marijuana and cocaine require no active treatment other than abstinence. The only exceptions to this occurs with chronic high dose cocaine snorting, binge freebase cocaine use and chronic intravenous cocaine use. Sedative-hypnotic stabilized patients are reduced 5-10% per day. Methadone-stabilized patients have their methadone stopped and are given clonidine 0.2-0.3 mg every two hours, whenever withdrawal symptoms occur as long as the systolic blood pressure remains above 70. This effectively treats all symptoms of opiate withdrawal except sleeplessness [151-153]. The polyaddicted patient is detoxified first from sedative-hypnotics and then from opiates as is described above.

FINAL PSYCHIATRIC AND TREATMENT DECISIONS

At any point during hospitalization it can be decided that a drug abusing patient's primary diagnosis is psychiatric and the patient will be transferred to an adult psychiatry unit. This is usually done after detoxification and a thorough psychiatric re-evaluation. We have seen the entire spectrum of psychiatric disorder from frank psychosis to major depression and bipolar illnesses occurring in drug abusing patients [154-156]. Neuroendocrine testing is included in suspected affective disorders [154,157] and a cosyntropin adrenal stimulation test may be used to help evaluate long term opiate abusers [131].

Triage to the appropriate treatment unit and appropriate psychiatric medication is determined by the predominant pathology encountered. It does not matter if the patient is transferred to the cocaine treatment unit, the opiate treatment unit, the alcohol treatment unit or a psychiatric treatment unit as long as secondary pathologies are not ignored. Detoxifying the patient, gaining the patients trust, recognizing and treating the medical, neurological and psychiatric causes and consequences of drug abuse are important first steps in recovery and prevention of relapse in drug abusing individuals. They do not cure the patient and his or her acquired chronic relapsing drug dependence illness. After the first steps described in this chapter, it is necessary to insist upon absolute permanent abstinence as a condition of further treatment. The nonambivalent staff, who are not themselves using drugs, will then be able to guide the patient from addiction to long term abstinence on a one day at a time basis.

REFERENCES

1. Dackis CA, Gold MS: Opiate addiction and depression—cause or effect? Drug Alcohol Depend 11:105-109, 1983
2. Gold MS, Byck R: Endorphins, Lithium, and Naloxone: Their Relationship to Pathological and Drug-Induced Manic-Euphoric States. NIDA Monograph 192-209, 1978
3. Gold MS, Pottash ALC, Extein I, et al: Anti-endorphin effect of methadone. Lancet 2:973, 1980
4. Gold MS, Pottash ALC, Sweeney DR, et al: Antimanic, antidepressant, and antipanic effects of opiates: Clinical, neuroanatomical, and biochemical evidence. Ann NY Acad Sci 140-150, 1982
5. Kleber HD, Gold MS: The use of psychotropic drugs in the treatment of methadone maintained narcotic addicts. Ann NY Acad Sci 311:81-98, 1978
6. Pottash ALC, Gold MS, Extein I: The use of the clinical laboratory. In LI Sederer (ed): Inpatient Psychiatry Diagnosis and Treatment. Williams & Willkins, 1982
7. Dackis CA, Pottash ALC, Annitto W, et al: Persistence of urinary marijuana levels after supervised abstinence. Am J Psych 139:1196-1198, 1982
8. Gold MS, Pottash ALC, Carman JS, et al: The role of the laboratory in psychiatry. In MS Gold, RB Lydiard, JS Carman (eds): Advances in Psychopharmacology: Predicting and Improving Treatment Response Boca Raton, FL, CRC Press, 1983
9. Jaffe JH, Martin WR: Narcotic analgesics and antagonists. In LS Goodman, A Gillman (eds): The Pharmacological Basis of Therapeutics. New York, Macmillan, Publishing Co, 1975
10. Ritchie JM: The aliphatic alcohols. In LS Goodman, A Gillman (eds): The Pharmacological Basis of Therapeutics. New York, MacMillian Publishing Co, 1975
11. Montgomery Jr EB: Neurologic emergencies. In JJ Freitag, LW Miller (eds): Manual of Medical Therapeutics. Boston, Little, Brown & Co, 1980
12. Wetli CV: Death from recreational cocaine use. In Symposium on Cocaine Proceedings, New York, May 3-4, 1982
13. Wetli CV, Wright RK: Death caused by recreational cocaine use. JAMA 241: 2519-2522, 1979

14. DiMaio VJM, Garriott JC: Four deaths due to intravenous injection of cocaine. Forensic Sci Int 12:119–125, 1978
15. Van Dyke C, Byck R: "Cocaine." Sci Am 246:127–141, 1982
16. Gold MS: Diagnosis and treatment of cocaine abuse–II. In Symposium on Cocaine Proceedings, New York, May 3–4, 1982
17. Byck R: Drugs and the treatment of psychiatric disorders. In LS Goodman, A Gillman (eds): The Pharmacological Basis of Therapeutics. New York, Macmillan Publishing Co, 1975
18. Jaffe JH: Drug addiction and drug abuse. In LS Goodman, A Gillman (eds): The Pharmacological Basis of Therapeutics, New York, Macmillan Publishing Co, 1975
19. Kreek MJ: Medical complications in methadone patients. Ann NY Acad Sci 311:110–134, 1978
20. Louria DB, Hensle T, Rose F: The major medical complications of heroin addiction. Ann Int Med 67:1–22, 1967
21. Ostor AG: The medical complication of narcotic addiction. Med J Aust 1:410–415, 448–451, 497–499, 1977
22. Becker CE: Medical complications of drug abuse. Adv Int Med 24:183–202, 1979
23. Sapira JD: The narcotic addict as a medical patient. Am J Med 45:555–558, 1968
24. Kurtzman RS: Complications of narcotic addiction. Radiol 96:23–30, 1970
25. Geelhoed GW, Joseph WL: Surgical sequelae of drug abuse. Surg Gynec Obstet 139:749–755, 1974
26. Ritland D, Butterfield W: Extremity complications of drug abuse. Am J Surg 126:639–731, 1973
27. Dawson CR, Whitcher SP, Proctor FI, et al: Ruminations. JAMA 230:728–731, 1974
28. Carter EF: Dental implications of narcotic addiction. Aust Dent J 23:308–310, 1978
29. Helpern M: Interim report on narcotic program, Aug 12, 1963, National Association for the Prevention of Addiction to Narcotics Newsletter Vol 2, 1964
30. Groth DH, Mackay GR, Crable JV: Intravenous injection of talc in a narcotics addict. Arch Pathol 94:171–178, 1972
31. Tomashefski JF, Hirsch GS, Jolly DN: Microcrystalline cellulose pulmonary embolism and granulomatosis. Arch Pathol Lab Med 105:89–93, 1981
32. Robertson CH, Reynolds RC, Wilson JE: Pulmonary hypertension and foreign body granulomas in intravenous drug abusers. Am J Med 61:657–664, 1976
33. Zeltner TB, Nussbaumer U, Rudin O, et al: Unusual pulmonary vascular lesions of intravenous injections of microcrystalline cellulose. Virchows Arch (Pathol Anat) 395:207–216, 1982
34. Anonymous: Cocapaste and freebase: New fashions in cocaine use. Drug Abuse and Alcoholism Newsletter 9 (3), 1980
35. Weiss RD, Goldenheim PD, Mirin SM, et al: Pulmonary dysfunction in cocaine smokers. Am J Psych 138:1110–1112, 1981
36. Wolters EC, Stam FC, Lousberg RJ: Leucoencephalopathy after inhaling "herion" pyrolysate. Lancet 2:1233–1236, 1982
37. Buchanan DR, Lamb D, Seaton A: Punk rockers lung: Pulmonary fibrosis in a drug snorting fire-eater. Br Med J 283:19–26, 1981

38. Lewis JW, Elliott JP, Obeid FN, et al: Complications of attempted central venous injections performed by drug abusers. Chest 78:4, 1980
39. Sanders B: Carotid triangle abscess secondary to heroin injection. J Oral Med 31:88-90, 1976
40. Merhar L, Colley DP, Clark RA, et al: Computed tomographic demonstration of cervical abscess and jugular vein thrombosis. Otolaryngol 107:313-315, 1981
41. Chillar RK, Jackson AL: Reversible hemiplegia after presumed intracarotid injection of Ritalin. N Engl J Med 304:1305, 1981
42. Klatte EC, Brooks AL, Rhamy RK: Toxicity of intra-arterial barbiturates and tranquilizing drugs. Radiol 92:700-704, 1969
43. Buckspan GS, Franklin JD, Novak GR, et al: Intra-arterial drug injury: Studies of etiology and potential treatment. J Surg Res 24:294-301, 1978
44. Lindell TD, Porter JN, Lanston C: Intra-arterial injections of oral medications. N Engl J Med 287:1132-1133, 1972
45. Wright CB, Lamoy RE, Hobson RW: Hemodynamic effects of intra-arterial injection of drugs of abuse. Surgery 79:425-431, 1976
46. Siegel S, Hinson RE, Krank MD, et al: Heroin "overdose" death: contribution of drug-associated environmental cues. Science 216:436-437, 1982
47. Rosenstein DL: Effect of long-term addiction to heroin on oral tissues. J Public Health Dent 35:118-122, 1975
48. Rosenstein DI, Stewar AV: Dental care for patients receiving methadone. J Am Dent Assoc 89:356-359, 1974
49. Colon PG: Dental disease in the narcotic addict. Oral Surg 33:905-910, 1972
50. Webb D, Thadepalli H: Skin and soft tissue poly-microbial infections from intravenous abuse of drugs. West J Med 130:200-204, 1979
51. Meislin HW, Lerner SA, Graves MH, et al: Cutaneous abscesses: Anaerobic and aerobic bacteriology and outpatient management. Ann Int Med 87:145-149, 1977
52. Sobel JD, Carrizosa J, Ziobrowski TF, et al: Polymicrobial endocarditis involving Eikenella corrodens. Am J Med Sci 282:41-44, 1981
53. Andy JJ, Sheikh MU, Ali N, et al: Echocardiographic observations in opiate addicts with active infective endocarditis. Am J Cardiol 40:17-23, 1977
54. Weinstein L, Schlesinger JJ: Pathonotomic, pathophysiologic and clinical correlations in endocarditis. N Engl J Med 291:832-837, 1974
55. Wright JS, Glennie JS: Excision of tricuspid valve with later replacement in endocarditis of drug addiction. Thorax 33:518-519, 1978
56. Child JA, Darrell JH, Rhys Davis N, et al: Mixed infective endocarditis in a heroin addict. J Med Microbiol 2:293-299, 1969
57. Reichman LB, Felton CP, Edsall JR: Drug dependence, a possible new risk factor for tuberculosis disease. Arch Int Med 139:337-339, 1979
58. Holzman RS, Bishko F: Osteomyecitis in heroin addicts. Ann Int Med 75:693-696, 1971
59. Gifford DB, Patzaus M, Ivler D, et al: Septic arthritis due to pseudomonas in heroin addicts. J Bone Joint Surg 57A:631-635, 1975
60. Ross GN, Baraff LJ, Quismorio FP, et al: Serratia arthritis in heroin users. J Bone Joint Surg 57:1158-1160, 1975
61. Norkrans G, Frosner G, Hermodsson S, et al: Multiple hepatitis attacks in drug addicts. JAMA 243:1056-1058, 1980

62. Arthurs Y, Doyle GD, Fielding JF: The effects of drug abuse on the natural history and progression of chronic active and chronic persistent hepatitis. Ir J Med Sci 150:104–112, 1981
63. Krugman S: The newly licensed hepatitis B vaccine. JAMA 247:2012–2015, 1982
64. Novick DM, Gelb AM, Stenger RJ, et al: Hepatitis B serologic studies in narcotic users with chronic liver disease. Am J Gastroenterol 75:111–115, 1981
65. Alexander M: Indictors of drug abuse-hepatitis. In LG Richards, LB Blevens (eds):   The Epidemiology of Drug Abuse: Current Issues. NIDA Research Monograph 10, 1977, pp 123-129
66. Schumacher RT, Trey C: Viral hepatitis types A, B and non-A/non-B: Current concepts. Ligand Quaterly 5:11–25, 1982
67. Estroff TW, Extein IL, Malaspina D: Hepatitis in suburban cocaine and opiate users. Presented at 136th Annual Meeting American Psychiatric Association, New York, April 20-May 6, 1983
68. Boughton CR, Hawkes RA: Viral hepatitis and the drug cult: A brief socio-epidemiological study in Sydney, Australia. NZ Med J 10:157–161, 1980
69. Blanck RR, Ream N, Conrad M: Hepatitis B antigen and antibody in heroin users. Am J Gastroeneterol 71:164–167, 1979
70. Serow SSW: Hepatitis in drug dependents. Aust Fam Physician 10:204–298, 1981
71. Miller DJ, Kleber H, Bloomer JR: Chronic hepatitis associated with drug abuse: Significance of hepatitis B virus. Yale J Biol Med 52:135–140, 1979
72. Cherubin CE, Schaefer RA, Rosenthal WS, et al: The natural history of liver disease in former drug users. Am J Med Sci 272:244–253, 1976
73. Fields HA, Bradley DW, Maynard JE: Non A/Non B hepatitis detection methodology: A review. Ligand Quarterly 5:28-32, 1982
74. Raimondo G, Gallo L, Ponzetto A, et al: Multicentre study of prevalence of HBV-associated delta infection and liver disease in drug addicts. Lancet 1:249–251, 1982
75. Masi RJ: Endogenous endophthalmitis associated with bacillus cereus bacteremia in a cocaine addict. Ann Ophthalmol 10:1367-1370, 1978
76. Getnick RA, Rodriques MM: Endogenous fungal endophthalmitis in a drug addict. Am J Ophthalmol 77:680-683, 1974
77. Waller BF, Brownlee WJ, Roberts WC: Self-induced pulmonary granulomatosis. Chest 78:90–94, 1980
78. Delaney P, Estes M: Intracranial hemorrhage with amphetamine abuse. Neurol 30:1125–1128, 1980
79. Dau PC, Weiner HL: Intracranial hemorrhage associated with amphetamine use. Neurol 31:922-923, 1981
80. Shukla D: Intracranial hemorrhage associated with amphetamine use. Neurol 32:917-918, 1982
81. Brust JCM, Richter RW: Stroke associated with addiction to heroin. Neurol Neurosurg Psych 39:194–199, 1976
82. Loizou LA, Boddie HG: Polyradiculoneuropathy associated with heroin abuse. Neurol Neurosurg Psych 41:855-857, 1978
83. Rumbaugh CL, Bergeron RJ, Fang HCH, et al: Cerebral angiographic changes in the drug abuse patient. Radiol 101:335-344; 1971
84. Hall III JH, Karp HR: Acute progressive ventral pontine disease in heroine abuse. Neurol 23:6-7, 1973

85. Ell JJ, Uttley D, Silver JR: Acute myelopathy in association with heroin addiction. Neurol Neurosurg Psych 44:448–450, 1981
86. Allister C, Lush M, Oliver JS: Status epilepticus caused by solvent abuse. Br Med J 283:1156, 1981
87. Takeuchi Y, Hisanaga N, Yuichiro O, et al: Cerebellar dysfunction caused by sniffing of toluene-containing thinner. Ind Health 19:163–169, 1981
88. Malm G, Lying-Tunell U: Cerebellar dysfunction related to toluene sniffing. Acta Neurol 62:188–190, 1980
89. Layzer RB: Myeloneuropathy after prolonged exposure to nitrous oxide. Lancet 2:1227–1230, 1978
90. Nevins MA: Neuropathy after nitrous oxide abuse. JAMA 244:2264, 1980
91. King MD, Day RE, Oliver JS, et al: Solvent encephalopathy. Br Med J 283:663–665, 1981
92. Tse DT, Ober RR: Talc retinopathy. Am J Ophthalmol 90:624–640, 1980
93. Friberg TR, Gragoudas ES, Regan CDJ: Talc emboli and macular ischemia in intravenous drug abuse. Arch Ophthalmol 97:1089–1091, 1979
94. Kresca LJ, Goldbert MF, Jampol LM: Talc emboli and retinal neovascularization in a drug abuser. Ophthalmol 87:334–339, 1979
95. Michelson JB, Whitcher JP, Wilson S, et al: Possible foreign body granuloma of the retina associated with intravenous cocaine addiction. Am Ophthalmol 87:278–280, 1979
96. Atlee, WE, Jr: Talc and corn starch emboli in eyes of drug abusers. JAMA 219:45–51, 1972
97. Olivero J, Bacque F, Carlton CE, et al: Renal complications of drug addiction. Urology 8:526–530, 1976
98. Kohler PF, Cronin RE, Hammond WS: Chronic membranous glomerulonephritis caused by hepatitis B antigen–antibody immune complexes. Ann Int Med 81:448–451, 1974
99. Eknoyan G, Gyorkey F, Dichoso C: Renal morphological and immunological changes associated with acute viral hepatitis. Kidney Int 1:413–419, 1972
100. Combes B, Shorey J, Barrera A: Glomerulonephritis with deposition of Australia antigen-antibody complexes in glomerula basement membrane. Lancet 2:234–237, 1971
101. Myers BD, Griffel B, Naveh D: Membrano-proliferative glomerulonephritis associated with persistent viral hepatitis. Am J Clin Pathol 59:222–228, 1972
102. Gutman RA, Striker GE, Gilliland BC: The immune complex glomerulonephritis of bacterial endocarditis. Med 51:1–23, 1972
103. Tu WH, Shearn MA, Lee JC: Acute diffuse glomerulonephritis in acute staphylococcal endocarditis. Ann Int Med 71:335–341, 1969
104. Friedman EA, Rao TKS, Nicastri AD: Heroin associated nephropathy. Nephron 13:421–426, 1974
105. McGinn JT, McGinn TG, Cherubin CE, et al: Nephrotic syndrome in drug addicts. NY State Med 74:92–95, 1974
106. Eknoyan G, Gyorkey F, Dichoso C, et al: Renal involvement in drug abuse. Arch Int Med 132:801–806, 1973
107. Kilcoyne MM, Gocke DJ, Meltzer JI: Nephrotic syndrome in heroin addicts. Lancet 1:17–20, 1972
108. Sreepada TK, Micastri AD, Friedman EA: Natural history of heroin-associated nephropathy. N Engl J Med 290:19–23, 1974

109. Eknoyan G, Gyorkey F, Dichoso C, et al: Nephropathy in patients with drug addiction. Virchows Arch (Pathol Anat) 365:1-13, 1975
110. Richter RW, Challenor YB, Pearson J, et al: Acute myoglobinuria associated with heroin addiction. JAMA 216:1172-1176, 1971
111. Schreiber SN, Liebowitz MR, Bernstein LH, et al: Limb compression and renal impairment (crush syndrome) complicating narcotic overdose. N Engl J Med 284: 368-369, 1971
112. Richlim DM, Saltzman DB, Willis J: Necrotizing angiitis and hepatitis in an amphetamine abuser. Del Med J 49:469-477, 1977
113. Allison SN: Arteriopathy and amphetamine abuse. Australas Radiol 23:173-175, 1979
114. Margolis MT, Newton TH: Methamphetamine ("speed") arteritis. Neuroradiol 2:179-182, 1971
115. Citron BP, Halpern M, McCarron M: Necrotizing angiitis associated with drug abuse. N Engl J Med 283:1003-1011, 1970
116. Koff RS, Widrich WC, Robbins AH: Necrotizing angiitis in a methamphetamine user with hepatitis B—angiographic diagnosis, five-months follow-up results and localization of bleeding site. N Engl J Med 288:946-947, 1973
117. Baker AL, Kaplan MM, Benz WX: Polyarteritis associated with australia antigen-positive hepatitis. Gastroenterol 62:105-110, 1972
118. Trepo CG, Zuckerman AJ, Bird RC, et al: The role of circulating hepatitis B antigen/antibody immune complexes in the pathogenesis of vascular and hepatic manifestations in polyarteritis nodosa. J Clin Pathol 27:863-868, 1974
119. Heazlewood VJ, Bochner F, Craswell PW: Hallucinogenic drug induced vasulitis. Med J Aust 1:359-360, 1981
120. Sergent JS, Lockshin MD, Christian CL: Vasculitis with hepatitis B antigenemia. Med 55:1-18, 1976
121. Trepo CG, Thivolet J, Prince AM: Australia antigen and polyarteritis nodosa. Am J Dis Child 123:390-391, 1972
122. Michalak T: Immune complexes of hepatitis B surface antigen in the pathogenesis of periarteritis nodosa. Am Pathol 90:619-632, 1978
123. Chalopin JM, Rifle G, Turc JM, et al: Immunological findings during successful treatment of HBSAG-associated polyarteritis nodosa by plasmapheresis alone. Br Med J 280:368, 1980
124. Behmard S, Sadeghi A, Moharei M, et al: Positive association of opium addiction and cancer of the bladder, Acta Cytol 25:142-146, 1981
125. Yellin AE: Ruptured mycotic aneurysm a complication of parenteral drug abuse. Arch Surg 112:981-986, 1977
126. Coleman DL, Ross TF, Naughton JL: Myocardial ischemia and infarction related to recreational cocaine use. West J Med 136:444-446, 1982
127. Halpern M, Citron P: Necrotizing angiitis associated with drug abuse. Am J Roentgenol 3:663-671, 1971
128. King J, Richards M, Tress B: Cerebral arteritis associated with heroin abuse. Med J Aust 2:444-445, 1978
129. Eisenman AJ, Fraser HF, Brooks JW: Urinary excretion and plasma levels of 17-hydroxycortico steroids during a cycle of addiction to morphine. J Pharmacol Exp Ther 132:226-231, 1961
130. Gold MS, Pottash ALC, Extein I: Evidence for an endorphin dysfunction in methadone addicts: Lack of ACTH response to naloxone. Drug Alcohol Depend 8:257-262, 1981

131. Dackis CA, Gurpegui M, Pottash ALC, et al: Methadone induced hypoadrenalism. Lancet 2:1167, 1982
132. Lafisca S, Bolelli G, Franceschetti F, et al: Hormone levels in methadone-treated drug addicts. Drug Alcohol Depend 8:229-234, 1981
133. Cicero TJ, Bell RD, Wiest WG, et al: Function of the male sex organs in heroin and methadone users. N Engl J Med 292:882-887, 1975
134. Mendelson JH, Meyer RE, Ellinghoe J: Effects of heroin and methadone on plasma cortisol and testosterone. J Pharmacol Exp Ther 195:296, 1975
135. Kolodny RC, Masters WH, Kolodner RM, et al: Depression of plasma testosterone levels after chronic intensive marijuana use. N Engl J Med 290:872-874, 1974
136. Hong CY, Chaput De Saintonge DM, Turner P: ⁹-Tetrahydrocannabinol inhibits human sperm motility, J Pharm Pharmacol 33:746-747, 1981
137. Hall RCW: Psychiatric Presentations of Medical Illness. New York, Spectrum Publications, 1980
138. Jefferson JW, Marchal JR: Neuropsychiatric Features of Medical Disorders. New York, Plenum Medical Book Co, 1981
139. Edwards N: Mental disturbances related to metals. In RCW Hall (ed): Psychiatric Presentations of Medical Illness. New York, Spectrum Publications 1980, pp 283-307
140. Estroff TW, Gold MS: Psychiatric misdiagnosis in psychopharmacology in the 1980's: Improvement of treatment response. In MS Gold, RB Lydiard, JS Carman (eds): Advances in Psychopharmacology: Predicting and Improving Treatment Response. Boca Raton, FL, CRC Press, 1984, pp 34-66
141. Golden NL, Sokol RJ, Hugnert BR: Maternal alcohol use and infant development. Pediatr 6:931-933, 1982
142. Clarren SK, Smith DW: The fetal alcohol syndrome. N Engl J Med 298:1063, 1978
143. Hutchings DE: Behavioral teratology: Embryonic and behaviorial effects of drugs during pregnancy. In G Gottlieb (ed): Studies on the Development of Behavior and the Nervous System. New York, Academic Press, 1978, pp 7-31
144. Hutchings DE: Neurobehavioral effects of prenatal origin: Drugs of use and abuse. In RA Schwarz, SJ Yaffe (eds): Drug and Chemical Risks to the Fetus and Newborn, New York, Alan R. Liss, 1980, pp. 109-114.
145. Hutchings DE: Behavioral Teratology: A new frontier in neurobehaviorial research. EM Johnson, DM Kochhar (eds): Handbook of Experimental Pharmacology. Berlin, Springer-Verlag, 1983
146. Strauss ME, Lessen-Firestone JK, Chavez GJ, et al: Children of methadone treated women at five years of age. Presented at the satellite meeting of the Committee on Problems of Drug Dependence on Acute and Protracted Effects of Perinatal Drug Dependence, Philadelphia, June 7, 1979
147. Chasnoff IG, Hatcher R, Burns WJ: Polydrug—and methadone—addicted newborns: A continuum of impairment. Pediatr 7:210-213, 1982
148. Eriksson M, Larsson G, Zetterstrom R: Amphetamine addiction and pregnancy. Acta Obstet Gynecol Scand 60:253-259, 1981
149. Marx JL: New disease baffles medical community. Science 217:618-621, 1982
150. Centers for Disease Control: Epidemiologic aspects of the current outbreak of Kaposi's sarcoma and opportunistic infections. N Engl J Med 306:248-252, 1982
151. Gold MS, Pottash ALC, Kleber HD: Outpatient clonidine detoxification.

Lancet 2:621, 1981
152. Gold MS, Pottash ALC, Sweeney DR, et al: Opiate withdrawal using cloni-
     dine. JAMA 243:343-346, 1980
153. Gold MS, Pottash ALC, Extein I: Clonidine: Inpatient studies from 1978 to
     1981. J Clin Psych 43(6):35-38, 1982
154. Gold MS, Pottash ALC, Sweeney DR, et al: Antimanic, antidepressant, and
     antipanic effects of opiates: Clinical, neuroanatomical, and biochemical evi-
     dence. Ann NY Acad Sci 398:140-150, 1982
155. Gold MS, Kleber H: Use of psychotropic drugs in the treatment of metha-
     done maintained narcotic addicts. Ann NY Acad Sci 311:81-98, 1978
156. Gold MS, Byck R: Endorphins, Lithium and Naloxone: Their Relationship
     to Pathological and Drug-Induced Manic-Euphoric States. Natl Inst Drug
     Abuse Res Monogr Ser (19): 192-209, 1978
157. Pottash ALC, Gold MS, Extein: The use of the clinical laboratory. In LI
     Sederer (ed): Inpatient Psychiatry Diagnosis and Treatment. Baltimore,
     Williams & Wilkins, 1983, pp. 205-221

CHAPTER 12

Evaluation of the Geriatric Patient

ALVIN J. LEVENSON and SUHA A. BELLER

The medical care of the U.S. elderly has been characterized by terms such as negative, nihilistic, and professionally antipathetic. Justification for such acrimony is reflected in several facts including: the elderly are often referred for disposal vs disposition; their complaints are often ignored, "tolerated," sedated, or responded to with "What do you expect at your *age*"?; additionally senility, a term without rational scientific basic use, remains a commonly employed diagnosis; and so on.

Psychiatry, as a specialty of medicine, is obviously not exempt from such misguided perspectives and intervention. An enormous quantitative and qualitative deficiency in mental health care delivery exists. Eighty to 93% of the 2½ to 5½ million elderly individuals requiring psychiatric treatment are receiving none at all. Those who do are often confronted with considerable defeatism. Psychpharmacologic palliation and control frequently form the mainstays of treatment; success is measured in decibels; little regard is paid to uncover reversible causes, to the production of remission, and to optimal rehabilitation. This chapter addresses the issue of evaluation of psychiatric illness in the elderly—specifically, diagnostic procedures useful to uncovering reversible causes for nonfunctional psychopathology.

Organic psychiatric states are common in later life compared to younger populations. These states may present in one or more of several ways: as an or-

Handbook of Psychiatric Diagnostic Procedures, vol. 2, edited by R. C. W. Hall and T. P. Beresford. Copyright © 1985 by Spectrum Publications, Inc.

ganic brain syndrome (OBS) in its pure cognitive, memory, and intellectual dysfunctional form; as a logical extension of the pure form (i.e., caused by the same physiologic insult which produced the "pure" form), manifested by lability of affect, sterotype, and pathologic resistance; as frightening or derogatory hallucinations or delusions; purely visual hallucinations, as well as tactile, kinesthetic, olfactory, and gustatory hallucinations, and as a retarded depression with history supporting an organic etiology (e.g., treatment with rawoulfia alkaloids).

The OBS (in its pure form) and its logical extensions are believed to be caused by an insult of sufficient magnitude to key critical areas of the cerebral cortex; the pathogenesis is less clear for the balance. Regardless, the brain is the target organ. Impairment pivots from the cerebral structures affected; nonfunctional psychopathology results most commonly from insult to the frontal and temporal lobes. In that light, appreciation of cause is fundamental to directed evaluation.

Two classes of causes exist for nonfunctional psychopathology—those that are irreversible and those that are not. Irreversible causes can be divided into three major categories—the primary neuronal degenerative states, the secondary neuronal degenerative states, and cancer. In the primary state, the initial pathogenetic insult begins intraneuronally; the neuron subsequently becomes hypofunctional and dies. Exemplary states include Alzheimer's, Pick's, and senile degenerative brain diseases, Huntington's chorea, and Jakob-Creutzfeldt disease. The most common causal primary degenerative state in the elderly is a combination of the Alzheimer's and senile degenerative forms, called senile dementia—Alzheimer's type (SDAT). In the secondary neuronal degenerative states, the insult begins extraneuronally and results in its eventual hypofunction and demise. The most common cause of the secondary state is cerebral atherosclerosis which reduced neuronal arterial perfusion. The most common primary cancer to affect the cerebral hemispheres in later life is the glioblastoma multiforme (predilection for the frontal an temporal lobes). Metastatic lesions of the brain arise more commonly in the elderly from the prostate, breast, colon, and stomach. The direct destructive role of the malignancy in perturbing cortical activity is considerably clearer than its distal effects on the brain. The most common irreversible cause of later and late life nonfunctional psychopathology is the primary state (50–70%). Cerebral atherosclerosis, contrary to populat opinion, constitutes only 12–18%; the balance is due to cancer (primary and metastatic).

There are multiple potential causes for reversible nonfunctional psychopathology. These include benign tumors, trauma, toxins, infection, metabolic disease, organ/systemic dysfunction, vascular disorders, and hydrocephalus. The most commonly occurring benign tumor affecting the cerebral cortex of the older individual is the meningioma. It has a predilection for the frontal lobes. The sequelae of head trauma, notably the hematoma, are not uncommon causes of nonfunctional psychopathology in the elderly. The more commonly occurring hematomas include the subdural and epidural types; subarachnoid hemorrhages occur with less frequency. The most common toxin implicated in producing organic psychiatric states is medication (prescription and over-the-counter types). The toxic effects are due usually to dosages which have not been adjusted downward for those of older age. Other toxins include alcohol, illicit drugs, and industrial pollutants. Toxins may cross the blood–brain barrier and affect the brain directly or act extracerebrally but nevertheless impact on brain function (e.g., antihypertensives producing hypotension and cerebral hypoperfusion). Infections may arise in the brain or meninges proper (e.g., encephalitis, cerebral abscesses, or meningitis) or travel to the brain from distant sites (septic, embolus, sepsis). Additionally, cerebral dysfunction may be produced by the effects of infection, notably fever* and dehydration. Metabolic dysfunction includes problem states such as dehydration, vitamin deficiency, starvation, electrolyte imbalance, altered thyroid hormone levels, etc. Organ/systemic problems involve disease in organs or major systems. As is well known, each system, or its component organ(s)/structure(s), support normal brain functions; abnormalities thus have a potentially harmful effect on cerebral function. Potentially reversible or treatable vascular lesions include the cerebrovascular aneurysm, arteriovenous malformation, and collagen vascular disease. The specific hydrocephalic state which affects the elderly most commonly is the normal pressure type. The lateral and third are the most frequently involved ventricles; cause is commonly not found.

Proof of existence of nonfunctional psychopathology is best done by means of standard (but thorough) mental status examination; older age should not mitigate its use. Where evidence of clinical abnormality does not support the "suspicions" of the evaluating physician, other means of assessing cognitive, intellectual function, and memory may be employed; these are in the form of psychological testing. Significantly, most of the parameters tested by these examinations are also covered in and uncovered by the standard, clinical mental status examination. Some of these tests are now briefly reviewed. The Wechsler Adult Intelligence Scale (WAIS) measures number of verbal and nonverbal intellectual functions. The Hooper Test assesses spatial visualization. The Benton Visual Retention Test evaluates nonverbal memory. The Inglis Paired-Association Learning Test measures memory. Of note, none of these alone is comprehensive enough to suffice as a complete diagnostic instrument.

Another diagnostic issue frequently receives consideration in the elderly–pseudodementia. In pseudodementia, the patient demonstrates cognitive, intellectual, and/or memory impairment; these manifestations are caused not by an organic but functional etiology. Functional psychopathology, such as the retarded depression may deprive the patient of interest and energy to answer questions correctly; incorrect answers secondary to severe anxiety and disorganization can be

---

*Increasing age brings about a variable decline in immune response. Consequently, the elderly individual tends to run lower temperatures and should not be regarded as less serious.

produced by an agitated depression and schizophrenia, respectively. Confusion about the accurate diagnosis of pseudodementia exists among many clinicians. Several tests may assist the discrimination, particularly the affective components—notably the Mini-Mental State, WAIS, Inglis Paired-Associate Learning Test, etc. It is the authors' opinion, however, that the differentiations should not be a compelling maneuver as *any* evidence of nonfunctional psychopathology must be evaluated as such, the goal being to find a reversible etiology. There is not truly a reliable way to accurately discriminate a functional etiology; to treat on the basis of an erroneous assumption with psychotropic medications or ECT may not only cloud but worsen existing, physiologic dysfunction. Further, a functional state may (and often does) accompany an organic disorder and therefore be unrelated etiologically; each state must be evaluated and treated individually (beginning with the organic condition).

The initial clinical approach of choice for suspected or actual nonfunctional psychopathology is the determination and correction of a reversible etiology. In addition to the standard history and physical examination, the authors recommend the following minimum etiologic screening evaluation; CBC with differential, liver function tests, BUN, Cr, Electrolytes, B_{12}, folic acid, thyroid function tests, Urinanalysis, urine screen for drugs and heavy metals, chest x-ray, EKG, EEG, and CT scan of the head. Additional laboratory evaluations should be ordered as indicated. The yield for each laboratory test has not been well validated in the elderly. In that light, however, several points are worthy of mention. Ten to 30% of organic brain syndromes (pure cognitive/intellectual/memory dysfunctional forms, as well as lability of affect, stereotypy, and pathologic resistance) are potentially reversible with timely interventions. The vast majority of other forms of nonfunctional psychopathology (e.g., characteristic of other forms of nonfunctional psychopathology (e.g., characteristic delusions and hallucinations) are usually reversible. Second, nonfunctional states do not represent normal aging; their presence therefore, demands evaluation for reversibility. The most common reversible etiology in the elderly is excess dosages of medications (including anesthesia). There is no reliable way to render such evaluations without adequate laboratory investigation. There is a tendency among clinicians to automatically assume that the presence of nonfunctional psychopathology in the elderly is irreversible; thus little or no attempts at evaluation and reversal are launched. This is a practice to be abhorred. As is well known, cerebral neurons are postmitotic. In the absence of reversal, sufficient neuronal death can convert of chronic illness.

The treatment of choice for nonfunctional psychopathology with a reversible etiology is reversal, regardless of one's age. Where functional co-exists with nonfunctional states, the latter should be treated first.

The pharmacologic treatment of irreversible nonfunctional states manifested by impairment in cognition, memory, and intellectual function can be subdivided into three groups—metabolic stimulants, the precursors of acetylcholine, and the so-called cerebral vasodilators. The first group includes medications such as methyl-phenidate (Ritalin®) or the ergot alkaloid preparation, Hydergine®, which pur-portedly act to stimulate/heighten the metabolic activity of the neurons. The use of the second group is predicated upon the notion that levels of a neurotransmitter, acetylcholine, have been found to be reduced in the brain of patients with Alz-heimer's disease. Thus, precorsors of acetylcholine, notably lecithin and deanol, have been tried. The third group presumably works by enlarging, or dilating the arteries of the brain, thus allowing more highly oxygenated blood to get to the brain tissue.

In general, these agents have proved largely ineffective in reversing the pure cognitive form of OBS although additional research is underway.* The reasons for suboptimal therapeutic outcome are numerous and include the following: first, dead neurons cannot be regenerated, regardless of stimulation, the administration of metabolic substrates, or increased oxygen concentration. Second, cerebral vaso-dilator is actually a misnomer in that this agent does not dilate arteries in the brain; it is in reality a dilator of peripheral arteries. Important also is the fact that the arteries in the brain are maximally dilated under hypoxic conditions. Further, the majority of irreversible OBS are caused by the primary degenerative states and not by reduced arterial blood supply. Major tranquilizers are not useful for reversing the pure form of an OBS; they can, however, cause cortical lesions. These agents are extremely efficacious, however, in producing remission of organic induced de-lusions, hallucinations, lability of affect, sterotype, and pathologic resistance.

The use of medications should never supplant a thorough evaluation to rule out a reversible cause; their prescription then should be confined to otherwise ir-reversible states. The appropriate form on nonorganic therapies must likewise be employed.

REFERENCES

1. Levenson AJ: The Neuropsychiatric Side Effects of Drugs in the Elderly. New York, Raven Press, 1979
2. Levenson AJ, Hall RCW: Psychiatric Manifestations of Physical Disease in the Elderly. New York, Raven Press, 1980
3. Levenson AJ: Aging and Mental Health. Health Values: Achieving High Level Wellness. 5:70–72, 1980
4. Levenson AJ: Geriatric Psychopharmacotherapy: Optimal Technique. Spring-field, IL, Charles C Thomas, 1982

---

*The ergot alkaloid preparation has been found somewhat effective in milder cases of the pure form; this is believed to be due to the fact that hypofunctional but not yet dead neurons were stimulated among other possible reasons.

5. Levenson AJ: Nonfunctional Psychopathology of Late Life. J Psych Tr and Eval 4:1, 1982
6. Weingarten CH, Rosoff LG, Eisen SV, et al: Medical Care in a Geriatric Psychiatry Unit: Impact on Psychiatric Outcome. J Am Ger Soc 30:738, 1982

CHAPTER 13

Diagnostic Approaches to Sexuality in the Medically Ill

THOMAS N. WISE and
CHESTER W. SCHMIDT, JR.

INTRODUCTION

The diagnosis of a sexual dysfunction in an individual with a medical disorder has gained attention since Masters and Johnson delineated a normal sexual response cycle. Early psychoanalytic investigators emphasized the ubiquitous nature of sexual fears, fantasies, and frustrations associated with both normal and abnormal psychosexual development. Treatment for sexual dysfunctions was considered within the context of neurotic illness and/or characterologic deficits. The development of current behavioral treatment methods utilizing both learning and psychodynamic principles are symptom focused and have achieved reasonably good results. Concurrently, development of specific medical and surgical procedures, such as the penile prosthesis, has restored sexual functioning in men with organic defects. Contemporary psychiatric competence includes the ability to assess sexual disorders both in the physically healthy and medically ill. This chapter will present an approach to the medically ill patient with a sexual dysfunction. By reviewing present diagnostic nomenclature of sexual dysfunctions in the healthy individual as well as reviewing the clinical assessment of sexual dysfunctions in healthy patients and those physically ill, the reader will learn a systematic approach to evaluating such problems.

Handbook of Psychiatric Diagnostic Procedures, vol. 2, edited by R. C. W. Hall and T. P. Beresford. Copyright © 1985 by Spectrum Publications, Inc.

The DSM-III divides psychosexual disorders in the physically healthy individual into three categories: disorders of sexual desire; disorders of sexual excitement; and disorders of orgasm. Additional categories, such as dyspareunia (pain upon intercourse), vaginismus, and premature ejaculation, fill out the common sexual dysfunctions. This nomenclature requires an understanding of the normal sexual response cycle.

THE SEXUAL RESPONSE CYCLE

It is useful to think of human sexual response as an evolving psychophysiologic event. Masters and Johnson have utilized graphs to the progression of sexual response (Figure 1). Kaplan modified Masters and Johnsons initial delineation of sexual physiology by viewing normal sexual response as a three-phased phenomena. The initial component is the *desire phase*. Desire appears to be an appetite drive that consists of fantasies and the actual desire for sexual activity. In addition to cognitive elements, there appears to ba a biologic component which produces libidinal drive. Disorders of the desire phase are poorly understood. Prototypically, the male with an obsessive-compulsive personality style may be seen with relatively little interest or motivation for sexual behavior, either autoerotic or with another partner. Disorders of sexual desire have been differentiated from sexual phobias by Kaplan. The sexually phobic individual is one for whom even the thought of sex arouses great anxiety, whereas in the disorder of sexual desire the individual is not interested and not made anxious by sexual thoughts and fantasies. It is important to note that inhibited sexual desire (302.71) in the DSM-III does not include diminished sexual drive in individuals with known organic pathology. Lowered sexual desire is a common symptom of Addison's disease, as well as postpartum pituitary necrosis. Increased sexual desire may be seen in manic depressive psychoses or as a toxic reaction to L-dopa medication.

The second phase of sexual responsivity is the *excitement phase*, characterized by penile tumescence in the male and vaginal lubrication in the female. Concurrent autonomic changes, such as increased heart rate and increased respiratory rate, are accompanied by development of a sex flush over the upper chest of women and nipple erection in both sexes. The excitement phase merges into a plateau phase as arousal increases. Within the male, testicular elevation occurs, whereas in the female clitoral turgidity increases as the clitoris retracts behind the symphysis pubis. The vaginal barrel characteristically constricts along the outer third to develop an organic platform. Voluntary contractions of large muscle groups occur. The excitement stage is generally of longer duration in women than in men. Disorders during this segment of the sexual response cycle include primary or secondary erectile dysfunction in males and the inability of females to complete or obtain adequate lubrication (inhibited sexual excitement−302.72). For individuals with physical

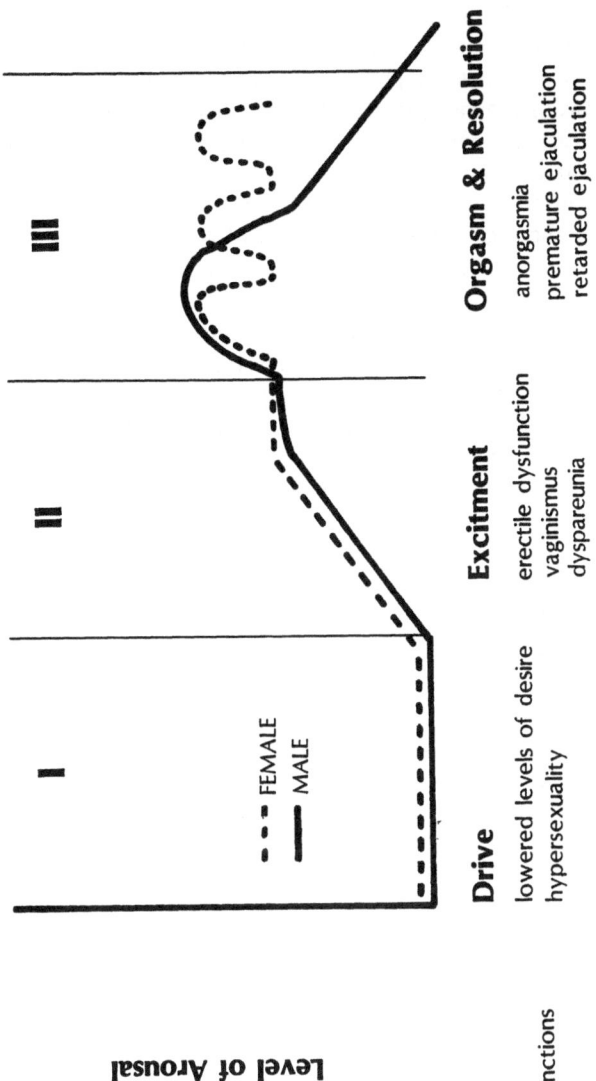

Figure 1.

illness, such as diagnoses cannot be made. Thus, for the male with impotence due to a diabetic neuropathy or the female following radiation treatment for cervical carcinoma with vaginal atrophy, the diagnosis must be considered the result of the physical condition. The final phase of the sexual response cycle is that of *orgasm*. In male emission production of the ejaculate fluid, ejaculation, and the propulsion of the semen, characterize the phase. In women, orgasm is characterized by rhythmic contractions of the vaginal canal. In both sexes, significant elevation of blood pressure and heart rate concurs with orgastic release and there is a highly pleasurable subjective release from the level of sexual tension experienced. Following orgasm, the resolution phase includes penile tumescence and resolution of vascular engorgement of the vaginal labia. The period of resolution depends upon both sex and age. Women are capable of multiple orgasms, whereas men usually require a refractory period that may last for 30 minutes in younger males and longer in older men. Thus, the major difference between the male and female sexual response is the ability for females to have multiple orgasms with minimal refractory periods. Sherfey has commented upon the sociobiologic aspects of these differences. Within the new nomenclature, inhibited female orgasm (302.73) and inhibited male orgasm (302.74) cannot be diagnosed if organic factors are present. Premature ejaculation (302.74), dyspareunia (302.76), and vaginismus (306.51), an involuntary spasm of the vaginal musculature that interferes with coitus, complete categorization of psychosexual disorders.

The clinician should be familiar with the physiology of normal sexuality in order to make a clinical assessment of the sexual dysfunctions in both the physically healthy and medically ill individual. The neurophysiology of sexual response in both the male and female is the end product of a complex interplay between the nervous, vascular, and endocrinologic systems.

Sexual desire depends upon a cortical response modified by psychologic factors. Hormonal input such as hypothalamic polypeptides may also influence the desire phase which motivates the actual sexual behavior experienced by the individual.

Sexual arousal in the male is initiated by sensory stimulation of the afferent pudendal nerve endings and by psychic or higher centers of cerebral cortex or diencephalon. Parasympathetic impulses are thought to cause dilation of the penile vasculature by relaxing valves in the arterioles of the corporal tissue, with concurrent inhibition of the vascular constrictive fibers, resulting in vascular engorgement and erection. The female analog of pelvic engorgement is vaginal lubrication.

The orgasmic phase in the male follows increasing stimulation via the sympathetic thoracolumbar center resulting in contraction of the muscles of the prostate and seminal vesicles and closure of the internal bladder. Sympathetic nerve response produces seminal fluid in the posterior urethral area, which in turn closes the bladder duct. The presence of fluid stimulated parasympathetic fibers which force contraction of the perineal muscles, resulting in ejaculation. The delivery system is complex, being implemented through squeezing of the seminal ducts, compression of the smooth musculature in the prostate gland, and shutting off of the bladder valves. The hypogastric nerve which carries sympathetic fibers, the pelvic nerves which carry parasympathetic efferents, and the pudendal nerve which carries voluntary nerve fibers contribute to emission. Any pathologic condition affecting the neural system described above can cause sexual dysfunctions, for example, autonomic neuropathy associated with diabetes, spinal cord lesions and surgical interference of these nerves following pelvic surgery.

Other neurologic lesions may create difficulties in male sexual response. Higher cortical lesions such as temporal lobectomy can affect sexual function. Both hyper- and hyposexuality are associated with temporal lobe epilepsy. Lesions in the cingulate gyrus may produce hypersexuality, whereas hypopituitarism may lead to decreased sexual function. Thus, appropriate neurologic, endocrine and vascular examination is mandatory when an organic basis of sexual dysfunction is suspected.

ASSESSMENT OF SEXUAL DISORDERS

The clinical assessment of a sexual dysfunction requires the ability to categorize and document sexual dysfunction within the broad context of the psychological status; physiologic capacity; and social set of the patient. One method of obtaining such data is the utilization of an open-ended interviewing technique which asks broad questions that allow the patient to describe the problems in a personalized fashion. Following open-ended queries, direct questions about sexual function may define specific areas that need to be covered. In this manner, the nature of the complaint as well as the individual's personality style are best revealed. Highly structured questioning may miss much important information regarding the patient's own perceptions of their difficulties. However, overall, the clinician thus must make an orderly and systematic assessment of the function of the individual and within the context of a sexual partnership, if present.

When rapport is established, detailed information can be gathered by reviewing the patient's last sexual experience. Information about the time, place and initiator of the sexual activity should be ascertained. The presence or absence of disorders of desire, arousal or orgasm can be reviewed in this specific context. From the last specific event to the relative frequency of sexual activities, the sexual history will naturally flow. Tactful review of the individual's sexual partners as well as autoerotic practices must be made.

The course of any disorder must be understood. Is the sexual dysfunction episodic; situationally induced, i.e., with specific sexual partners; or related to other factors such as the presence of absence of drugs or alcohol? What are the patient's fantasies during sexual activity, both with a partner and during autoerotic practices? Many patients will initially feel embarrassed about relating such material but it is important to cover this material. Often, dysfunctions will concur with psychosocial difficulties or physical problems. Delineation of the presence of an affair by either the patient or the patient's partner, or the development of a serious illness must be elucidated. In order to fully understand the sexual complaint, the clinician must carefully review all phases of the sexual response cycle. Does desire fluctuate? Are there any problems in achieving arousal and orgasm? Notation of medicines which may modify such physiologic responses is essential.

The next step in the evaluation is a review of the development of attitudes and early sexual experiences. How did the patient learn about sexuality? Was such information gleaned from peers, family or school? What was the nature of the individual's first sexual experiences, such as masturbation, nocturnal emission or menarche? Were they prepared for such experiences? How did they cope with erotic drives during adolescence? What was the nature of their first sexual activities with partners? Were these heterosexual or homosexual? Were they frightening or pleasurable? What traumatic sexual events, if any, occurred? Have individuals been seduced, traumatized or raped during sexual activities. For female patients, review of menstrual histories is important. The presence or history of venereal disease is also important to note. Data about the mechanical sexual functioning is important but must be complemented by the patient's own psychological reactions to sexuality and interpersonal relationships. The clinician must remember that the patient is more than a mechanical sexual being and that sexual functioning serves as a medium for pleasure, both autoerotically as well as interpersonally. Thus, patients ability to relate both sexually and emotionally must be investigated.

Following review of the sexual dysfunction within the context of the patient's past and present sexual attitudes and experiences, a full psychosocial history is completed. This part of the evaluation focuses on the individual's developmental history. Finally, a formal mental state examination is mandatory to document the presence of signs and symptoms of a coexisting psychiatric disorder.

In the circumstance of a patient with both a sexual disorder and a physical illness, it is necessary to understand how the individual is coping with the illness itself in order to appreciate the relationship between the illness and sexual function. To accomplish this, the clinician must observe how the patient recounts his symptoms, ideas about etiology of the illness and reactions to the discomfort and inconvenience that the disease has created. The physician should review data regarding the patient's independent and dependent functioning. Does the patient begin to intellectualize and isolate fearful aspects of the illness, or is there evidence of anxiety, depression, or denial when talking about the actual limitations and discomfort of any disease state. Certain patients are comfortable with the passive position that a physical disease may cause in order to rationalize the difficulties in sexuality that the sick role created. Many patients dislike the limitations imposed by illness. For them, sexual dysfunction becomes a distressing aspect of the illness. This aspect of the evaluation requires a characterization of individuals as to their predominant personality styles to better understand how they cope with illness and a coexisting dysfunction. Obsessional patients often require more information about the illness whereas the hysterical or dramatic individual responds more to compliments and global support strategies. These patients often have trouble tolerating rigid methodical treatment regimens and need support, direction, and continuing encouragement. The patient who is dependent also requires more support. Thus, assessment of sexual dysfunctions in healthy and physically ill patients requires review of the nature of the sexual complaint, the sexual response cycle, psychosocial development, the individual's characteristic way of coping with stresses in general, and a mental status examination.

SPECIAL CONSIDERATIONS IN THE ASSESSMENT OF SEXUAL DYSFUNCTIONS IN THE MEDICALLY ILL

The medical history should focus on the presence of the symptoms or history of vascular, endocrine, neurologic diseases, or use of pharmacologic treatment which may affect sexual function (Table 1). Use of tranquilizers, neuroleptic medication, and previous surgical procedures, including urologic or gynecologic surgery, must be identified. In absence of specific diagnostic information, careful attention should be directed to the presence of shortness of breath, weakness, sensory difficulties, motility problems, polydipsia dnd polyuria. Family history for chronic diseases is also important. The evaluation will often require appropriate laboratory testing for endocrinologic disorders including fasting blood sugar, assays of follicle-stimulating hormone, luteinizing hormone and testosterone. Measurement of the thyroid axis may also be necessary [1]. Doppler studies measuring blood flow as well as pelvic angiography may be indicated.

Neurologic assessment includes review of the motor, sensory, and autonomic nervous system, as well as cortical function. The integrity of the lumbosacral spinal pathways is essential to sexual functioning and may be determined by the following tests: S1-S2 may be evaluated by intact motility of the small muscles of the foot. S2-S4 may be evaluated by the ability to contract and relax both the internal and external anal sphincter, ascertained by digital examination of the anus to test the initial contraction and relaxation of the external sphincter. The finger should then be advanced to test the internal sphincter tone. S2-S4 may be further tested by the bulbocavernosus reflex which involves inserting a gloved examining finger into the anus, allowing initial contraction, relaxation and squeezing the glans penis while the finger remains in the anus. The intact reflex promotes contraction of the anal sphincter. Absence of anal sphincter contraction is common even in normal subjects, requiring electromyographic studies to further investigate the potency of the sacral cord segments. S2-S5 is tested by the presence of perianal sensations [2]. Physical inspection of the distribution of body hair, such as the presence or

Table 1. Highlights of Physical Examination of Sexually Dysfunctional Patient

Endocrine system	— hair distribution gynecomastia thyroid gland
Vascular system	— patency of peripheral pulses
Stigmata of alcoholism	— hepatomegaly, or atrophic liver peripheral neuropathy
Genitourinary system	— Prostate (in male) Pelvic examination (in female)

Nervous system
1. Sacral Innervation

S_1-S_2	— mobility of small muscles of the foot
S_2-S_4	— internal, external anal sphincter tone bulbocavernosus reflex (in male)
S_2-S_5	— perianal sensation

2. Peripheral sensation
3. Deep tendon reflexes
4. Long tract signs

absence of a normal beard in men as well as the precence of hirsutism in women, distribution of body fat, or presence of gynecomastia in the male may indicate an endocrine disorder. Thyroid status should be assessed by noting the individual's ability to tolerate temperature changes, as well as appetitive and energy levels. Direct examination of the thyroid gland is indicated in addition to laboratory screening of thyroid function.

CASE FORMULATIONS

To organize data obtained from clinical assessment of a patient with a sexual dysfunction and a medical illness, the clinician may wish to consider three areas of function. First, what are the psychologic effects of an illness; second, what are the actual performance limitations produced by the illness in respect to sexual functioning (Table 2); and, finally, what impact does the illness have on the enjoyment of sexuality. This review obviously must be conducted with an application to the context of an individual's current life situation. Even though sexual function is often organically compromised by either acute or chronic disease, there may be additional determinants to the sexual dysfunction. Illness aspects of disease promote psychological changes such as regression. Impairments secondary to a disease may result in a narcissistic assault upon the patient, altering their social role expectations and lowering their self-esteem. For example, a young woman with severe

Table 2. Features That May Differentiate Organic from Psychologic Impotence

	Organic	Psychogenic
Course of Disorder	Insidious	May be acute, episodic, situational
Presence of early morning erection	weak	present
Erection with masturbation	no	yes
Taking antihypertensive medication	often	rarely
Diabetes mellitus	often	rarely
Presence of depression	yes	yes
Alcoholism	yes	rarely

psoriasis may react to her external disfigurement by sexual promiscuity or by sexual withdrawal. Such behavior can be considered a psychologic reaction to a disease state and not a strict sexual dysfunction. In contradistinction, a man with ulcerative colitis and a colostomy may become demanding of his wife in multiple aspects of their relationship, promoting sexual withdrawal of the wife who becomes angry and embittered by her husband's behavior. In such a situation, the husband may be fully capable of sexual functioning on an organic basis but has major interpersonal impediments to such activity. Pain from diffuse metastatic lesions as well as shame from physical changes due to disease states may modify an individual's sexual enjoyment but not sexual potential. Although the enjoyment factor overlaps with the psychologic reaction to an illness, it allows the clinician to systematically assess the patient's abilities and limitations [3]. Physical illness markedly affects and changes one's basic plans for life, a condition described as "life trajectory" [4]. The loss of sexual function in an 80-year-old man may be as important as it is to a 23-year-old woman. The consequences of function may differ in the 23-year-old woman, who has yet to have children, is faced with the possibility of a hysterectomy whereas the male has many grandchildren. It is important to emphasize that in addition to individual evaluation of the patient, assessment and cooperation of the sexual partner, if available, is very helpful. The clinician will often need to include the sexual partner in ongoing assessment and treatment of various disabilities.

CARDIOVASCULAR DISEASE

Cardiovascular disease covers a wide range of pathologic entities that affect both the heart and peripheral vasculature.

Peripheral Vascular Disease

Organic Limitations Peripheral vascular occlusion may limit blood supply to the pelvic area causing microvascular and neuropathic changes resulting in erectile dysfunction within the male and probably some organically based arousal disorders in females. Leriche's syndrome, occlusion of the bifurcation of the abdominal aorta, can result in erectile dysfunction secondary to a general insufficient genital blood supply. The precise role of peripheral vascular disease upon sexual function in females is not yet understood.

Enjoyment Factors Pain secondary to deficient peripheral vascular circulation may make sexuality less enjoyable by distracting the patient. The presence of wounds and ulcers which fail to heal may create shame and embarrassment as well as difficulties in mobility.

Psychological Factors Some patients with Buerger's disease do not comply with medical treatment [5]. These patients tend to be dependent and dissatisfied and often continue to use cigarettes and tobacco products which advances the progression of their disease. They tend to be complaining, demanding, aggressive and negativistic. They keep supportive individuals at a distance. Patients with intermittent claudication can become depressed and dissatisfied because of the progression of their disease. Depressive symptoms must be evaluated and treated.

Cerebrovascular Accidents

Organic Limitations The poststroke victim may require antihypertensive medication such as alpha-methyldopa or guanethidine which inhibits erectile functioning. Following a cerebrovascular accident, intact sexual functioning may be limited especially if lesions have caused deficient bowel and bladder control. Erectile dysfunction may also be a concurrent indicator of central nervous system damage [6].

Enjoyment Factors Decreased sensory and motor abilities are the most common sequelae of cerebrovascular accidents. Hemiplegia and anesthesia can diminish sexual enjoyment. Speech loss and visual difficulties further impair sexual enjoyment and communication. Motor weakness and unstable joints decrease mobility. Thus sexual activity may not be spontaneous and will require planning and assistance to achieve something as specific as proper positioning to engage sexually.

Psychological Factors Stroke victims frequently experience depression and use denial. Their depression is often a reaction to the loss of sensory and motor function and enforced dependency, but may also be an organic response to the stroke. Some cerebrovascular lesions result in aphasias and agnosias which may cause the stroke victim to become guarded and paranoid as he becomes increasingly frustrated with his inability to communicate.

Coronary Artery Diseases

Organic Limitations Sexual functioning is generally preserved in patients with coronary artery disease who do not have widespread peripheral vascular disease. The cardiovascular demands of sexual intercourse have been outlined by Hellerstein [7]. Blood pressure during intercourse generally rises to no more than 160 mm. Hg systolic with a concurrent heart rate of 150 beats per minute. Tolerance of vigorous walking around a city block equates with the physiologic demands of sexual intercourse. If the postcoronary patient can perform that level of activity, he may resume intercourse three to four months following the acute infarct. Specific problems in the postcoronary patient, such as persistence of anginal pain, may require utilization of beta-blockers and sublingual nitrates prior to intercourse. Patients with congestive heart failure are usually treated with cardiac glycosides that may lower testosterone and increase estrogen, causing lowered sexual drive and erectile problems in men [8].

Enjoyment Factors The presence of anginal pain and dyspnea upon exertion, as noted, may clearly diminish enjoyment of sexuality. Headaches from sublingual nitrates may also modify the enjoyment factor of intercourse.

Psychological Factors Studies suggest that few patients are counseled regarding sexual functioning following an infarct despite the fact that a majority of males fear their ability to perform sexually following a coronary occlusion and at one year follow up, persist in these worries [9]. The presence of sexual dysfunctions including erectile difficulties and premature ejaculation are frequently found. These dysfunctions often appear to be on a psychogenic basis and relate to the anxiety about the illness itself. Organic causes of dysfunction should be ruled out but, following this, psychological factors must be reviewed and treated. Although most studies have focused upon men with heart disease, Abramov reported that 100 females following myocardial infarction had a much higher incidence of orgasmic difficulty than a controlled population [10]. The angorasmia was felt to be due to psychologic factors.

Treatment Considerations Recognizing the patient's fears about sexual activity following a myocardial infarction is mandatory. Both patient and spouse should be included in such a discussion. If a patient does not bring up the role of sexuality, the clinician must tactfully inquire if this has been a worry. Resumption of sexual activities has been recommended 8–12 weeks following acute infarct. During this interval, the patient and spouse should be warned that they may have disagreements over various minor issues which are displacements of the psychologic issues arising from the infarct and their responses to it. Gradual resumption of sexual activity is advisable utilizing sexual activities such as touching exercises prior to actual intercourse. Utilization of the male superior position may increase isometric tension which increases cardiovascular demand. Thus, alternate positioning, such as side-by-side, may be advisable. Sexual problems which develop should be dealt with by the primary physician with appropriate referral when necessary.

Hypertensive Cardiovascular Disease

Organic Limitations Drugs commonly used for treatment of hypertension, such as alpha-methyldopa and guanethedine, have been reported to cause erectile dysfunction and inhibition of ejaculation [11]. Ganglionic-blocking agents, such as mecamylamine, may also cause erectile dysfunction. Even diuretics have been implicated in causing erectile dysfunction. The effects of these medications on females is not too well understood [12].

ARTHRITIS

Arthritis, either inflammatory or degenerative disease of the joints, covers a wide spectrum of specific disorders which may occur at any age. Juvenile forms of arthritis may severely disfigure a young adolescent whereas degenerative joint disease can incapacitate and immobilize the older individual.

Organic Limitations

Functional limitations from arthritis most commonly occur due to lack of mobility of the hips, knees or back which may make intercourse difficult because of mechanical impediments to mobility. Bilateral hip contractures may make intercourse impossible as well as interfere with genital hygiene. Medications used for treatment of arthritis may further compromise sexual functioning. Steroid medication used in rheumatoid arthritis may further compromise sexual functioning. Steroid medication used in rheumatoid arthritis may render males impotent.

Enjoyment Factors

The pain from musculoskeletal joint disease can inhibit organic enjoyment. The stiffness common to many forms of arthritis may further make the physical activity in sexuality problematic. The disfiguring aspects of the disease itself, whether joint disfigurement or the effects of steroid such as moon-facies, truncal obesity and hirsutism provoke shame and diminish self-esteem. Sjogren's syndrome, which accompanies rheumatoid arthritis, inhibits mucosal secretions and can cause atrophic vaginitis or male urethritis, making intercourse painful. Fatigue associated with the prolonged pain of degenerative joint disease, may further diminish enjoyment of sexual activity.

Psychological Factors

The depression which accompanies the constant pain from arthritis as well as the shame from physical disfigurement changes diminish one's self-esteem about himself and can lower libidinal drive. The psychological changes of steroid medication such as depression or severe cognitive factors also may compromise sexual functioning.

Treatment Considerations

In order to enhance sexual functioning, attention must be paid to alleviation of arthritic pain [13]. Salicylates and other anti-inflammatory agents may diminish discomfort and increase mobility. Many individuals with rheumatoid arthritis note that certain periods of the day correlate with greatest mobility and comfort. It is during this time that individuals may best engage in sexual activity. Good communication patterns between the arthritic patient and their sexual partner is necessary. In juvenile arthritic patients, it is necessary to be aware of fears pertaining to peer group relationships, self-worth as well as sexuality.

OBESITY

Obesity severely compromises an individual's health status and may be considered a pathologic entity.

Organic Limitations

The few studies of morbidly obese individuals suggest that there are few, if any, sexual dysfunctions in the obese and hyperobese which are a direct result of the weight problem [14]. Nevertheless, individuals who are severely overweight do experience difficulties such as shortness of breath during intercourse. Potency problems in obese men and orgastic difficulties in women appear to be no more common than in a normative population.

Enjoyment Factors

The body image distortion of the hyperobese may severely compromise an individual's self-esteem and lead to depression. The obese adolescent male may be ashamed of gynecomastia and refrain from heterosexual activities and sexual experiences. The hyperobese woman appears to have more frequent sexual opportunities than her male counterparts. This may be due to the obese woman's utilization of sexual activity as an attractive facet of her femininity. The pendulous tissue mass of the obese male may foster fears of inadequate penis size. Another factor diminishing organic enjoyment of sexuality is the difficulty in finding an adequate position for intercourse because of the large body mass.

Psychological Factors

Obesity has been suggested to be a defense against sexuality by psychoanalytic theorists. This may occur in a selected group of individuals and may prevent their engaging in sexual activity. Frequently, however, depression from isolation and stigmatization of an unattractive body image results in withdrawal and limited social and sexual opportunities.

Case: A 32-year-old single woman stated that she wished to be "skinny" and noted "I've been overweight since I was six years old and it's no fun. Society doesn't like fat people; you get discriminated against in dating and jobs." The patient worked as an administrative assistant in a major corporation but felt that she would have further vocational opportunities if she were thinner. When initially seen, the patient weighed 295 lbs. despite her 5'6" frame. She noted she had been overweight her whole life and had tried all forms of dieting without success. Her eating pattern consisted of nighttime snacking. An outgoing individual, she had many friends—both men and women—but rarely dated. She reported continuing humiliation beginning in adolescence because of her size. Despite her weight, she felt that her pleasant personality allowed her to have some friends. Her job required her to work closely with people and she functioned quite well in this capacity. Her first intercourse occurred when she was in college and she subsequently had occasional sexual experiences on dates. She noted that her weight clearly made her socially unattractive. She would frequently go out with men who were also obese. Her sexual response included full orgasm. She gave no history of any psychologic difficulty but noted that she rarely expressed anger because she constantly needed to please people to compensate for her appearance which she described as "grotesque." The patient underwent an uneventful ileal bypass procedure and began to lose weight. After 18 months, she had lost 120 lbs. Her appearance markedly improved and she began to have an active social life. It was during this time that she noted confusion in how to relate to men sexually. Her limited social and sexual activity prior to her weight loss rendered her vulnerable when she began to date. Psychotherapy was utilized to help her monitor her feelings and discuss what she wanted from an interpersonal relationship. She also needed to establish a more appropriate self-esteem based on a body image that was far different from her massively obese status.

Comments

This woman appeared to be a capable and intelligent individual with a pleasant personality. She used humor, minimization and suppression to deal with her appearance. In essence, she was stigmatized by her abnormal physical appearance. This limited a socialization and educational process in learning how sexuality is used in interpersonal relationships. Therapy was directed towards this aspect.

Treatment Considerations

For the obese individual, the major focus of treatment must be on achieving a lowered body weight. This is usually a difficult task which results in repeated dieting via various methods ranging from modified protein fasts to more drastic surgical techniques such as ileal bypass or gastric stapling in the morbidly obese individual. The vast majority of overweight individuals, however, engage in chronic dieting. As the obese individual loses weight, sexual opportunities become more available. This may be come a problem if the individual has no previous sexual experience and is made anxious by new intimate relationships.

CHRONIC PULMONARY DISEASE

Chronic obstructive pulmonary disease ranks only second to coronary artery disease in its prevalence in adult males of middle age. A heterogeneous group of conditions including chronic obstructive pathology as well as asthmatic disease are denoted when referring to chronic obstructive pulmonary disease.

Organic Limitations

Recent studies have demonstrated that chronic obstruction to airways may be associated with low testosterone values [15]. Thus, arterial hypoxia is directly related to testosterone depression. Symptomatically, this may result in impotence in the male with chronic obstructive airway disease. No data is available regarding arousal or orgasmic response in women with similar pulmonary pathology. One study demonstrated 17% of a sample of men with chronic lung disease were impotent on an organic basis [16].

Enjoyment Factors

Fatigue and dyspnea upon exertion is common in individuals with chronic pulmonary disease and may severely limit sexual enjoyment. In advanced pulmonary disease, the use of auxilliary oxygen as well as muscular wasting may create motor problems during sexual activity. The physical requirements during intercourse have also been cited as provocateurs of asthmatic attacks in a selected population of patients.

Psychological Factors

Depression resulting from the chronic incapacitation of pulmonary disease may limit libidinal drive.

Treatment Considerations

Premedication for individuals with exercise-induced asthma will modify any pulmonary symptoms induced during sexual activity. For those individuals with chronic obstructive disease, utilization of various positions to minimize exertion will often be necessary to maximize sexual enjoyment. Awareness of the sexual partner's feelings and role is imperative for successful counseling because of the sexual partner is often angry at the pulmonary patient's inability to stop tobacco use.

DIABETES

Diabetes mellitus affects over two million adults and adolescents. The disease forces the patient to carefully regulate his diet and medicate himself with parenteral insulin.

Organic Limitations

Diabetes, although an endocrine disorder, has serious affects on the small vessles, nervous system, and kidneys. The progressive neuropathy found in many diabetics will eventually render almost one-half of diabetic men impotent. The erectile dysfunction appears to be unrelated to the severity or duration of the diabetes. There is no evidence that plasma testosterone is affected. Confusion exists regarding the sexual functioning of the female diabetic. Early studies by Kolodny noted that there was a positive correlation with orgastic dysfunction in female diabetics and with the duration and severity of the diabetes [17]. Recently, Ellenberg has repeated this study and found *no* diminution of libido or orgastic potential in the female diabetics with peripheral neurologic changes [18]. Autonomic neuropathies found commonly in diabetes may cause retrograde ejaculation in the diabetic male. This can produce a serious problem in patients who wish to procreate. Specific urologic techniques have been developed to allow extraction of semen for insemination.

Enjoyment Factors

Complications of diabetes may result in renal failure, blindness, skin changes due to diabetic lipodystrophy and pain from peripheral neuropathies. Sensory limitations may limit sexual enjoyment due to discomfort and general malaise. Shame about leg ulcers and poorly healing abrasions may further modify sexual enjoyment. The adolescent who suffers from diabetes may feel ostracized and different because of the dietary limitations and stigmatization of his peer group marking him as different. This may result in social withdrawal or paradoxically, promiscuity to prevent abandonment.

Psychological Factors

The diabetic patient may be depressed for a variety of reasons. As noted, the young diabetic may feel ashamed and different. The adult with sequelae may be depressed due to the actual limitations of the disease such as the visual loss, need for hemodialysis, or pain secondary to peripheral vascular disease. These may all limit libidinal drive and make sexual activity difficult.

Case: A 52-year-old woman was seen in consultation because of marital difficulties. The patient was a juvenile diabetic who carefully controlled her disease since its discovery at the age of 4. The patient was raised in an affluent family who treated her, as she noted, "like a China doll who had been cracked but repaired." As an adolescent she dated frequently but had minimal sexual experience because her moral standards required this. The patient went away to college, enjoyed her social life but had limited sexual experiences which did not include intercourse. She eventually married and on her honeymoon, she found her first experience with intercourse very frightening. Her husband noted that she put a towel under herself to prevent "dirtying the bed." The patient explained that she was not sure what to expect and did this as perhaps a nervous gesture. She was orgastic and enjoyed subsequent activity but never could be the initiator of intercourse. The patient's marital relationship drifted towards increasing isolation from her husband and she frequently visited her parents in a nearby city. Her husband cared for her materially and medically, yet showed little sexual interest. The patient eventually developed complications from her diabetes including painful peripheral dysthesias and nonhealing abrasions. Her lack of sexual interest magnified her isolation and low self-esteem. When she complained, her husband reacted with anger. He openly admitted that he feared hurting her but he also felt that she had been a spoiled young woman who had never been able to fully separate from her family and had never been interested in sex. He rationalized his lack of sexual attention by stating they never could discuss sexual matters. Marital counseling was presceribed where sexuality was taken up as one part of their marital difficulties.

Comments

The illness effects of diabetes upon personality development is still unclear but it appears that certain individuals such as the woman in the above ·case are overprotected. This leaves them vulnerable in their marital relationships.

Treatment Considerations

In males with diabetic nephropathy and impotence, the use of silastic implant is often indicated. Either silastic rods or fluid pump prosthesis have been successful in restoring sexual function. In patients who have maintained their diabetic status poorly, nutritional malnourishment and fatigue may inhibit sexual functioning. Restoration of control is needed to restore sexual functioning. In those patients who are depressed, antidepressants and psychotherapy are indicated to restore sexual expression in the absence of organic limitations [19].

RENAL DISEASE WITH HEMODIALYSIS AND TRANSPLANTATION

Chronic renal disease often requires maintenance hemodialysis. The individual is dependent upon routine hemodialysis by a "kidney" machine. In addition, severe limitations of fluid and food are necessary to maintain life. Other patients may be treated with kidney transplantation.

Organic Limitations

Individuals undergoing chronic renal dialysis commonly experience sexual dysfunctions. In one series, 45% of men undergoing hemodialysis reported diminished potency [20]. The source of diminished potency appears to be related to dysfunction between the pituitary–Leydig cell axis resulting in testosterone depletion [21]. Exogenous testosterone could restore sexual function but would accelerate atherosclerosis so it cannot be used. Following renal transplantation, many patients report restoration of sexual potency, suggesting uremia and/or hemodialysis itself cause the sexual disorders. Transplantation patients may also be subject to dysfunction secondary to the many medications such as corticosteroids and immunosuppressant agents that they must take.

Enjoyment Factors

Women being hemodialyzed report sexual dysfunctions which appear more psychologically based. The resultant fatigue, chronic malaise and interpersonal difficulties associated with hemodialysis impact on sexual function. Orgastic potential with masturbation appears to be intact although orgasm during intercourse is less commonly achieved [22]. The chronic stresses associated with hemodialysis adversely affects the enjoyment aspect of sex in both sexes.

Psychological Factors

Hemodialysis fosters dependence and causes depression in some patients. Both conditions may limit sexual interest. However, other patients who have the need to be considered attractive and loved may become preoccupied with their sexuality. Partners of hemodialysis patients may be fearful of harming the patient and may withdraw sexually from the patient.

Treatment Considerations

Sexual function is important to some patients and not to others, so it must be assessed on a case-by-case basis. Discussion with the patient and sexual partner is necessary in order to clarify the current roll of sexual function within the partnership. Since posttransplant patients may also experience sexual difficulties, albeit on an organic basis, the psychological meaning of having another person's kidney and its relationship to sexual function may need to be explored.

Case: A 42-year-old married man was seen complaining of depressed mood, difficulty sleeping, and periods of tearfulness. A juvenile diabetic, the patient had maintained himself carefully on insulin and dietary limitations. Four years before consultation, the patient was found to be uremic and for two years was being hemodialyzed. The patient had married at 25 and had two children. The patient continued to work. His wife had begun a new career shortly before him beginning hemodialysis. In addition to the stress from this chronic treatment which included substantial disruption of the family schedule in order to permit the patient to continue working as well as receive his necessary life support, the patient and his wife begain bickering over minor matters. Frequently she was not home when he returned from his dialysis treatments at night. The patient noticed a gradual loss of ability to maintain an erection. Eventually he experienced total erectile impotency when making love to his wife although he was able to masturbate to ejaculation with a flaccid penis. Evaluation revealed the patient had abnormal cystometrogram, absent ankle jerks and a nocturnal penile tumescence test showed no erectile episodes. The erectile dysfunction was diagnosed as being secondary to a peripheral neuropathy. Unfortunately, the patient's general medical condition precluded implantation of a penile prosthesis and marital counseling was needed to maintain the precarious balance between the patient and his wife.

Comments

The stress of a serious, chronic illness alone may destabilize a marriage but the added stress of a sexual dysfunction can further disrupt the relationship. Conjoint counseling should focus on alternate forms of lovemaking such as mutual masturbation or oral-genital activity provided these activities are acceptable to the couple. Realistic goals should be established by both the therapist and the patient (couple).

DERMATOLOGICAL CONDITIONS

Organic Limitations

All the venereal conditions—chancre, herpes, condyloma on penis or vulva—can cause pain. Dermatologic conditions which are nonvenereal rarely cause organic limitations on sexual functions.

Enjoyment Factors

Dermatologic conditions which cause decreased functioning of mucosal or serosal tissues may cause pain during sexual activity. Vaginitis, vaginal atropy, urethritis, and various neoplastic growths on the genitals may cause pain, adversely affecing sexual enjoyment. Just as important, the sense of disfigurement and shame associated with dermatologic lesions such as hirsutism, baldness, scarring, open lesions, itching rashes, may decrease ones sense of sexual attractiveness. Acne vulgaris, a very common lesion, frequently decreases patient's self-esteem, resulting in sexual withdrawal. Some patients respond to a disfigurement with sexual promiscuity.

Psychological Features

Embarrassment and disfigurement contribute to the development of depressive symptoms. Adolescents and young adults who have severe acne are especially prone to alienation and depression. A reaction to this may be sexual promiscuity or aggressiveness.

Treatment Considerations

The clinician who treats patients with dermatologic conditions should be aware of the psychological impact of skin disfigurement [23]. Those conditions affecting the sexual organs should be evaluated for the affect on sexual functioning. Patients with vaginal atrophy and decreased lubrication should be instructed to use a nonpetroleum lubricant rather than jellies which may provide a nidus for infection. Patients with acne vulgaris may need counseling for the emotional problems associated with the condition which will augment compliance with treatment.

CHRONIC LOW BACK PAIN

Low back pain secondary to degenerative disc disease or injury is common and may result in sexual dysfunction.

Organic Limitations

Low back pain is rarely associated with organic sexual problems [24]. Occasionally pain, coupled with a neurogenic bladder may be associated with a pathologic condition which includes organically based sexual dysfunction. Medications utilized to control pain, narcotics, qualgesics, antidepressants and phenothiazines, individually or in common, may cause disorders of desire or arousal when used in heavy doses or abused.

Enjoyment Factors

Patients with chronic pain are susceptable to depressive symptoms. Preoccupation with their disorders, increased dependency, social withdrawal and low frustration tolerance, all of which adversely affect their ability to relate in general and to engage sexually.

Treatment Considerations

Attention must be paid to the medications used with regard to level of dosage and abuse liability. If analgesics and narcotics appear to inhibit sexual functioning, dosages must be lowered or discontinued. If certain positions cause pain, alternate positions should be tried. The most important aspect of managing chronic pain patients, however is awareness of the impact of the chronic nature of the pain on the patient and the need to teach the patient to cope with the discomfort. If this goal can be achieved with increased physical activity and less medication, sexual functioning may become a more enjoyable activity.

CANCER

Cancer is the most feared disease process by both laymen and health professionals. Advances in medical chemotherapy, radiation therapy and surgical techniques have extended the survival rate of the cancer victims. The quality of life, including sexual functioning, becomes an important aspect of the patient's existence with neoplastic disease. Rehabilitation rather than just palliation is often a major goal. The focus of psychosocial treatment has shifted from acute care to a longitudinal approach which assists the patient in reentering their social and occupational systems in order to maximize potential abilities. Since each neoplasm has its own idiosyncratic impairing features, common neoplastic conditions will be considered separately.

Breast Cancer

Organic Limitations Mastectomy following carcinoma of the breast obviously impairs tactile pleasure from breast caressing. Nipple stimulation is ablated unless there is preservation of areolar tissue in breast reconstruction. Decreased desire, impaired arousal and orgastic inability may result from chemotherapy. Dyspareunia may result from vaginal epithelial atrophy when estrogens are withheld in postmenopausal women.

Enjoyment Factors Anger and discouragement are common affects associated with the narcissistic blow of breast neoplasia and can modify sexual functioning [25]. Pain and discomfort from the incisional scar or swelling and edema of an arm due to blocked lymphatic drainage may aggrevate this discomfort, further limiting sexual enjoyment. Shame secondary to disfigurement may limit sexual interest.

Psychological Factors A minority of women with breast cancer develop psychiatric conditions severe enough to be defined as clinical syndromes. Nevertheless, many women become transiently discouraged or depressed. These symptoms may affect their relationships. Couples in which there is discussion in the meaning of a mastectomy prior to surgery and frequent visiting during hospitalization have fewer postsurgical sexual problems and less marital discord. The withdrawal of spouse or sexual partner may enhance the patient's sense of shame.

Treatment Considerations Witkin recommends that immediately following a mastectomy, the spouse be present as the mastectomy wound is unbandaged and inspected. This provides a professional setting in which the husband may view the site of the absent breast and help allay both the husband's and the woman's fears and anxieties. Rapid resumption of sexual activity has also been recommended as a means of avoiding sexual problems which often foster lack of self-esteem in these patients. Cosmetic reconstructive breast surgery following mastectomy is increasingly available.

Case: A 54-year-old woman who had been treated for carcinoma of the breast was referred for psychiatric evaluation following a tearful visit with her radiation therapist. The patient complained that her husband was uncaring and acted in a cruel and vengeful manner. The incident leading to the psychiatric referral was a beach holiday with her husband and 20-year-old daughter. The patient, who underwent a modified radical mastectomy, felt conspicuous in a bathing suit despite the fact that a breast prosthesis was cosmetically acceptable. She began to fear that her husband was overly interested in her daughter. When seen for psychiatric evaluation, the patient was an attractive woman who stated that the loss of a breast was "the most dreadful thing that had ever happened to me." The patient had experienced a very difficult life. Born in Europe, she had had a difficult time during the war and lived in a city constantly overrun by invading armies. She subsequently married a serviceman, immigrated to America and lived a comfortable life. Upon discovering that she had a breast lump, she went to her doctor and decided upon surgery without asking for her husband's advice. She did not want her husband to see her surgical scar nor did he make any request to discuss this situation. Prior to her illness, their sexual retionship had been good but since the mastectomy, frequency decreased markedly. Her husband was a passive man who was confused about her anger and unable to express his anger towards her behavior. Psychiatric evaluations revealed the patient had a narcissistic character disorder. The mastectomy had upset a precariously balanced emotional equilibrium. Treatment focused on the patient's narcissistic wounds. The couple was also seen conjointly.

Comments Jamison et al [26] have described the psychologic implications of mastectomy. The significance of a perceived assault upon one's body image following breast amputation are exemplified by the above case. Awareness of the patient's past psychosocial history assists the health professional in assessing the extent to which a patient's self-esteem has been damaged. The clinican should encourage the patient to discuss dysphoric feelings or thoughts, provide specific information and, if need be, recommend psychotherapy.

Prostatic Cancer

Organic Limitations   The various treatments for prostatic cancer differ in their effects upon sexual functioning [27]. Potency is lost in only 10% of patients who undergo transurethral resection for well differentiated and localized adeno-carcinomas of the prostate. If radiotherapy is utilized, impotency increases to 50%. Estrogenic hormonal therapy may lower libido but potency is preserved in most individuals undergoing 'hormonal treatment. Orchiectomy for metastatic prostatic lesions may also create erectile dysfunction.

Enjoyment Factors   The pain from metastatic prostatic lesions of the skeletal system may diminish enjoyment of sexual activity. Gynecomastia secondary to estrogenic therapy may cause shame and inhibit sexual expression.

Psychological Factors   The discouragement and depression from the neoplastic disease itself as well as severe pain, if present, may modify libido and inhibit sexual activity. Despite the fact that prostatic cancer often occurs in older individuals, many of these patients still have sexual interests and recognition of their psychologic and sexual needs is mandatory.

OSTOMIES

The surgical creation of an abdominal wall stoma is sometimes required for both neoplastic and severe inflammatory bowel disease.

Organic Limitations

The ileostomy created for treatment of various neoplastic conditions of the large and small bowel may cause organic erectile dysfunction [28]. This is especially common in surgical procedures which require extensive dissection of lymph node and vascular tissue which ablate the autonomic nervous system in the lower abdomen and pelvis. Men who undergo posterior abdominal perineal resection are generally impotent. Women who have this procedure have been noted to have decreased fertility as well as dyspareunia. Individuals with inflammatory bowel disease who have ostomy surgery generally have intact sexual ability. Medication utilized for severe inflammatory bowel disease, however, such as steroids or immunosuppressives, may cause erectile dysfunction.

Enjoyment Factors

Many ostomy patients are embarrassed by their surgery unless they have the opportunity to discuss their feelings. Fears of stool leakage and appearance of the stoma itself may seriously detract from sexual enjoyment and thereby create marital tension. Women tend to avoid their husband's help and often request aid from other women such as nurses or ostomy therapists. The partners of ostomy patients should be included in counseling efforts.

Psychological Factors

Depressive symptoms, secondary to either inflammatory bowel disease or neoplasm, are often coupled with the fear and stigma of the ostomy. Paradoxically, individuals with inflammatory bowel disease often feel physically much better after surgery if the disease process has been resolved. The effects of medication such as steroids must also be considered in patients who become depressed and dysphoric following surgery.

Treatment Considerations

Use of ostomy therapists and ostomy clubs are of great help to patients. If depression and inability to utilize the ostomy appliances persist, referral for psychiatric evaluation and treatment may be necessary. The best preventive measure, however, is active involvement of the sexual partner in viewing and helping learn about the ostomy appliance. Discussion about sexual functioning is often necessary. For patients whose sexual functioning has been affected by surgery, counseling, and/or prosthesis (for men) should be considered.

ULCERATIVE COLITIS,

Case: A 24-year-old single woman was seen for depression and lack of energy. The patient noted that she had begun having cramping and rectal bleeding at 15. This condition was diagnosed as ulcerative colitis which persisted despite traditional medical interventions. The patient underwent a surgical removal of her large bowel and establishment of a colostomy. Her medical condition rapidly improved with regard to weight gain, energy level, and resolution of body changes due to reduction of steroid medication. She completed college and began to work in a health related profession. A very attractive individual, she was frequently pursued by men but was unable to establish a lasting relationship. The patient admitted to being ashamed about her colostomy. She could not bring herself to tell suitors about her condition and feared sexual involvement. The patient's sexual experience had been limited to superficial petting. The patient was seen in psychotherapy in which the issues and psychological meanings of the colostomy were explored. She eventually was able to establish a sexual relationship which included intercourse. It made little difference to her lover that she had a colostomy.

Comments

Colostomy is particularly stressful for adolescents or young adults. Support, encouragement, and utilization of peer groups assists patients in overcoming the fear of social ostracization and stigmatization from this procedure [3].

MULTIPLE SCLEROSIS

Multiple sclerosis is a demyelinating disease of the nervous system which affects young adults. Characterized by remissions and exacerbations, the symptomatology frequently includes both sensory and motor defects.

Organic Limitations

Men with multiple sclerosis frequently have erectile dysfunction [29]. The presence of abnormal sweating phenomena as well as defective lumbosacral spinal reflexes are correlated with total or partial impotence. The longer an individual has suffered from multiple sclerosis, the greater the chance there will be for sexual dysfunction. In addition to the autonomic nervous system pathology, testicular atrophy has been observed in affected males. This may be due to abnormal lumbar sympathetic function which impairs vascular supply to the testes and results in compromised interstitial cells of Leydig in the male gonads. Women with multiple sclerosis report a qualitative change in their orgastic response. No controlled studies have been done to demonstrate the incidence of orgastic dysfunction in women with multiple sclerosis.

Enjoyment Factors

Patients with multiple sclerosis may have sufficient motor impairment to limit sexual functioning. More commonly, extreme fatigue may modify sexual activity. Compromised bowel and bladder function may also diminish sexual enjoyment unless care is taken to evacuate both bowel and bladder prior to sexual activity. Sensory defects occurring during acute attacks and residual sensory losses may further diminish sexual enjoyment.

ALCOHOLISM

Ingestion of alcoholic beverages, a common social "lubricant," when abused may cause serious medical problems. The affects of alcohol on sexual functioning are significant [3]].

Organic Factors

Alcohol has a biphasic affect upon sexual functioning. Low blood levels of alcohol (25 mg%) may increase sexual arousal. Moderate blood level alcohols (less than 50 mg%) disinhibit individual's belief systems and modify psychological defenses against sexuality and aggression. Thus, alcohol may diminish an individual's sexual control and lessen guilty attitudes towards sexuality. Clinical manifestations of intoxication may be sexual aggressiveness in males which may be viewed as rape (Rada) and promiscuity in women. Consequences of uncontrolled sexual behavior can be unwanted pregnancies. Blood levels of alcohol greater than 75 mg% depress and impair erection and ejaculation.

Organic Limitations

In addition to the acute affects of alcohol, chronic alcoholism is a disease which affects the peripheral nervous system, the central nervous system and the liver. Impotence is a frequent finding in chronic male alcoholics. The role of peripheral neurologic changes is a major factor. In addition, many chronic alcoholics with cirrhosis have gynecomastia and testicular atrophy. Despite these signs, there is usually a normal plasma estradiol. The initial alcohol induced hypoandrogenicity may continue until chronic irreversible liver damage produces irreversible testicular germ cell injury. Chronic alcohol ingestion in women has been reported to result in increased lowered sexual desire and anorgasmia. Acute alcohol ingestion lowers blood flow to the vaginal area which may be analogous to the finding that high blood alcohol levels diminish erectile response in males.

Enjoyment Factors

The chronic alcoholic may be decidedly repulsive to his sexual partner with the presence of alcohol upon his breath and disheveled demeanor. The physical consequences of alcoholism, such as gynecomastia, have been reported to be a source of shame to individuals who have retained or regained their potency (Bjork report). Likewise, women suffering from chronic alcoholism may find their physical deterioration a source of shame.

Psychological Factors

Chronic alcoholism has been associated with numerous psychologic characteristics. The passiviity, dependency and depression common in individuals addicted to alcohol can modify sexual functioning and the ability to relate to another partner. Chronic alcoholics, both men and women, report problems finding suitable sexual partners. This is often due to diminished capacity for interpersonal relationships.

General Treatment Aspects

Sexual rehabilitation of individuals suffering from chronic alcoholism demands directly confronting the problem of alcoholism and the promotion of sobriety. Drugs utilized for the treatment of alcoholism may cause problems. Antabuse has been reported to cause impotence. All neuroleptic medications have been reported to cause a variety of sexual impairments. Sexual and marital counseling are useful adjuncts in the treatment of alcoholism.

PREGNANCY

Although not a disease, pregnancy, delivery and the postpartum period are significant medical experiences, the sexual effects of which are important [31] to both wife and husband.

Organic Limitations

Fears of fetal harm are common in expectant mothers. In fact, prepartum coitus is well tolerated until the last trimester. The role of prostaglandins in semen may stimulate uterine contractions and thus make intercourse without a condom inadvisable in the latter part of a pregnancy. Immediately postpartum the tissue trauma to the perineal and vaginal areas due to delivery precludes intercourse until four to six weeks postpartum.

Enjoyment Factors

Sexual activity may be limited in the first trimester due to nausea and breast swelling which makes breast caressing painful. Fear of injury to the baby may also diminish enjoyment of sexual activity. During the latter stages of pregnancy, the abdominal girth may require utilization of new positions such as side-by-side for comfortable intercourse. Postpartum fatigue from infant care as well as nursing may diminish libidinal drive.

Psychological Factors

Postpartum depressions diminish libidinal drive and preclude effective sexual response. It has been suggested that an unexpected caesarean delivery may make the mother feel less of a "complete" woman. This appears to be true in only a selected group of patients. Untoward reactions to the birth of a child, however, should be investigated and treated. In these situations, sexuality is only one part of a complex reaction to the birth of a child. The nursing mother may feel less sexually responsive because of investment in the nursing process. The role of prolactin in limiting libidinal drive is not clear. An essential variable in the role of sexuality during pregnancy and during the postpartum period is the perceptions of the husband. Men with vulnerable psychologic characteristics may feel abandoned or threatened by the introduction of a new member to their family. This can provoke withdrawn behavior. The clinician must be aware of this possible development.

UROLOGIC SURGERY

Mechanical derangements, such as hypospadias, where the urethral meatus is abnormally located, may make vaginal penetration difficult. Procedures to correct this difficulty may create erectile dysfunction. Peyronies disease is a painful deformity of the penis due to fibrous tissue within the tunica albuginea. Surgical treatment involves dermal grafting which may result in impotence. Priapism is the painful prolongation of an erection. It is caused by blood dyscrasias such as sickle cell disease or leukemia, neoplastic disease, and drugs such as phenothiazines, antihypertensives, or anticoagulants. The condition may lead to tissue destruction and erectile dysfunction. Surgical treatment to detumesce the penis via a saphenous vein shunt will often cause impotence. Treatment for carcinomas of the prostate depends upon the degree of neoplastic invasion of the prostatic capsule. Transurethral resection will often cause retrograde ejaculation but potency will be maintained in 90% of cases. Retropubic prostatectomy, however, for more extensive malignancies, will usually (80-90%) ablate potency. Radiation therapy for prostatic cancer may also cause impotency (about 50% of cases) due to damage to the parasympathetic nervous plexus. Estrogen therapy for metastatic prostate cancer may lower libido and render the patient impotent.

Enjoyment Factors

The mechanical inability to successfully penetrate the vaginal canal in severe hypospadias produces shame and distress. Urinary spray due to the abnormal urethral opening further embarrasses the individual. Individuals with Peyronies disease are also embarrassed. Patients with priapism are agitated and distressed by the pain and persistence of the erection. Patients with prostatic cancer on estrogen therapy may be threatened by the gynecomastia.

Psychological Factors

Depression and sexual inhibition may result from any of these urologic situations. The limitations on enjoyment and actual functional limitations increase distress.

Case: A 57-year-old man suffered from recurrent episodes of painful priapism. Initially these prolonged erections were treated mechanically by aspiration utilizing an 18-gauge needle. The patient's alcoholism was primarily responsible for the priapism since evaluation for blood dyscrasias and neoplastic disease was negative. The patient finally underwent a saphenous vein bypass and was rendered impotent. He previously prided himself on his appearance and his ability to seduce women. He became increasingly despondent about his inability. He became depressed and eventually committed suicide.

Comment

This case illustrates a severe psychological reaction to erectile dysfunction following surgery. It also demonstrates the inherent danger of necessary urologic procedures. Although any suicide is overdetermined, this individual became increasingly obsessed regarding his impotence and, in the setting of a severe depression, focused all his attention upon his sexual dysfunction.

Treatment Considerations

Impotence from any of these causes may be treated by surgical prothesis. Some patients will not be candidates for such a procedure because of their debilitated medical state or need for various treatments such as anticoagulation. Careful psychological assessment and follow-up is recommended if urologic procedures cause impotence.

SEIZURE DISORDERS

Epileptic seizures of any variety, whether petit mal, grand mal, or temporal lobe, often lead to fear and uncertainty in the patient due to the loss of control and the unpredictable nature of the disorder. Since epilepsy represents a neurophysiologic disorder of the cerebral cortex, there may be some direct effect on higher centers involved in sexuality. The exact relationship is presently unclear. Temporal lobe epilepsy has been associated with a variety of sexual difficulties including problems in sexual drive, potency and paraphilias [32].

Enjoyment Factors

The patient with epilepsy has been said to be vulnerable to both personality and psychiatric disorders. The episodic nature of the disorder as well as the fear of loss of control may contribute to personality development. Shame and stigmatization complicate interpersonal relationships. Until recently, patients with seizure disorders had to apply for a legal dispensation in order to marry. Thus, our culture has had difficulty in relating to individuals with seizure disorders. These psychosocial factors may inhibit sexuality generally but especially if seizures occur during sexual experiences.

Psychological Factors

Patients with temporal lobe epilepsy have been described to have contentious, aggressive personalities which make for difficult interpersonal relationships. In addition, intellectual impairment may occur secondary to brain damage following surgical correction of seizure disorders or inability to control seizures. Patients with well controlled epilepsy are not at risk for cognitive impairment or psychiatric disorders which impair sexual function [33].

GYNECOLOGIC SURGERY

Surgical procedures which involve the genitalia and reproductive organs of women often have an emotional as well as mechanical or hormonal effect upon sexual function.

Organic Limitations

The specific gynecologic procedure will determine the organic limitations upon sexual functioning. Major surgical procedures such as pelvic exenteration may destroy the vaginal canal [34]. In some cases, the vaginal canal can be reconstructed, allowing intercourse although removal of clitoral tissue can result in anorgasmia. Hysterectomy for cervical carcinoma involving removal of the cervix with subsquent vaginal shortening and stenosis [35].

Enjoyment Factors

Disfigurement from genital surgery may cause shame in the patient or disgust in the sexual partner. Radiation implants for uterine carcinoma may stimulate fantasies in the sexual partner that he will be radiated if he engages in sexual activity. Following oophorectomy, the steroid deprivation may create vaginal epithelial thinning which can result in an atrophic vaginitis and dyspareunia.

Psychological Factors

Depression following major or minor gynecologic procedures originates in reaction to the actual disease state and surgery but also in the fantasies associated with the cause of surgery. Patients may blame former sexual activities as etiologic reasons for their disease. Such thoughts can aggrevate depression and shame, resulting in decreased sexual desire.

Treatment Considerations

Women with vaginal shortening have reported elongation of the vaginal canal following regular intercourse. Fantasies about the impact of radiation implants must be elicited and discussed with both the patient and her sexual partner if normal sexual activity is to be resumed. Discussion of the fantasies and fears regarding the etiology and course of any gynecologic carcinoma is necessary to prevent morbidity. The sexual partner should be included in counseling whenever possible.

CLINICAL INTEPRETATION OF LABORATORY FINDINGS

Evaluation of a sexually dysfunctional individual involves integrating psychologic, social and biologic data. A full psychosocial data base must complement physical observations and physiologic laboratory examinations. The presence of psychologic distress in the form of depression, a major mental disorder, or organic brain syndromes does not provide *prima facie* evidence for psychologic causes to a sexual dysfunction. Individuals may react to sexual difficulties with emotional distress. Social difficulties and interpersonal conflict are also commonly found in a wide variety of sexual difficulties. A causal, reactive or correlative phenomena cannot always be determined on initial evaluation. Nevertheless, it is essential to fully document psychologic and social aspects of the individual even in the presence of multiple abnormal laboratory findings.

Interpretation of a variety of physiologic findings may help the clinician confidently diagnose a sexual dysfunction as organic or psychogenic. Far more is known about male sexual dysfunction than sexual difficulties in women. Abnormalities in the physical examination, as noted earlier, should alert the clinician to utilize appropriate laboratory investigations. Difficulties in the vascular, neurologic, or endocrinologic systems may cause sexual difficulties. Absent peripheral pulses or limb hypothermia on physical examination should alert the physician for a more careful study of this system. Advanced technology has allowed more sophisticated evaluation of the vascular system. Measurement of penile blood pressure may document vascular pathology. Penile blood pressure may be measured by development of a ratio between the penile pressure to arm pressure. These data are not sufficient in themselves to confirm an organic cause to erectile dysfunction. Utilization of ancillary tests such as Doppler evaluation to measure blood flow are also important [36]. If results from the previous examinations are ambiguous, utilization of more invasive procedures may be necessary. Utilization of arteriography of the pelvic and genital vascular system may define certain dysfunctions. Thromboses of the dorsal and deep penile arteries may promote impotence in an otherwise healthy individual, but can only be documented via invasive arteriography [37].

The nocturnal penile tumescence test is increasingly utilized to document organic contributions to male impotence [38]. This investigation, done contemporaneously with an EEG, documents appropriate episodes of sleep to allow measurement of change in penile circumference at both the top and base of the penis; change in length of an erection and measurement via a pressure gauge of penile buckling pressure. Abnormalities in any one of these measures may indicate an inadequate erective ability which may indicate organic dysfunction. Specifically, erections may develop an adequate circumferential change but buckle easily under pressure and thus be inadequate for penile penetration. Utilization of each of the measures within the NPT evaluation is necessary to properly assess the study.

Investigating the central nervous system, the clinician will use various physical observations. Subtle changes within the autonomic nervous system such as the absence of pulse variation during full inspiration or sluggish pupillary response may indicate early autonomic pathology. Use of a cystometrogram may also demonstrate bladder dysfunction due to parasympathetic nerve dysfunction. As noted, measurement of the bulbocavernosus reflex will also demonstrate the integrity of the sacral reflex arc. Other nervous system examination findings such as absent ankle reflexes and areas of sensory dysfunction indicate nervous system difficulties. Such neuropathies may be strong evidence that an underlying disease state is causing a sexual dysfunction. Common etiologies include medications which affect the anticholinergic system; alcohol, or diabetes.

Evaluation of the endocrine system also relies upon physical observation and laboratory investigation. An abnormal fasting blood sugar should prompt the clinician to more vigorously investigate the possibility of diabetes mellitus. Measurement of serum testosterone is also a common laboratory value gathered for males with erectile dysfunction. For the adult male, the normal range for serum testosterone is 350-800 ng/dl [39]. Elevated testosterone levels may be found in hyperthyroidism [40]. Conventional treatment of this endocrine disorder will restore potency. Elevated testosterone is also found in an unusual condition of 5-alpha-reductase deficiency which occurs in infertile men with normal secondary sexual characteristics.

Low serum testosterone generally indicates a defect in the hypothalamic-pituitary-gonadal axis. The clinical task is to find which segment of the axis is dysfunctional. In the setting of low testosterone and high gonadotropin levels, primary hypogonadism is often the disease state [41]. If gonadotropin levels are low or low-normal, hypothalmic-pituitary disease may be the primary condition. Serum prolactin levels must then be measured. Hypoprolactinemia is a treatable form of male hypogonadism and responds to bromocryptine [42]. This condition is often due to pituitary adenomas which are best evaluated utilizing computer tomography as opposed to sella turcica tomograms.

Little is known about analogous states in females which may be due to pituitary or hypothalmic disease states. At this point in time, only a few research centers have availability of vaginal plethysmography which is the female analog of the nocturnal penile tumescence test [43].

In summary, clinical investigation of the sexually dysfunctional patient involves cooperation between the specialist in vascular angiography; the endocrinologist; the investigator of the peripheral nervous system and the psychiatrist.

Summary

The preceding data have cataloged the affects of common medical and surgical conditions upon sexual activity. Each patient reacts to their illness in part on the basis of their prior emotional strengths and weaknesses. Reactions are modified by the seriousness of the disease itself, the specific treatment and the interpersonal support systems. Thus, the role of sexuality in any given patient is dependent upon prior sexual functioning, the nature of the disease itself and the affect of treatment on the patient and partner. The clinician should not impose his own sexual values upon the patient when offering counseling. The role of sexuality must be placed within the broad context of each patient's existence. Counseling should thus focus on the patient's psychological reaction to the illness as well as the intrinsic limitations of sexual functioning secondary to pathologic features of the illness and treatment side effects from medication and/or surgery.

REFERENCES

1. Blaivas JG, O'Donnell TF, Gottlieb P, et al: Comprehensive laboratory evaluation of impotent men. J Urol 124:201-204, 1980
2. Bors E, Blinn KA: Bulbocavernosus Reflex. J Urol 182:128-129, 1959

3. Wise TN: Sexuality in the aging and incapacitated. Psych Clin North Am 3: 173–176, 1980
4. Viederman M, Perry III SE: Use of a psychodynamic life narrative in the treatment of depression in the physically ill. Gen Hosp Psych 2:177–185, 1980
5. Farberow NL, Nehamkis AM: Indirect self-destructive behavior in patients with Buerger's disease. J Pers Assess 43:86–96, 1979
6. Renshaw D: Sexual problems in the stroke patient. Med Aspects Hum Sex 9: 68–73, 1975
7. Hellerstein HK, Friedman EH: Sexual activity and the postcoronary patient. Arch Intern Med 125:987–999, 1970
8. Neri A, Aygen M, Zukerman Z, et al: Subjective assessment of sexual dysfunction of patients on long-term administration of Digoxin. Arch Sex Behav 9: 343–347, 1980
9. Krop H, Hall D, Mehta J: Sexual concerns after myocardial infarction. Sex and Disability 2:91–97, 1979
10. Abramov LA: Sexual life and sexual frigidity among women developing acute myocardial infarction. Rsychosom Med 38:418–425, 1976
11. Seagraves RT: Pharmacologic agents causing sexual dysfunction. J Sex Marit Ther 3:177–186, 1977
12. Moss HB, Procci WR: Sexual dysfunction associated with oral antihypertensive medication. Gen Hosp Psych 4:121–130, 1982
13. Richards JS: Sex and arthritis. Sex and Disability 3:97–99, 1980
14. Wise TN: Sexual functioning in the hyperobese. Obesity/Bariatric Med 6: 84–85, 1977
15. d'A Semple P, Watson WS, Beastall GH, et al: Diet, absorption and hormone studies in relation to body weight in obstructive airways disease. Thorax 34: 783–788, 1979
16. Kass I, Updegraff K, Muffly RB: Sex in chronic obstructive pulmonary disease. Med Aspects Hum Sex 6:33–35, 1972
17. Kolodny RC: Sexual dysfunction in diabetic females. Diabetes 20:557–559, 1971
18. Ellenberg M: Sexual function in diabetic patients. Ann Intern Med 92:(2 PT 2): 331–333, 1980
19. Abel GG: Impotence in Diabetes. Presented at American Psychosomatic Society, Boston, 1981
20. Levy NB: Sexual adjustment to maintenance hemodialysis and renal transplantation: National survey by questionnaire: Preliminary Report. Trans Am Soc Artif Intern Organs 19:138–143, 1973
21. Chen JC, Vidt DG, Zorn EM, et al: Pituitary-Leydig cell function in uremic males. J Clin Endocrinol 31:14–17, 1970
22. Milne JF, Golden JS, Fibus L: Sexual dysfunction in renal failure. A survey of chronic hemodialysis patients. Int J Psych Med 8:335–345, 1977
23. Johnson SM: Sexual dysfunction and dermatologic changes. Med Aspects Hum Sex 10:157–160, 1976
24. Maruto T, Osborne D: Sexual activity in chronic pain patients. Psychosomatics 19:531–537, 1978
25. Witkin MH: Psychosexual counseling of the mastectomy patient. J Sex Marital Therapy 4:20–28, 1978
26. Jamison KR, Wellison DK, Pasnau RO: Psychosocial aspects of mastectomy: The woman's perspective. Am J Psych 135:432–436, 1978

27. von Eschenbach AC: Sexual dysfunction following therapy for cancer of the prostate, testis, and penis. Front Radiat Ther Oncol 11:42–46, 1978
28. Dlin BM, Perlman A, Ringold E: Psychosexual response to ileostomy and colostomy. Am J Psych 126:374–381, 1969
29. Lundberg PO: Sexual dysfunction in patients with multiple sclerosis. Sex and Disability 1:218–219, 1979
30. Gad–Luther I: Sexual dysfunctions of the alcoholic. Sex and Disability 3:273–276, 1980
31. Butler JC, Reisner DR, Wagner NN: Sexuality during pregnancy and postpartum. In R Green (ed): Human sexuality Baltimore, Williams & Wilkins, 1979, pp 176–191
32. Blumer D, Walker AE: Sexual behavior in temporal lobe epilepsy. Arch Neurol 16:37–43, 1967
33. Standage KF, Fenton GW: Psychiatric symptom profiles of patients with epilepsy. Psychol Med 5:152–160, 1975
34. Brown RS, Haddox V, Posada A, et al: Social and psychological adjustment following pelvic exenteration. Am J Obstet Gynecol 114:162–171, 1972
35. Decker WH, Schwartzman L: Sexual function following treatment for carcinoma of the cervic. Am J Obstet Gynecol 83:401–5, 1962
36. Montague DK: The evaluation of the impotent male, In A H Bennett (ed): Management of Male Impotence, Baltimore, Williams & Wilkins, 1982, pp 52–61
37. Gray RR, Keresteci, St Louis, et al: Investigation of impotence by internal prudendal angiography. Radiol 144:733–780, 1982
38. Karacan I, Moore CA: Nocturnal penile tumescence: An objective aid for erectile dysfunction. In AH Bennett (ed): Management of Male Impotence, Baltimore, Williams & Wilkins, 1982, pp 62–72
39. Chen JC, Zorn EM, Halberg MC, et al: Antibodies to testosterone 3 bonne serum albumin applied to assay fo serum 17-beta-ol-androgens. Clin Chem 17:581–584, 1971
40. Spark RF: Neuroendocrinology and impotence. Ann Intern Med 98:103–105, 1983
41. Spark RF, White RA, Connolly PB: Impotence is not always psychogenic: newer insights into hypothalamic-pituitary-gonadal dysfunction. JAMA 243:750–755, 1980
42. Prescott RWG, Kendall–Taylor P, Hall K, et al: Hyperprolactenemia in men: Response to bromocriptine therapy. Lancet 1:245–249, 1982
43. Beck JG, Sakheim DK, Barlow DH: Operating characteristics of the vaginal photoplethysmograph. Arch Sex Behav 12:43–58, 1983

Laboratory Assessment of the Paraphilias and Their Treatment with Antiandrogenic Medication

FRED S. BERLIN and
FREDERICK W. SCHAERF

INTRODUCTION

Recently, Wirth and Folstein of The Johns Hopkins Hospital studied a group of patients with severe kidney disease who needed to receive chronic hemodialysis maintenance care [1]. For such patients compliance with oral water and salt intake restrictions is considered essential in order to maintain optimal health. However, even though patients were repeatedly admonished by the staff to keep their weight gain between dialysis treatments at or below 0.3 kilograms per day, as shown in Figure 1, most patients failed to do so. The amount of weight gained was a function of the amount of excess fluid consumed, which in turn appeared to be a function of the degree of thirst any given patient experienced. Wirth and Folstein concluded that limits to fluid intake set by physicians may not suffice, because they differ from those set by the patients' own physiology.

When persons attempting to restrict their fluid intake or to diet state that they are unable to do so on their own, they are generally believed, and an effort

Handbook of Psychiatric Diagnostic Procedures, vol 2, edited by R. C. W. Hall and T. P. Beresford. Copyright © 1985 by Spectrum Publications, Inc.

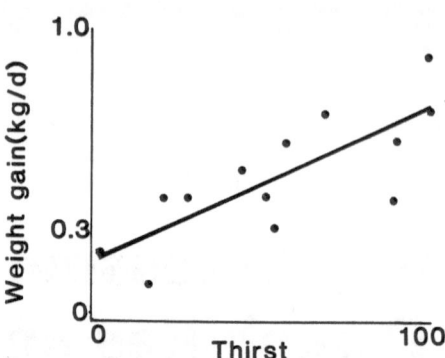

Figure 1. Water-induced weight gain as a function of self-reported thirst (as measured on a 100 mm visual analog scale) in 13 patients without kidneys on chronic renal dialysis. The requested maximum daily weight gain was 0.3 kg. The greater the thirst, the more the weight gain.

is made to provide qualified assistance to them. Similarly, when persons fail in their efforts to give up cigarette smoking, such failure is usually viewed with understanding and concern. When patients with anorexia nervosa binge-eat, or induce vomiting, it is generally accepted that they need help in order to become better able to control their own actions. The same can be said of compulsive handwashers.

On the other hand, when sexual behaviors are considered, a much different perspective is often proposed and invoked. Thus, it is usually taken for granted that "sex offenders" are invariably bad or evil people and that they could change if only they wanted to and would try their best to do so. It is possible that in some instances these assumptions may be wrong, and that instead concepts such as the medical diagnosis and treatment of "sex offenders" should be considered.

Following are verbatim excerpts from letters written by a convicted rapist. This man was found on laboratory examination to have an elevated level of follicle-stimulating hormone. He was subsequently treated with antiandrogenic medication. His example will be used as a starting point for the following discussion of the laboratory assessment and biologic treatment of "sex offenders."

"Sir, I am 32-years-old and in the penitentiary for several rapes. All my life I've felt I wasn't normal. . . . being the sex maniac I've been . . . messed up in sexual thought and behavior for God only knows how long. Since I was 4- or 5-years-old, sex has been 90% of my thoughts. After I was married I would have sex with my wife every night, then I would go masturbate. Sex was all I could think of.

The rapes started when I (saw) a naked woman through a window. Since that time its been 8 or 10, maybe more. The only way to stop the thoughts was to have sex or ejaculate. Sometimes I masturbated. After (each rape) I felt ashamed. I tried to stop and could for a month or longer, but ended up doing it again. It was as if I was being driven. I know it (doesn't) sound true or logical, but at a certain point, I could not control myself. I don't know why, if my true feelings was to be decent and good, why was I filthy and bad. I couldn't really control my mind on sexual things. The only things against the law I've ever done is because of sex. I don't like to hurt people.

Prior to antiandrogenic medication treatment, a number of paraphiliac patients have insisted that they lacked the capacity to consistently resist sexual temptations on their own. During hormone treatment, many of the same men have reported an increased capacity for self-control, and their subsequent behavior seems to confirm the validity of their assertions. This suggests that they acquired a capacity for self-control following hormonal treatment not previously present.

The compulsive rapist quoted above has now begun antiandrogenic medication treatment. He finds it helpful, as have others who have received this kind of medication. His comments about the effects of treatment, which are suggestive of a relationship between the hormone milieu of the brain and subjective mental experiences, follow.

In here (prison) the bad things stopped. You can't do them here, but the self hate and confusion inside me did not. I was still unable to control my sexual thoughts. Then, I started the shots. The feeling I now have is a feeling I cannot express in words. I have always known right from wrong, but now I can do right when I want to. I can stop ugly thoughts from ruling my life, and I can concentrate on other things. I wish I could explain how it feels to be able to put bad thoughts aside. I could not do this before. I just can't believe the effects of the shots is (due to) psychological factors. I feel I still have psychological problems, but the control I now have in this area of my (mental) life due to the medication leads me to feel that, perhaps, some physical part of my problem was involved much more than I thought possible. If they (others) believe it or not, it ain't going to stop me from continuing to take it."

He continues receiving antiandrogenic medication treatment in prison where he is serving a life sentence.

DIAGNOSTIC INDICATIONS FOR THE USE OF ANTIANDROGENIC MEDICATIONS

A person is considered a sex offender by virtue of having behaved in a particular way—e.g., by having exposed himself publicly. However, similar behaviors can be enacted for a variety of reasons. Not all sex offenses (a legal concept) are the reflection of a "sexual deviation disorder," or paraphilia (a medical concept). Table 1 lists those conditions considered in DSM III to be paraphilias (sexual deviation disorders) [2]. Antiandrogenic medications are used to treat those sex offenders whose behaviors are either the expression of an unusual and troublesome sexual appetite (eg., homosexual pedophilia—a sexual appetite for young boys), or as in the case just presented, seem less than fully controllable through the application of willpower alone [3]. These two possibilities are by no means mutually exclusive. Antiandrogenic medications may have a role to play as sexual appetite suppressants in the treatment of each of the paraphilias listed in Table 1, since many such patients experience difficulty in resisting the temptation to act upon unacceptable erotic urges.

Diagnosis of a sexual deviation syndrome can be made by inquiring about a person's thoughts, feelings, and behaviors. Individuals with "deviant" sexual interests ordinarily experience repeated erotic fantasies about engaging in unconventional forms of sexual activity. Asking about masturbatory fantasies can be revealing in this respect because erotic arousal for the purpose of masturbation may be difficult in the absence of erotic mental imagery [4]. The homosexual pedophile frequently fantasizes about young boys, whereas the heterosexual exhibitionist often has recurring thoughts and urges to expose himself to women. The male transvestite is preoccupied with the idea of cross-dressing in female clothing. Measures of penile tumescence and other forms of polygraphic data have also been used to try to document unconventional sexual ideas [5], but clinically we have found this unnecessary. Usually diagnosis of a sexual deviation syndrome can be made simply by gaining the patient's confidence and asking him to describe the nature of his erotic interests and behavior.

A sex offense could represent the expression of any of a number of psychiatric conditions including schizophrenia (in which phenothiazine treatment rather

Table 1.   Categories of Paraphilia ("Sexual Deviation") as
Listed in DSM-III

1. Pedophilia

2. Exhibitionism

3. Transvestism

4. Voyeurism

5. Zoophilia

6. Erotic sadism

7. Erotic masochism

8. Other (numerous others, including paraphilic, or compulsive, rape)

than antiandrogens might be warranted), mania (in which lithium carbonate might prove helpful), or dementia. The use of antiandrogenic medications is not considered appropriate with all sex offenders [3].

In assessing sex offenders and to learn more about their motivations and how best to deal with them, one can ask a number of questions. What are the various states of mind which people experience that may lead them to commit a sexual offense? Is the nature of one's sexual orientation and interests to some extent independent of characterological traits (such as concern or lack of concern for others)? What environmental or biologic factors, are associated with the development of unconventional sexual interests? What happens in the brain during erotic arousal? Is it possible, through a combination of psychologic counseling and pharmacotherapy, to provide effective treatment to men who experience unconventional, or uncontrollable, sexual appetites? Some of these questions can be addressed with the aid of laboratory tests or by the application of standardized scientific methods for determining therapeutic efficacy.

The remainder of this chapter will focus primarily upon three issues. (1) What is the rationale for using laboratory tests to try to elucidate the contribution made by biologic factors to sexual appetite and behavior and what are these tests? (2) What laboratory procedures can be used to learn more about regional brain activity and how it relates to erotic arousal? (3) What is the conceptual rationale and what laboratory tests need to be employed when using antiandrogenic medications to try to treat sex offenders? Methods for performing some of the relevant tests, when to use them, how to interpret the results, and how to place them into a proper clinical perspective will also be detailed.

LABORATORY TESTS TO ASSESS FOR BIOLOGICAL FACTORS THAT MAY PREDISPOSE TOWARDS PARAPHILIAC BEHAVIOR

Some laboratory tests have helped us to learn more about organic factors associated with the presence of unusual sexual appetites and about biological "risk factors" which may predispose to difficulty in controlling sexual behavior. There is a great deal of animal and human research relevant to these and related issues.

Persons vary in sexual orientation and in the nature of their sexual desires. Although in the past, most psychiatric theories have postulated that differences in sexual interests are primarily the product of early life experiences, this hypothesis has not been proven. In animals, biologic factors play a major role in influencing sex-related activities. Most dog owners, for example, are well aware of the fact that female dogs become sexually responsive to male dogs only while in "heat" (estrus). At such times, in response to the odor of chemical substances that are secreted by the female, which can be measured in a laboratory, the males themselves become much more sexually assertive.

The degree and manner by which biologic factors, measurable in the laboratory, influence human sexuality is not entirely clear. This issue has been discussed by several researchers in *The Psychobiology of Sex Differences and Sex Roles* [6]. Goy and McEwen have suggested that biologic factors may contribute more to human sexual experience and behavior than previously appreciated [7]. In support of such a contention Money has published data which suggest that females exposed prenatally to high dosages of androgen may, as adults show patterns of psychosexual development more typically seen in males [8]. Recently Pillard summarized data suggesting there may be a genetic predisposition towards male homosexuality [9].

In 1982 researchers reported finding frequent lutenizing hormone abnormalities in a group of transsexuals [10]. Other research conducted in Czechoslovakia suggested that the development of sexually "deviant" behavior, such as sadomasochism, exhibitionism, or fetishism seemed sometimes to be correlated with brain injury or cerebral infection occurring during the first few years of life [11]. Unfortunately, in clinical situations involving the evaluation of men with unconventional sexual interests such as exhibitionism, pedophilia, raptophilia, transvestism, or voyeurism, genetic and other biologic factors have frequently gone unassessed.

With such information in mind, we performed a variety of laboratory tests on a group of paraphilic men [3]. Several areas of biologic functioning appeared particularly relevant. Genetic karyotyping was thought to be important since the genes which determine anatomical sexual gender are contained on the X and Y chromosomes. Endocrine assessment was considered necessary since certain hormones are suspected to be of relevance to sexual phenomenology including testosterone, follicle-stimulating hormone (FSH), luteinizing hormone (LH), estrogens, and progesterone. We studied brain structure by means of computerized axial tomography (CT scan), and brain-wave activity by electroencephalogram (EEG) recordings.

Table 2. Recommended Laboratory Tests
in Looking for Biologic Abnormalities
in Paraphilic Patients

1. EEG
2. CT Scan
3. Testosterone
4. Estrogens
5. Progesterone
6. FSH
7. LH
8. Chromosomal karyotyping and analysis

A complete neurologic and physical examination should also be performed.

The series of laboratory tests shown in Table 2 (exluding estrogens and progesterone) was performed on a group of men meeting the DSM-III diagnostic criteria for paraphilia [2]. In 34 of 41 assessed cases, one or more significant biologic or clinical abnormalities were detected. These abnormalities (Table 3) included structural brain damage, hormonal irregularities, and chromosomal anomalies such as Klinefelter's syndrome. The finding of Klinefelter's syndrome in a number of homosexual pedophiles was particularly interesting since it is unclear whether Klinefelter's patients should be thought of as men with an extra X chromosome, or as women with an extra Y chromosome [2].

Although the biologic abnormalities found in this group of paraphilic patients occurred with greater frequency than would have been expected on a chance basis alone, similar tests were not performed on a group of men with conventional heterosexual interests. Future research should include such control groups in looking for associations between biologic pathologies and the nature of an individual's sexual orientation and behavior. Researchers concerned with such issues may wish to employ the tests in Table 2 on their paraphilic patients to continue documenting the frequency of biological abnormalities in this population.

LABORATORY PROCEDURES

Measurement of Serum Testosterone

The measurement of androgen concentrations in blood (specifically testosterone concentrations) not only provides the clinician information about gonadal function, but also, along with serum FSH and LH values, can provide data on the competence of the whole hypothalamic-pituitary-testicular axis. Disturbances of this homeostatic regulatory system may be associated with the presence of unusual sexual interests or with difficulties in exercising adequate behavior control over sexual appetite.

Plasma androgen concentrations have been measured in many ways. While such methods as enzymatic conversions to estrogen, double isotope derivative procedures, gas liquid chromatography, and competitive protein binding techniques have all been used, the development of the radioimmunoassay in 1969 has provided the best method to measure androgens in biological fluids [12]. Aulelta and others have explained how to suitably equip a laboratory in order to carry out radioimmunoassays of testosterone levels [13].

As shown in Figure 2, the measurement of testosterone levels in peripheral plasma by radioimmunoassay requires three basic elements: antibodies, radioactively labeled testosterone, and a plasma sample (usually first purified as described below) containing the unknown quantity of testosterone to be measured.

Initially the radioactively labeled hormone (the tracer) is added in excess to the antibody (AB) in a buffered solution. This tracer then binds to the antibody.

Table 3. Abnormal Laboratory and Clinical Findings in a Group of
Patients with Various Sexual Disorders

Patient Diagnosis	Associated Findings
1. Erotic sadism	Occulomotor abnormality suggestive of basal ganglion dysfunction. Unexplained gait disturbance.
2. Homosexual pedophilia	Dyslexia, childhood lisp requiring speech therapy.
3. Homosexual pedophilia	Cortical atrophy, grand mal seizures, recurrent slow delta waves and sharp activity over frontal brain regions on EEG.
4. Hypersexuality	Elevated testosterone, family history of adrenogenital syndrome.
5. Homosexual pedophilia	Klinefelter's syndrome, Mosaic (90% 47XXY, 10% 46XY). Elevated FSH and LH. Low testosterone.
6. Homosexual pedophilia	Strabimus, childhood learning disorder.
7. Heterosexual pedophilia	Schizophrenia.
8. Exhibitionism	Elevated testosterone, prior history of coma X several months following head trauma, grand mal seizures.
9. Heterosexual pedophilia	Cortical atrophy ($2°$ to trauma), right sided partial hemiparesis, visual spacial deficits.
10. Homosexual pedophilia	Elevated testosterone.
11. Heterosexual pedophilia	Near total blindness due to brain damage.
12. Heterosexual pedophilia	Elevated testosterone, mild ventriculomegaly and cortical atrophy most pronounced in areas of right sylvian fissure (by CAT scan), elevated 24 hour urine pregnanediol (3.1. Normal is less than 2.5 mg).
13. Homosexual pedophilia	Elevated LH. Generalized muscular hypotonia.
14. Paraphilic rape	Elevated testosterone, grand mal seizures.
15. Homosexual pedophilia	Elevated testosterone.

Normal (2 standard deviation) *testosterone* range in men = *275 to 875* ng/100 ml. Normal *FSH* in males = *9 to 369* ng/ml. Normal *LH* in males = *22 to 78* ng/ml. No associated abnormalities were detected in 7 other patients with sexual disorders who were also assessed.

When the unknown sample is added, it displaces some of the radioactively labeled tracer from the antibody in proportion to the amount of hormone in the sample. The radioactively labeled tracer which is displaced is referred to as the "free hormone." After ample incubation time, this free hormone can be removed from the bound hormone and the amount of radioactivity that it emits can be measured by a scintillation counter. By comparing this count to those obtained from samples containing known quantities of hormone, one can calculate, using standard curves, the amount of hormone that was present in the sample of serum tested.

In order to perform a radioimmunoassay procedure, it is first necessary to obtain antibodies to testosterone. Because testosterone is of too low a molecular weight to act as an antigen by itself, it must first be linked to a larger protein molecule in order to evoke an antibody response. The necessary antibodies are usually

Table 3. (continued)

Patient Diagnosis	Associated Findings
16. Hypersexuality	Cortical atrophy, cortical blindness, mild mental retardation.
17. Voyeurism	Elevated LH.
18. Homosexual pedophilia	Mosaic chromosomal pattern (97.5% XY, 2.5% XX), large heterochromatic region at centromere of autosome number 19 (polymorphic variant), low LH.
20. Homosexual pedophilia	46 XY, inversion 9 (p+, q⁻) Chromosome pattern. High LH.
21. Homosexual pedophilia	47 XXY chromosome pattern. Elevated testosterone, FSH.
22. Paraphilic rape	Elevated FSH.
23. Exhibitionism	Elevated LH.
24. Homosexual pedophilia	Low LH.
25. Heterosexual pedophilia	Elevated testosterone, FSH, and LH.
26. Homosexual pedophilia	Klinefelter's syndrome. Elevated FSH and LH. Low testosterone.
27. Heterosexual pedophilia	Elevated testosterone.
28. Homosexual pedophilia	Elevated testosterone.
29. Voyeurism	Elevated testosterone and LH.
30. Hypersexuality	Elevated testosterone, structural brain damage.
31. Homosexual pedophilia	Elevated testosterone, FSH and LH. EEG abnormality.
32. Transexualism and transvestism	Klinefelter's syndrome. Low testosterone.
33. Homosexual pedophilia	Elevated testosterone.
34. Homosexual pedophilia	Klinefelter's syndrome. Elevated FSH and LH. Low testosterone.

produced by injecting rabbits or sheep with testosterone linked with bovine serum ablumin (BSA). This procedure yields a high titer of immunogens which have a high affinity for testosterone and dihydrotesterone but which will not cross-react with estrogens, progestens, or other steroids [12]. Testosterone antibodies are commercially available or they may be made by injecting rabbits or sheep with commercially available testosterone—BSA conjugates [13].

The second element needed to perform a radioimmunoassay procedure is radioactively labeled testosterone. At one time tritiated steroids were used for this purpose. However, these are now generally being replaced by radioiodinated steroid derivatives. I^{125} labeled steroids give a high level of sensitivity and their radioactive output is easily countable. They can also be used in the presence of high antiserum dilutions [14]. I^{125} labeled testosterone is readily available commercially; its

282

BERLIN AND SCHAERF

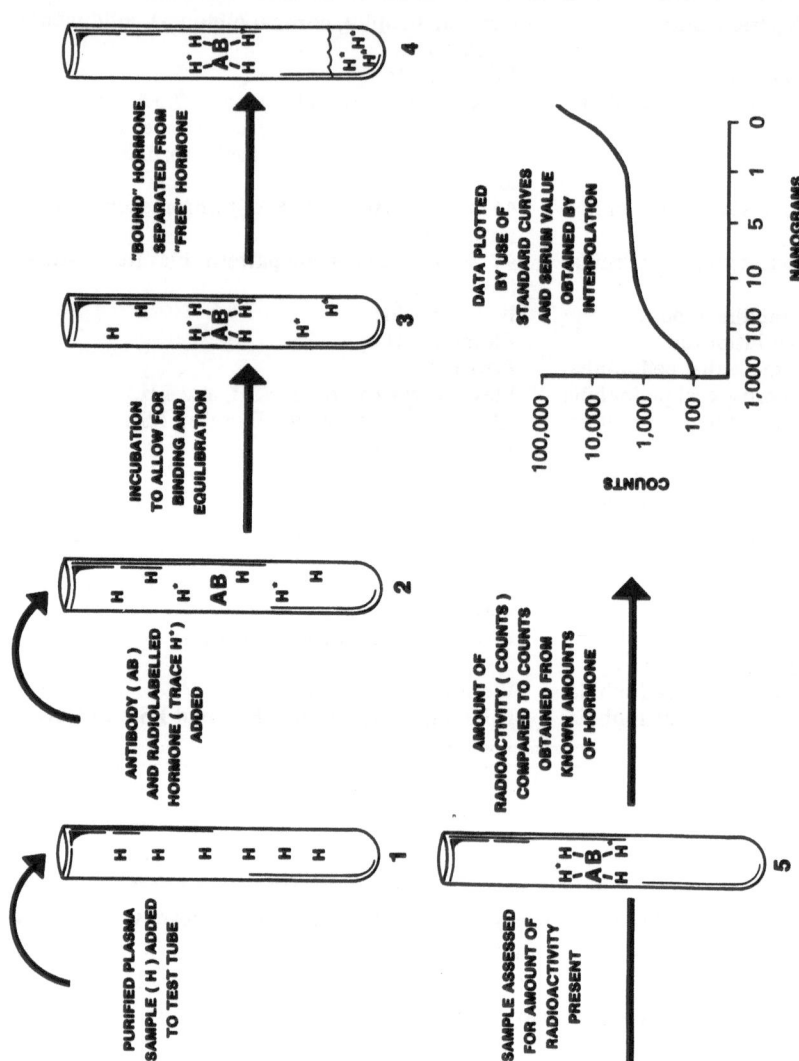

Figure 2. Measurement of testosterone levels by radioimmunoassay (following purification).

inclusion in radioimmunoassay kits has made measurements using this ligand routine.

The third element needed in doing radioimmunoassays is a sample of serum containing testosterone. Most radioimmunoassays are capable of measuring testosterone levels in as little as 0.5 ml of serum. However, ordinarily for ease of collection a 10 ml glass stoppered tube containing sodium heparin is used. In most hopsitals, heparinized tubes contain a green topped stopper. Ideally, blood should be obtained before 8 AM since marked diurnal variations in plasma testosterone levels have been reported and sampling at this time ensures determinations during peak levels [15]. Fasting samples are not necessary, and no commonly prescribed drugs (with the exception of sex steroids) seem to interfere with this assay.

In order to obtain accurate testosterone measurements, the sample of the patient's blood must have first been purified (before having been exposed to the mix of testosterone antibodies and radioactively labeled testosterone) to rid the plasma of proteins and other steroids such as dihydrotestosterone which would interfere with binding to the antibody. This is usually done by extracting one ml of the sample with an organic solvent and then purifying it by standard chromatographic methods [12]. Most antibodies are unable to distinguish testosterone from dihydrotesterone because they cross-react with both steroids.

Once plasma testosterone levels have been determined from a given patient's blood, the results can be compared to data obtained from a control population. It must be cautioned that in some centers the normal range of testosterone has been determined by sampling a population of presumably healthy men (usually between the ages of 20 and 60), sometimes numbering as few as 20. By convention, any value falling within the two standard deviation range of such a sample is then considered normal. As shown in Table 4, at our hospital, the two standard deviation range of testosterone in men is between 275 and 875 ng/100 ml of blood. The mean is 575 ng/100 ml with a standard deviation of ± 150. Any value above 875 is considered elevated. It is usually good practice to repeat any abnormal value at least once to ensure the accuracy of the finding.

There are a number of medical conditions associated with low levels of testosterone. Adrenal, gonadal, or pituitary tumors are the known major medical causes for excessively elevated androgen levels.

Measurement of FSH and LH

Serum FSH and LH levels can also be obtained by using radioimmunoassay methods. In this case, antibodies generated against gonadotropins must be employed. Radioiodinated hormones can again be used as tracers.

In obtaining blood to determine FSH or LH levels, a 10 ml nonheparinized (red capped) tube is generally used. A nonheparinized tube is used because this assay makes use of the serum rather than the plasma fraction of blood. The sample of blood may be obtained at any time, but early morning is preferable. Once again

Table 4. Normal (Two Standard Deviation) Ranges of Blood Levels in Men
and Women of Testosterone, FSH, and LH

	Men	Women
Testosterone	275–875 ng/100 ml	23–75 ng/100 ml
FSH	9–367 ng/ml	97–425 ng/ml (except midcycle)
LH	22–78 ng/ml	15–99 ng/ml (except midcycle)

normal values are considered to be those falling within the two standard deviation range as established by using a group of apparently healthy adults as the reference population. Our normal two standard deviation range for males for serum FSH is between 9 and 367 ng/ml and for serum LH is between 22 and 78 ng/ml. Moudgel and others give a complete description of radioimmunoassay methods for measuring the amount of FSH and LH (as well as the amount of estrogens and progesterone) present in blood [16].

Karyotyping

It is now reasonably well established that patients with particular kinds of chromosomal anomalies are more at risk for unconventional sexual appetites, feelings of gender dysphoria, or commission of a sex offense than persons whose chromosomal pattern is nonpathological [17]. Karyotyping, a procedure first used in the late 1950s, consists of the visual examination of chromosomes and the determination of their number and structure [18]. Most individuals have 23 homologous pairs, or 46 chromosomes, in each somatic cell of their body. Each chromosome contains about 100,000 genes. Twenty-two pairs are similar in appearance in males and females and are termed autosomes, while the 23rd pair, the so-called "sex chromosomes," determine anatomic gender. If a fertilized oocyte is to become a male, ordinarily the 23rd chromosome pair will by an XY; if it is to be a female, that pair will by an XX.

In order to perform karyotyping, 3 to 5 ml of blood is collected in a heparinized test tube. The blood is used in order to obtain leukocytes. This sample should be kept at room temperature and may sit overnight before being processed.

Briefly summarized, the karyotyping procedure consists of placing leukocytes in a 3 day tissue culture with phytohemmagglutin, an extract of the red bean. This substance stimulates the white cells to divide in culture by 72 hours. Once mitosis has begun, a dilute solution of colchicine is added which stops mitosis at metaphase. This allows the visualization of chromosomes under a microscope after the

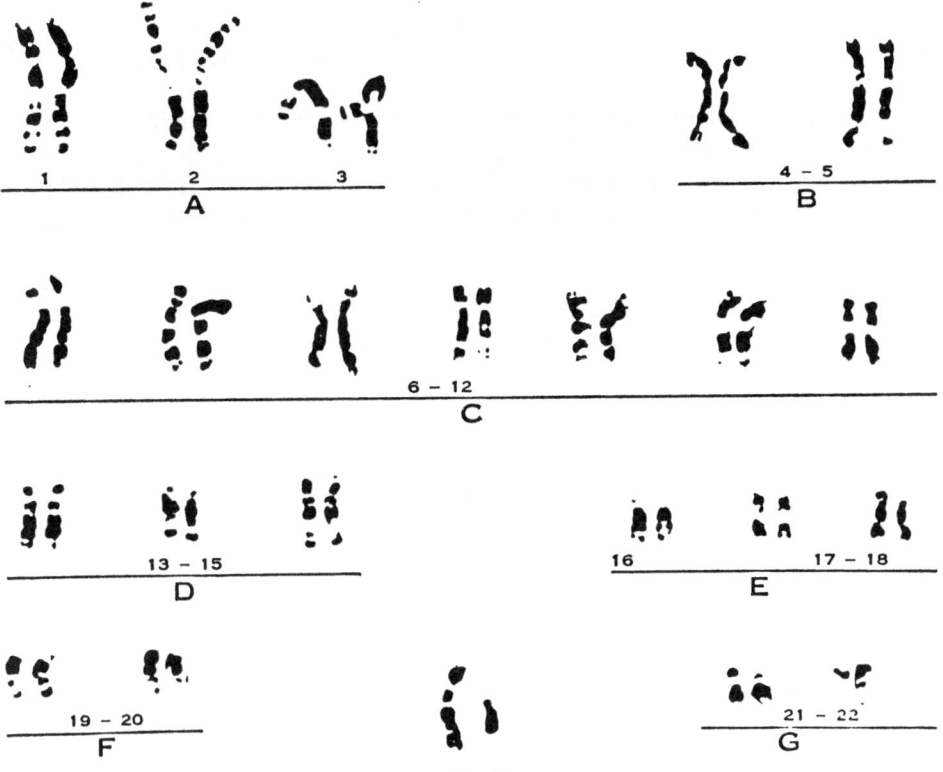

Figure 3.   A normal male (46 XY) karyotype.

cells have been fixed and stained. Photographs of the chromosomes are then taken. The chromosomes are cut from the photographic print, matched into homologous pairs, mounted on cardboard and analyzed for number as well as structure. A normal male karyotype is shown in Figure 3.

Techniques such as banding and autoradiography have been developed to identify specific abnormalities *within* a given chromosome. These additional procedures increase the expense of chromosomal analysis. Complete instructions for culturing human leukocytes, composing karyotypes, and interpreting the results can be found elsewhere [18,19].

Chromosomal karyotyping and analysis reports whether the number of chromosomes present are normal in quantity and whether within each chromosome there are abnormalities of the constituent gene segments.

THE PETT SCANNER AS AN INVESTIGATORY PROCEDURE:
WHAT HAPPENS IN THE BRAIN DURING EROTIC AROUSAL?

There is reason to believe that the brain differs from one region to another in metabolic activity during sexual arousal. As discussed below, and elsewhere in this text, the recent development of the PETT scanner provides a new technology that may be capable of documenting such differences [20,21]. Thus, the PETT scanner may be able to provide knowledge about (1) how this "organ of thought and feeling," the brain, functions at such times, and (2) whether the brains of persons who experience unconventional sexual appetites, or who have difficulty controlling their sexual behaviors, function differently than the brains of persons who seem less troubled in these ways.

It is already known that certain brain structures (eg., the area preoptica in the hypothalamus) accumulate relatively large amounts of sex related hormones such as testosterone, whereas other areas (such as the limbic system) do not [22]. It is also known that stimulation or ablation of *specific* brain areas can lead to dramatic changes in the amounts of such hormones released into the blood stream [23]. In addition, stimulation, or ablation, of specific brain regions in animals is correlated with obvious changes in the frequency of various kinds of sexual behavior [24]. Damage to certain areas of the brain in humans has also been associated with the development of aberrant sexual activity [25]. It seems likely then that certain areas of the brain may be more involved than others during erotic arousal.

Lesions made in the area preoptica of the hypothalamus, an area particularly rich in sex hormone receptors, have been shown to lead to a decrease in the frequency of sexual behavior in animals, without affecting either perceptual-motor capabilities or circulating testosterone levels [26]. Estrogen applied locally to specific hypothalamic sites in male rats (but not other sites) leads to a lordotic response, i.e., a backward elevation of the pelvis that facilitates female intercourse [27]. Testosterone implants in certain hypothalamic sites can reactivate mating behavior in castrated male animals, but similar implants in other brain sites cannot [28]. Electrical stimulation of the dorsal part of the lateral area preoptica causes almost uninterrupted mounting and frequent ejaculations in male rats [29].

As long ago as 1939 Kluver and Bucy described a syndrome in cats produced by bilateral lesions to the temporal lobes that resulted in intensified indiscriminate sexual behavior [30]. Schreiner and Kling have shown that this "hypersexual" activity can be abolished by castration but reinstituted with testosterone replacement therapy, suggesting that the behavior is sex hormone related [31]. They have also demonstrated that lesions applied to specific sites in the ventromedial nucleus of the hypothalamus can likewise abolish this "hypersexual" activity.

In 1966 a team of neurosurgeons performed sterotactic brain surgery on a homosexual pedophile, making a lesion in the ventromedial nucleus of the hypothalamus in the same area that Schreiner and Kling had ablated in cats [32]. The patient subsequently indicated that his erotic fantasy life was virtually abolished, and that he had lost his pedophilic urges. Orthner reported that substantial sex drive reduction had been achieved in 34 sex offenders treated neurosurgically by making lesions in analogous brain regions [33]. Although these claims of therapeutic success have been questioned by some, Freund feels that these surgical teams may have obtained genuine success [34]. A recent governmental task force appointed to consider the topic of psychosurgery in the United States concluded that it may have therapeutic promise [35]. If PETT scanning, or similar techniques, can confirm that certain areas of the brain do indeed selectively increase in metabolic activity in association with erotic arousal, and, if it suggests that these areas differ depending upon the nature of one's sexual interests, a more rational basis for providing therapy to those persons who experience unconventional erotic urges potentially harmful to themselves or others may eventually become possible.

ANALYSIS OF PETT SCANNING RESULTS

PETT scanning requires that a patient be administered a small amount of radioactively labeled material such as C-11 deoxyglucose. A computer attached to Geiger counter type sensors placed around the patient's head then produces a series of cross sectional pictures of the brain which vary in color according to the amount of glucose being utilized at any given anatomic site (Figure 4). PETT scanning can be performed twice on any given patient; first prior to and then during erotic arousal with a penile transducer being used to confirm arousal.

Table 5 summarizes categories of data that can be generated by performing PETT scanning before and during erotic arousal on men with conventional and unconventional sexual interests. That table also includes categories that could be generated by repeating PETT scanning after initiation of antiandrogenic medication treatment.

PETT scan results of the sort which would fit into such a table can be reported (either based upon the visual observations of an experienced radiologist or by means of direct analysis of the computer-stored data) in terms of the relative density of radioactive output per defined area of the brain. When these assessments are based upon visual observations, they reflect an assessment of the type and intensity of a particular color as seen on the computer-produced picture of a given brain region. However, such subjective assessments are unnecessary because observations from a given brain region (or Pixel) can be quantified by actually totaling the counts of radioactivity from that region and then comparing them to counts from other regions or to counts from the brain as a whole. Various regions of the brain can be systematically compared in this way. Thus, each of the cells in Table 5 can be compared with one another for any given brain region, with differences in mean group densities between men with conventional vs unconventional sexual interests

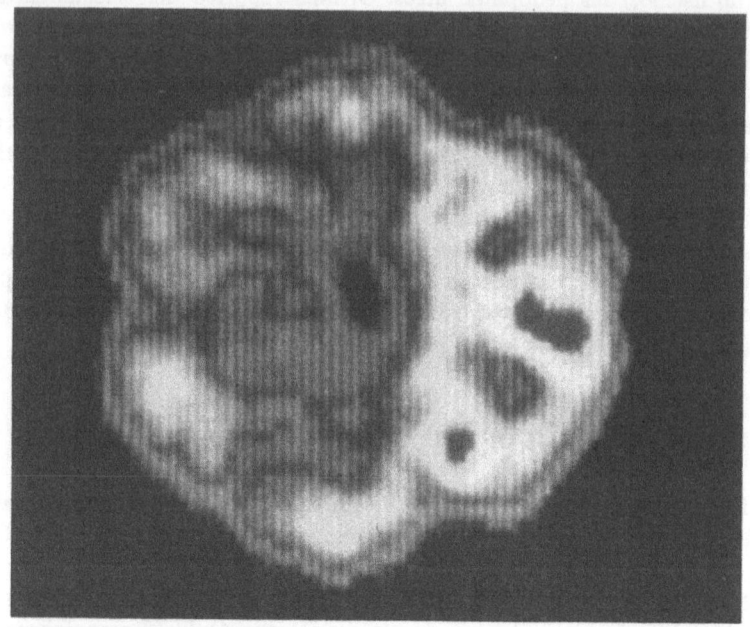

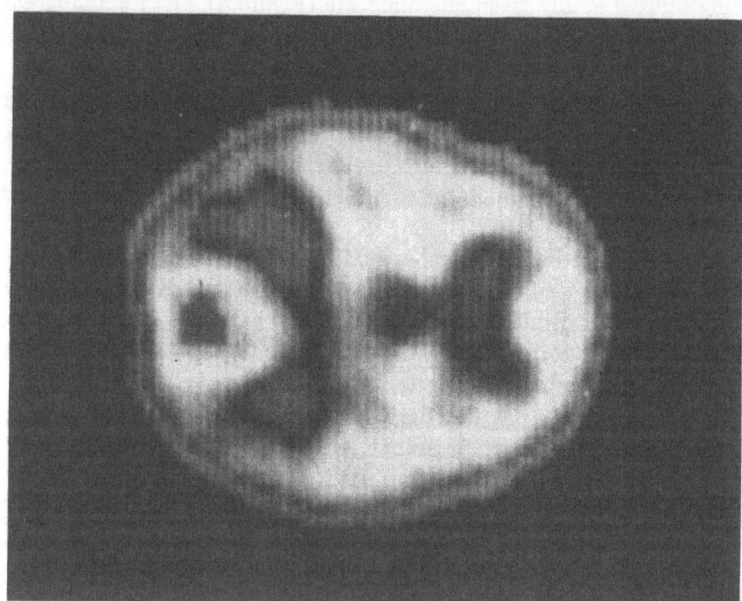

Figure 4.   A cross-sectional picture of the brain at two levels produced by PETT scanning.

Table 5. Summary of Categories of Data That Can Be Generated by Performing PETT Scanning

			Participant number	Before antiandrogenic medication is given	After antiandrogenic medication is given
Persons with unconventional sexual interests	E P V T O	Prior to sexual arousal	A_1 A_n		
	E P V T O	During sexual arousal	A_1 A_n		
Persons with conventional sexual interests		Prior to sexual arousal	B_1 B_n		
		During sexual arousal	B_1 B_n		

E, exhibitionist; P, pedophiles; t, transvestites; v, voyeurs, O, other paraphilias

being assessed for statistical significance. When comparisons are made between data obtained prior to and during sexual arousal, each study participant can be used as his own control. If a sufficient number of men in each category of paraphilia (exhibitionism, pedophilia, voyeurism, etc.) can be obtained, statistical comparisons can be made among these groups as well.

In studies where participants are asked only to *imagine* erotically stimulating imagery in order to attain a state of sexual arousal, a different pattern of regional brain activity may occur then would be the case in the presence of olfactory, visual, tactile, or other forms of erotic sensory stimulation. Regional brain metabolism during sexual climax (as opposed to during the arousal or desire phases) may also be different. Although at present only radioactively labeled glucose is ordinarily used in performing Pett scanning, in the future labeling of testosterone, FSH, or LH may also be possible.

PETT scanning may help provide answers to the following questions. Are there differences between groups of patients (eg., heterosexual exhibitionists vs homosexual pedophiles) in regional brain metabolism when *not* sexually aroused? What areas of the brain become metabolically active during sexual arousal? Do these areas differ among persons who experience different sexual interests? What are the effects upon brain metabolism during sexual arousal of various sorts of sensory inputs such as visual, auditory, or olfactory stimulation? Does metabolic brain activity change during sexual climax? What are the effects of antiandrogenic medication treatment upon regional brain metabolism during sexual arousal?

RATIONALE FOR USING TESTOSTERONE-LOWERING METHODS TO TREAT PARAPHILIAS: EVIDENCE OF EFFICACY

Sex offenders make up a significant proportion of many prison populations at major expense to the public. Thus, the question of whether or not persons who experience unconventional erotic desires, such as pedophiles, exhibitionists, and some rapists can be helped by antiandrogenic medication treatment is important.

It is known from simplest phenomenology that people do not decide voluntarily what will arouse them sexually. Recently Abel reported that prior to therapy a number of rapists seemed unable to prevent themselves from obtaining an erection while listening to descriptions of coercive sexual acts, whereas most non-rapists could [36]. Quincey showed that some rapists can be distinguished from nonrapists by the ratio (as measured by penile plethysmography) of their erotic arousal while listening to descriptions of coercive versus noncoercive sexual acts [5]. Abel's and Quincey's data suggest two possibilities. (1) Some men may rape as a consequence of difficulty suppressing their sexual urges. (2) Some rapists may become relatively more aroused than other men by coercive (as opposed to non-coercive) sexual acts. If this is so, treatments which lower sexual appetite may be helpful.

One of the early methods used in an attempt to decrease sexual appetite was bilateral orchiectomy which lowers the hormone testosterone. In animals, although individual differences in the rate of change in sexual behavior following orchiectomy are frequent, castration invariably results in an eventual decrease in most forms of sexual activity [34].

Several studies have looked at the recidivism rate of sex offenses following castration in humans. Unfortunately, few such studies stipulated whether the sex offenders treated in this manner had previously been experiencing unconventional erotic urges. Nevertheless, these studies are relevant to the question of whether or not treatment with antiandrogenic medication is likely to be helpful.

Sturup and others conducted over 4,000 follow-up examinations on 900 castrated sex offenders in Denmark over a 30-year-period and reported that only

1.1% definitely recidivated [37]. If unclear cases were included, the recidivism rate was 2.2%. Wiffels reported comparable findings [38]. Ficher Van Rossum reported similarly low rates on 307 Swedish patients [39]. Bremer found a 7.3% recidivism rate after 5 years among a group of 41 castrated sex offenders who, prior to treatment, had had a recidivism rate of 58% [40]. Additional data regarding the effects of castration upon recidivism are presented in an excellent review article by Freund [34]. Although there has been some debate about how to interpret these data, Freund concluded that this form of treatment, which is intended as a means of therapeutic sex drive reduction to facilitate self control, and not as punishment, has been successful.

Besides documenting changes in recidivism rate, a number of investigators have obtained self-reports from castrated sex offenders regarding potency. In many cases, following castration some degree of erotic desire and the capacity to perform sexually remained [39]. Freund pointed out that this does not necessarily present a problem in terms of treatment, however, since the surgery fulfills its intent if it decreases the sex drive sufficiently to enable the patient to refrain from acting upon unacceptable erotic urges [34].

Two medications which have been used as sexual appetite suppressants are medroxyprogesterone acetate (MPA) and cyproterone acetate (CPA). Like castration, both lower testosterone levels. However, unlike castration neither results in a compensatory elevation of FSH or LH by the pituitary gland, suggesting that they may have a direct effect upon brain activity.

Langerin and colleagues have reported two double-blind studies using MPA [41]. In both cases MPA seemed to lower sexual libido. However, the dosages employed, route of administration, duration of treatment, and outcome measures utilized were not comparable to most clinical antiandrogenic treatment protocols. A double-blind investigation using CPA reported successful reductions in "deviant" sexual interests and libido, but a pharmacologically active placebo medication was not used for comparison purposes [42].

Table 6 shows changes in sexually "deviant" behavior in a group of 20 chronic paraphilic patients treated in a non-blind study with medroxyprogesterone acetate [43,44]. Fifteen percent of patients (3 of the 20) showed recurrences of deviant activity while taking the medication, indicating that it is not 100% effective. On the other hand, 85% of these men were apparently totally without further legal involvements while receiving medication, sometimes for periods as long as several years. Some patients in this study were self-referred, but most were referred by a physician or attorney subsequent to legal apprehension.

Most of the patients reported upon in Table 6 were not hospitalized to initiate treatment and were not required as a condition of probation to take medication. In time, many became noncompliant, sometimes because they believed themselves cured. Currently, most of our patients are hospitalized for 3 or 4 weeks at the beginning of therapy and subsequent outpatient compliance has improved dramatically.

Table 6. Changes in Paraphilic Behavior During and After Treatment With Antiandrogenic Medication[a]

Patient	Age (years)	Diagnosis	Average frequency of sexually deviant behaviors before treatment[b]	Drug treatment		Occurrence of sexually deviant behaviors	
				Length	Maximum dosage	During treatment	After treatment
1	34	Homosexual pedophilia	Once/week	5 years, 9 months	500 mg/week	None	Treatment dropout; no relapse less than 1 year after treatment
2	31	Homosexual pedophilia	Twice/month; 1 known arrest	1 year	300 mg/week	None	Treatment dropout; relapsed less than 1 year after treatment
3	30	Heterosexual exhibitionism	Twice/week	10 months	250–300 mg/week	None	Treatment dropout; relapsed more than 1 year after treatment
4	34	Homosexual masochism	4 times/week	3 months	200 mg/week	None	Treatment dropout; relapsed less than 1 year after treatment
5	27	Bisexual pedophilia	Twice/week	3 months	400 mg/week	None	Treatment dropout; relapsed more than one year after treatment
6	43	Transvestism; homosexual incest	7 times/week; 2 incidents	1 year, 4 months. intermittently	150 mg every other week	None	Relapsed less than 1 year after treatment
7	52	Heterosexual sadism	Once every 2 weeks for 25 years	3 years, 5 months	600 mg/week	None	Treatment continues; no relapses
8	29	Homosexual pedophilia	Twice/week; 6 arrests in 6 years	10 months	500 mg/week	None	Treatment dropout; relapsed less than 1 year after treatment
9	36	Homosexual pedophilia	Once every 2 months; 4 arrests in 6 years	2 years	500 mg/week	None	Treatment continues; no relapses
10	56	Homosexual pedophilia	Once/week; 14 arrests in 29 years	3 years, 9 months	300 mg/week	Relapsed	Treatment continues
11	40	Homosexual pedophilia	Twice/week; 7 known arrests	4 years, 2 months	400 mg/week	None	Treatment continues; no relapses
12	45	Voyeurism; heterosexual pedophilia	Twice/week; 5-8 arrests; numerous institutionalizations	5 years, 3 months	300 mg/week	None	Relapsed less than 1 year after treatment; treatment now resumed

	Age	Type	Frequency/History	Duration	Dose	Relapse	Outcome
13	27	Homosexual pedophilia	Twice/week since age 10	5 years, 9 months	200 mg/week	None	Treatment completed; no relapse more than 1 year after treatment
14	41	Homosexual pedophilia	Once/month; numerous arrests; 4 convictions; 4 reported parole violations	3 years, 8 months	500 mg/week	Relapsed	Treatment continues
15	37	Homosexual pedophilia; exhibitionism	Record unclear; probably several incidents/year	3 years, 9 months	350 mg/week	None	Treatment completed; no relapse less than 1 year after treatment
16	26	Homosexual pedophilia	Once/week	1 year, 1 month	200 mg/week	None	Treatment dropout; relapsed more than 1 year after treatment
17	24	Heterosexual voyeurism	Once/month	1 year	400 mg/week	Relapsed after alcohol consumption	Treatment continues; in prison
18	40	Heterosexual exhibitionism	Five times/day since age 11; first arrest at age 21; numerous others	2 years, 2 months	200 mg/week	None	Treatment dropout; relapsed less than 1 year after treatment
19	29	Heterosexual exhibitionism	Twice/week	2 years, 1 month	250 mg/week	None	Treatment dropout; relapsed less than 1 year after treatment
20	46	Heterosexual exhibitionism	Four times/week; binges of 20/day	2 years, 3 months	300 mg/week	None	Treatment continues; no relapses

aSexually deviant behavior was considered to have occurred if the patient was accused of having or admitted having a deviant sexual contact (for example, an episode of public genital exposure). Any occurrence of such behavior was scored as a relapse once treatment had been initiated, even if it did not come to the attention of the law as an official complaint.

bBased on institutional records and patients' statements.

cStudy participants who stopped taking medroxyprogesterone acetate did so against medical advice, except in the cases of patients 13 and 15. Some patients were irregularly compliant with medication even during the period when it was being prescribed.

The data presented in Table 6 show clearly that in most cases when paraphilic patients discontinue medications they relapse. This supports the hypothesis
that this form of treatment is neither a cure nor a temporary catalyst to be used
until psychotherapy can become effective. Rather, for the majority of patients, the
medication appears to act as a sexual appetite suppressant. If deviant hungers are
allowed to return, most patients seem again to be at risk. In a few cases, patients
have reported that MPA fails to significantly decrease their sexual drive. Why this
should be so is not known. Currently we are treating approximately 70 paraphilic
patients on an outpatient basis with a combination of group therapy and antiandrogens. Less than 10% have recidivated, and none have committed a physically violent crime.

ANDROGENS AND FACTORS RELATED TO THEIR MEASUREMENT

Thus far the discussion has concerned (1) what laboratory tests can be used to
look for biologic pathologies in paraphilic patients, (2) PETT scanning as a potential procedure for documenting what goes on in the brain during erotic arousal, and
(3) the rationale for and efficacy of using testosterone-lowering methods to treat
some "sex offenders." In closing, a discussion of androgens and antiandrogens and
of the laboratory protocol used to assess for possible side effects of testosterone-
lowering treatments will be presented.

Classically, an androgen is defined as a substance which stimulates the growth
of the male reproductive tract [45]. These substances, all of which are steroids, are
secreted 90% by the testes and 10% by the adrenal cortex [46]. Testosterone is the
major androgen produced by the testes of man, and it is also the androgen present
in highest concentration in the peripheral bloodstream [47]. Testosterone is the
hormone which causes the fetus to take on a male appearance. It is also the androgen which increases in males at puberty resulting in increased growth of facial and
pubic hair, deepening of the voice, thickening of bodily muscles, and increased
sexual interests.

The biochemical pathways of androgen biosynthesis by the testes are now well
established as shown in Figure 5. Essentially, steroid metabolism in the testes consists of distinct steps requiring specific enzymes and their cofactors [48]. Whether a
hormonal endproduct such as testosterone is produced depends upon the presence
or absence of the necessary enzymatic components within the tissues of a particular
organ.

Cholesterol is the key precursor of all steroid hormones synthesized by the
testes. This cholesterol can originate from the circulation, or be synthesized from
acetate by Leydig cells in the testes themselves.

Once produced and secreted, testosterone can undergo two additional biochemical conversions. (1) It can be reduced to 5 alpha-dihydrotesterone (DHT) by

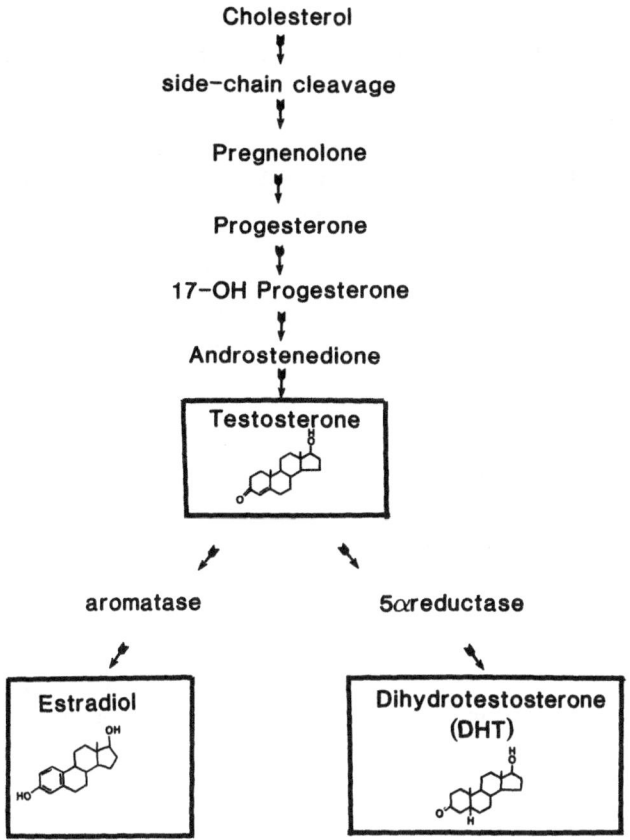

Cholesterol

side-chain cleavage

Pregnenolone

Progesterone

17-OH Progesterone

Androstenedione

Testosterone

aromatase   5αreductase

Estradiol   Dihydrotestosterone
                                             (DHT)

Figure 5. Biochemical pathways of androgen biosynthesis by the testes.

a intracellular enzyme known as 5-alpha-reductase. DHT, which is an even more potent androgen than testosterone, is the biologically active intracellular androgen in some tissues. It is present in the brain cells of many species and it may play a role in the functioning of the central nervous system [49]. (2) Alternatively, testosterone (as well as androstenedione) can be converted to estrone and estradiol respectively (rather than to DHT). The series of reactions by which testosterone is converted to estradiol is collectively referred to as aromatization. Many tissues including brain, skin, fat, and liver are capable of converting androgens to estrogens, and it has been shown that the majority of blood estradiol and estrone comes from the aromatization of circulating androstenedione and testosterone [50]. Up to 60 mg/day of estrone and 40 mg/day of estradiol are produced in normal healthy men [51].

Once synthesized, testosterone enters the systemic circulation bound mainly to serum proteins. These proteins include testosterone estradiol binding globulin (TeBG), which binds 30% of serum testosterone, albumin (which binds 67%), and other plasma proteins, which transport the remainder of bound hormone. Only about 2% of circulating testosterone is free in the plasma [52].

Classically, it has been taught that in order for a hormone to be physiologically active, it must be present in the blood stream in pure form, free from serum binding globulins or other proteins that ordinarily transport substances through the circulation. Recently, however, this formulation has been questioned, and it is now uncertain whether it is the free or bound component of a hormone circulating through the plasma which is actually responsible for its biologic effects in some instances. Thus, as described earlier, in the Hopkins laboratory total plasma testosterone (ie., bound plus free) is ordinarily ascertained. This value is a good indicator of an individual's androgenic status, and it is easily measured. Tests currently available to assess free hormone are time consuming, cumbersome, and frequently inaccurate.

Like other steroid hormones, androgens are metabolized by the liver and the breakdown products are eventually secreted by the kidneys (in the form of glucuronides or sulfates) into the urine [12]. A small amount of testosterone (about 6%) enters the enteroheaptic circulation and is excreted into the feces [51].

Total plasma testosterone values obtained from patients with severe liver disease may be somewhat depressed. This is so because the carrier proteins to which most of the testosterone present in the circulatin binds are produced by the liver, and they may be produced in lesser amounts in severe liver disease. Thus, the protein-bound component of total plasma testosterone will be lower. In addition, a malfunctioning liver may have a reduced ability to clear normally present amounts of testosterone from the plasma. This can result in a transient elevation of testosterone which in turn will suppress FSH and LH production by the pituitary, thereby in the long run lowering testosterone production by the testes.

The measurement of urinary ketosteroids reflects mainly adrenal function. Therefore, urinary 17-ketosteroid determinations are not clinically useful indicators of testicular function [51].

ANTIANDROGENS AND THE LABORATORY PROTOCOL

The first compound used clinically to antagonize the biologic actions of male sex hormones was diethylstilbesterol. It was initially used in 1943 for its antiandrogenic effects in the treatment of prostatic cancer [53]. It and similar compounds have found clinical us in such conditions as hirsutism, precocious puberty, virilization, acne, male pattern baldness, and breast carcinoma. Some antiandrogens have been proposed as possible male contraceptives [54]. Compounds used as antiandrogens include estrogens and progestins, as well as several nonsteroidal substances.

The ideal antiandrogen for clinical use would be a substance that possesses low toxicity, high potential as a "sexual appetite suppressant," and negligible feminizing effects. One compound which may come close to meeting these three criteria is medroxyprogesterone acetate (Depo-provera). Its chemical structure is shown in Figure 6.

Medroxyprogesterone acetate (MPA) is a potent synthetic progestin. When used as a sexual appetite suppressant, this hormone can be injected intramuscularily in doses as high as 800 mg/week. The ususal starting dosage is 500 mg/week. Following injection, this depot medication binds to muscle and is slowly released into the bloodstream, where it maintains fairly constant serum levels. The dosage can be titrated to avoid impotence and the medication is not feminizing. The 100 mg/ml concentration has greater bioavailability and is less painful when injected than is the 400 mg/ml solution. No more than 250 mg/ml should be administered into a single injection site.

The major side effects of MPA are weight gain and mild lethargy, but cold sweats, nightmares, myalgia, dyspnea, hyperglycemia, azospermia, hypertension, and breast cancer in female beagle dogs have all been reported. Hypertension sometimes becomes sufficiently problematic as to require concommitant treatment. Currently it is believed that the side effects produced in humans are fully reversible after the drug is discontinued, but MPA has not been in clinical use long enough to be certain that this will remain true.

The mechanism by which MPA lowers serum testosterone has been the subject of a number of recent studies. It appears that MPA works in several ways. It is known, for example, that MPA inhibits gonadotropin release from the pituitary

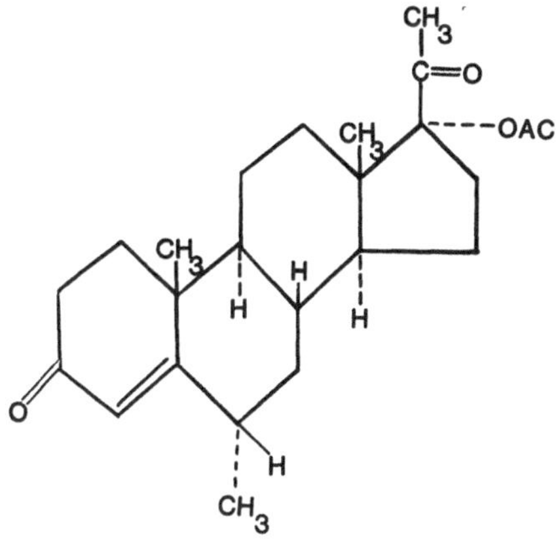

Figure 6.   Chemical structure of medroxyprogesterone acetate (Depo-provera).

gland [55,56]. MPA also increases the metabolic clearance rate of testosterone and increases hepatic testosterone reductase activity, thereby facilitating removal of testosterone from the plasma by the liver [57,58]. Besides lowering testosterone, MPA decreases spermatogenesis [59,60].

MPA may bind to peripheral androgen receptors on various target organs and it may also interfere with the conversion of testosterone to the more potent androgen, DHT. Some of the possible sites, and mechanisms of action, of MPA are depicted schematically in Figure 7.

Apparent changes in sexual appetite resulting from injections of MPA may be related more to its central effects upon the brain than to its effect upon circulating serum testosterone levels. This is supported by the observation that some patients report a subjective decrease in sexual appetite when the dosages of MPA given are beyond those which would lower serum testosterone any further. When MPA is used to increase sexual self-control, dosage levels should be adjusted according to the patient's subjective reports of changes in the intensity and frequency of unacceptable erotic preoccupations rather than by monitoring serum testosterone levels.

Ordinarily, prior to initiating antiandrogenic medication treatment baseline levels of FSH, LH, and testosterone should be assessed and follow-up tests should be conducted every six months to document current levels. Every six months an SMA-12 should also be performed to be certain blood sugar, kidney function, and liver functions are stable and not adversely effected by the treatment regime. Blood pressure and body weight should be monitored weekly. This protocol, along with recommended dosage and injection instructions, is summarized in Table 7. In our clinic as part of their treatment protocol men receiving MPA to facilitate self-control of sexual behavior are also expected to attend weekly group therapy sessions intended to try to reinforce their efforts to succeed. Group therapy sessions and medication injections are seen as a form of maintenance treatment rather than being seen as curative.

FUTURE CONSIDERATIONS

Because of the complex interaction of the hypothalamus, pituitary gland, and the testes, many possibilities exist for pharmacologic interruption of testosterone production or for preventing its utilization. As shown in Figure 8, testosterone production by the Leydig cells of the testes is controlled by LHRH which is produced by the hypothalamus and stimulates the release of LH by the pituitary gland. (Sperm production by the testes may also be controlled by FSH production from the pituitary gland and by another hormone produced by the testes itself called "inhibin," which inhibits FSH production).

Male sexuality seems related to the interaction (both constitutional and ac-

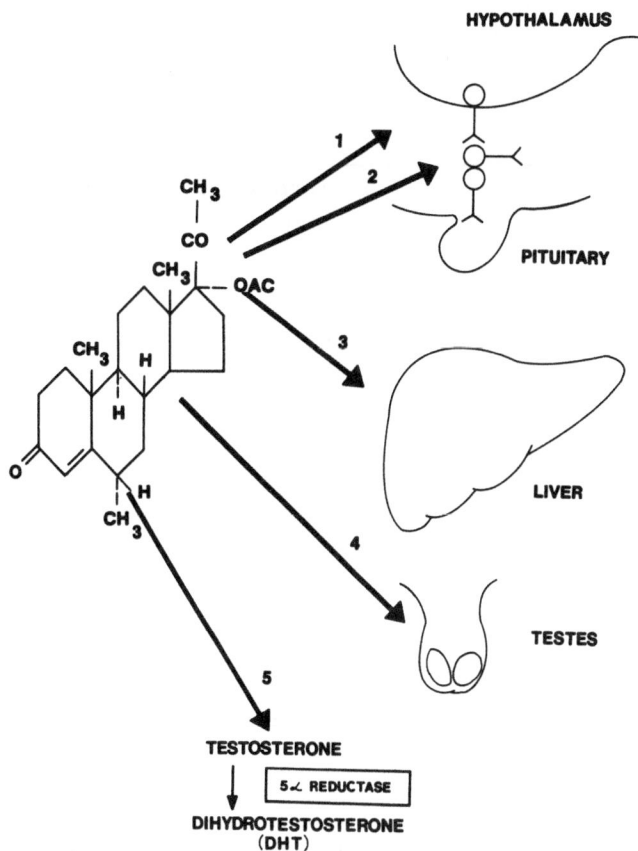

Figure 7. Possible sites of action of medroxyprogesterone acetate. (1) hypothalamic and higher cortical center inhibition; (2) inhibition of FSH and LH release from the pituitary gland; (3) increased hepatic testosterone reductase activity and increased metabolic clearance rate of testosterone by the liver; (4) decreased spermatogenesis and decreased testosterone production; (5) inhibition of the conversion of testosterone to DHT in various tissues and organs, including the central nervous system.

quired) between the central nervous system and the endocrine system. This interaction apparently develops rapidly in early prenatal life in monkeys, guinea pigs, and humans, and during the immediate postnatal period in rats [61]. At those times testosterone secretion from the testes causes actual structural brain changes believed responsible for the development of gender specific sexual behaviors in

Table 7. Recommended Protocol When Employing Antiandrogenic
Medication to Treat Paraphilic Patients

Assessement prior to initiating antiandrogenic treatment	Assessments during antiandrogenic treatment	
1. Testosterone	1. Testosterone	
2. FSH	2. FSH	
3. LH	3. LH	
4. SMA$_{12}$	4. SMA$_{12}$	once every 6 months
5. CBC	5. CBC	
6. Physical examination	6. Physical examination	
7. Blood pressure	7. Blood pressure	
8. Body weight	8. Body weight	once/week
	Major side effects: weight gain, hypertension,	
	Minor side effects: hot flashes, cold sweats, lethargy, myalgias.	

Recommended starting dosage of medroxyprogesterone acetate:
(A) 500 mg IM once/week
(B) 100 mg/cc concentration (rather than 400 mg/cc)
(C) no more than 250 mg into a single injection site
(D) After 4 weeks titrate dosage according to patient's subjective reports.
    (1) increase (up to 800 mg/week) if sexual urges are still too intense
    (2) decrease if problems with side effects or sexual potency
Most of our patients are presently maintained at the 500 mg/week level.

animals and for the suppression in males of the monthly surge of FSH that is ordinarily seen in females [49]. Thus, some biologic changes possibly relevant to
the regulation of sexual behavior may occur prenatally, making subsequent alterations difficult. Nevertheless, better methods of lowering troublesome sexual urges
may be possible. For example, studies have shown that LHRH agonists can suppress testosterone production when given chronically [62]. The mechanism seems
to involve supersaturation of receptors to the point where they no longer function. Since LHRH acts at the pituitary level, entry via the nasal route is possible.
The use of LHRH nasal sprays in human females to treat infertility has been reported, but use in males to decrease testosterone production awaits clinical trials
[63,64]. LHRH antagonists have also been synthesized, and they too hold promise for use in inhibiting testosterone formation [65].

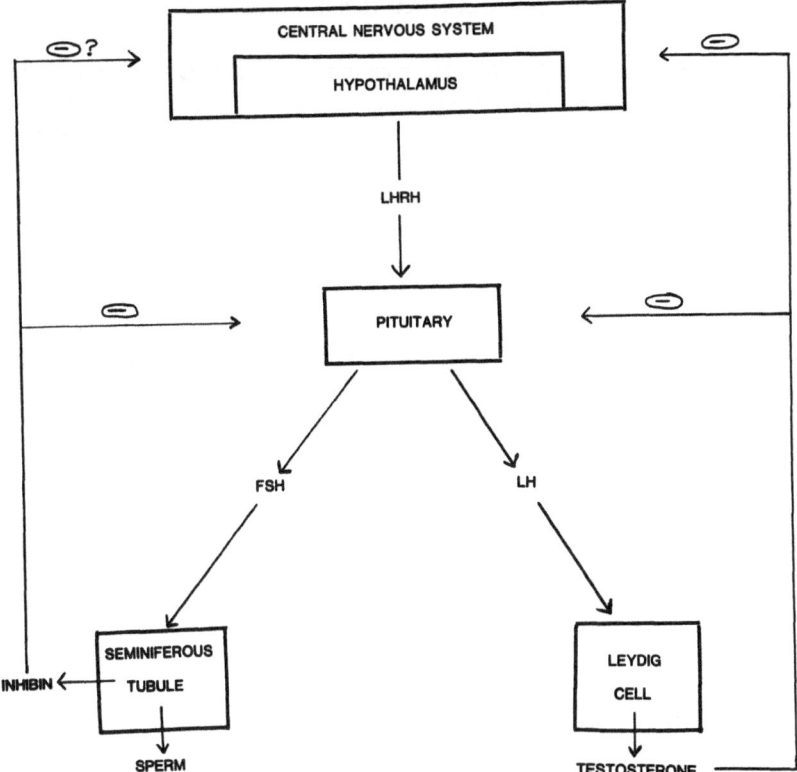

Figure 8. Homeostatic relationship between the hypothalamus, pituitary gland, and testes.

There is evidence that sometimes testosterone exerts biologic effects on the brain only after being converted in the central nervous system to estrogen via aromatization [49]. Aromatizable androgens, for example, can increase the frequency of mounting and lordosis in rabbits; nonaromatizable androgens cannot. ATD, an inhibitor of the anomatase enzyme (which converts testosterone to estrogen) blocks testosterone-stimulated copulatory behavior in rats. Thus, theoretically, in the future it may be possible to block the aromatization of testosterone to estrogen centrally, thereby inhibiting testosterone's action in the brain itself. This might have the benefit of avoiding side effects (such as azospermia) resulting from lowering testosterone production peripherally. The clinical application of this method awaits additional animal trials which will reveal whether aromatose inhibitors can enter the brain and inhibit the conversion of testosterone to estrogens in those areas thought to be related to sexual phenomenology and behavior.

CONCLUDING COMMENTS

Human experience and behavior, including sexual experience and behavior, results from the complex interaction of constitutional factors, willpower, and environmental inputs. Although it is difficult to define the concept of willpower, phenomenologically it is possible to describe what one means in using such a term. When it comes to appetites (or drives) such as hunger, thirst, pain, the need for sleep, or sex, biologic regulatory systems exist which may cause an individual to experience desires to satisfy those hungers which cannot invariably be successfully resisted by means of willpower alone.

Although this chapter has stressed the application of laboratory procedures, it is possible to provide antiandrogenic medication treatment to any interested man experiencing difficulty controlling his sexual behavior through willpower alone, even without performing the tests in question and even if he shows no evidence of a biologic abnormality. Clinical experience suggests that when this form of medication treatment is given to cooperative patients in conjunction with regularily scheduled maintenance group therapy sessions by a well trained caring staff, treatment success is frequently possible. Furthermore, in many instances, this appears to be a just and humane course to follow.

REFERENCES

1. Wirth JB, Folstein MF: Thirst and weight gain during maintenance hemodialysis. Psychosomatics 23:1125-1134, 1982
2. American Psychiatric Association: Diagnostic and Statistical Manual of Mental Disorders, 3rd ed. Washington, DC, APA, 1978
3. Berlin FS: Sex offenders: A biomedical perspective. In J Greu, IA Stuart (eds). Aggression: Current Perspectives in Treatment. New York, Van Nostrand Reinhold, (in press)
4. Evans PR: Masturbatory fantasy and sexual deviation. Behav Res Ther 6:17-49, 1968
5. Quincey VL, Chaplin TC, Varney G: A comparison of rapists' and non-sex offenders sexual preferences for mutually consenting sex, rape, and phyiscal abuse of women. Behav Assess 3:127-135, 1981
6. Parsons JE: The Psychobiology of Sex Differences and Sex Roles. New York, McGraw-Hill, 1980
7. Goy R, McEwen BS: Sexual Differentiation of the Brain. Cambridge, MA, MIT Press, 1977
8. Ehrhardt AA, Epstein R, Money J: Fetal androgens and female gender identity in the early treated adreno-genital syndrome. Johns Hopkins Med J 122:160-167, 1980
9. Pillard RC, Poumandere J, Carretta RN: Is homosexuality familial? A review, some data, and a suggestion. Arch Sex Behav 10:465-475, 1981
10. Boyer RM, Aiman J: The 24-hour secretory pattern of LH and the response to LHRH in transsexual men. Arch Sex Behav 11:157-169, 1982

11. Kolarsky A, Freund K, Machek J, et al: Male sexual deviation associated with early temporal lobe damage. Arch Gen Psychiatry 17:735–743, 1967
12. Migeon C, Forest ME: Androgens in biological fluids. In B Rothfeld (ed): Nuclear Medicine *in vitro*. Philadelphia, Lippincott, 1983
13. Auletta FJ, Caldwell BV, Hamilton GL: Androgens: Testosterone and dihydro-testerone. In B Jaffe, H Behrman (eds): Methods of Hormone Radioimmuno-assay. New York, Academic Press, 1978, pp 715–726
14. Painter K, Niswender G: Radioiodinated steroid hormones—general principles. In B Jaffe, H Behrman (eds): Methods of Hormone Radioimmunoassay. New York, Academic Press, 1978, pp. 727–739
15. DeLacerda L, Kowarski A, Johanson AJ, et al: Integrated concentration and circadian variation of plasma testosterone in normal men. J Clin Endocrinol Metab 37:366, 1973
16. Moudgal NR, Idhar KM, Madhwaraj HG: Pituitary gonadotropins. In B. Jaffe, H Behrman (eds): Methods of Hormone Radioimmunoassay. New York, Academic Press, 1978, pp 173–195
17. Baker HJ, Stoller J: Can a biological force contribute to gender identity? 124:1653–1658, 1968
18. Yumis JJ: New Chromosomal Syndromes. New York, Academic Press, 1977
19. Hack M, Lawce H: The Association of Cytogenetics Technologists Cytogenetics Laboratory Manual. San Francisco, University of California Press, 1980
20. Phelps M: Positron computed studies of cerebral glucose metabolism in man: Theory and application in nuclear medicine. Semin Nucl Med 11:32–49, 1981
21. Ter-Pogossian MM, Raichle ME, Sobel BE: Positron emission tomography. Sci Am 10:169–181, 1980
22. Hutchinson JB: Biological Determination of Sexual Behaviors. Toronto, John Wiley & Sons, 1978
23. Whalen RE: Brain mechanisms controlling sexual behavior. In FA Beach (ed): Human Sexuality in Four Perspectives, Baltimore, Johns Hopkins University Press, 1976
24. Raisman G, Field PM: Sexual dimorphism in the preoptic area of the rat. Science 173:731–733, 1971
25. Orthner H: Textbook of Stereotaxy of the Human Brain. Albuquerque, NM, University of New Mexico Press, 1979
26. Christensen LW, Nance DM, Garski RA: Effects of hypothalamic and preoptic lesions on reproductive behavior in male rats. Brain Res Bull 2:137–141, 1977
27. Whalen RE, Luttge WG, Gorgalka BB: Neonatal androgenization and the development of estrogen responsivitity in male and female rats. Horm Behav 2:83–90, 1971
28. Kierniesky NC, Gerall AA: Effects of testosterone propronate on the brain on the sexual behavior and peripheral tissue of the male rat. Psychobiol Behav 11:633–640, 1973
29. Malsbury CW: Facilitation of male rat copulatory behavior by electrical stimulation of the medial preoptic area. Psychobiol Behav 7:797–805, 1971
30. Kluver H, Bucy PC: Preliminary analysis of functions of the temporal lobes in monkeys. Arch Neurol Psychiatry 42:979–1000, 1939
31. Schreiver L, Kling A: Behavioral changes following paleocortical injury in rodents, carnivores, and primates. Fed Proc 12:419:128, 1953
32. Roeder FD, Muller D, Orthner H: The stereotaxic treatment of pedophilic homosexuality and other sexual deviations. In E Hitchcock, L Laitienn, K Vaernet (eds): Psychosurgery, Springfield, IL, Charles C. Thomas, 1972

304   BERLIN AND SCHAERF

33. Sweet WH, Obrader S, Martin-Rodriguez JG: Neurosurgical Treatment in Psychiatry, Pain, and Epilepsy, Baltimore, University Park Press, 1977
34. Freund K: Therapeutic sex drive reduction. Acta Psych Scand 62 (suppl):1-39, 1980
35. Cullington GJ: Psychosurgery: National commission issues surprisingly favorable report. Science 194:299-301, 1976
36. Abel G: Evaluating objective methods of determining arousal. Treatment for Sexual Aggressiveness News, 5:1,3-4, 1972
37. Sturup GK: Castration: The total treatment. In HPL Resnik, ME Wolfgang (eds): Sexual Behaviors: Social, Clinical and Legal Aspects. Boston, Little Brown & Co, 1972, pp 361-382
38. Wiffels AJAM: Het castratie Vraagstuk. Nach der englischen zusammenfassung. Leyden, 1954
39. Sturup GK: Treating the "Untreatable" Chronic Criminals at Herstedvester. Baltimore, The Johns Hopkins University Press, 1968
40. Bremer J: Asexualization: A Follow-up Study of 244 Cases. New York, MacMillan Publishing Co, 1959
41. Langerin R, Paitch D, Hucker S, et al: The effect of assertiveness training, provera, and sex of therapist in the treatment of genital exhibitionism. J Behav Ther Exp Psychiatry 10:275-282, 1979
42. Cooper AJ: A placebo controlled trial fo the antiandrogen cyproterone acetate in deviant hypersexuality. Compr Psych 22:458-465, 1981
43. Berlin FS, Meinecke CF: Treatment of sex offenders with antiandrogenic medication: Conceptualization, review of treatment modalities and preliminary findings. Am J Psych 138:601-607, 1981
44. Berlin FS, Coyle GS: Sexual deviation syndromes. Johns Hopkins Med J 149:119-125, 1981
45. Kochakian CD: Definition of androgens and proteins of anabolic steroids. Pharmacol Ther [B] 1:149-177, 1975
46. Murad F, and Haynes, Jr., RC, Androgens and anabolic steroids. In AG Gilman, LS Goodman, A Gilman (eds): Pharmacological Basis of Therapeutics, New York, MacMillan, 1980
47. Bardin C, Wayne C: Pituitary-testicular axis. In S Yen, R Jaffe (eds): Reproductive Endocrinology. Philadelphia, WB Saunders, 1978
48. Eikens B, Kristen B: Biosynthesis and secretion of testicular steroids. In RO Greep, E Astwood (eds): Handbook of Psychology. Section 7, Volume 5. Washington, DC, American Psychological Society, 1975
49. McEwen B, Davis P, Parsons B, et al: The brain as a target for steroid hormone action. In W Cowon (eds): Annual Review of Neuroscience, Palo Alto, CA, Annual Reviews Inc, 1979
50. Bardin C, Wayne C, Paulsen CA: In RH Williams (ed): The Testes. Textbook of Endocrinology, Philadelphia, WB Saunders, 1981
51. McDonald PC, Grodin DM, Sitteri PK: Dynamics of androgen and oestrogen secretion. In DT Baird, JA Strong (eds): Gonadal Steroid Secretion. Edinburgh, Edinburgh Universtiy Press, 1971
52. Nisula BC, Dunn JF: Measurement of the testosterone binding parameters for both testosterone estradiol binding globulin and albumin in individual serum samples. Steroids 34:771-791, 1971
53. Huggins C, Hodges CV: Studies on prostatic cancer. I) The effect of castration of estrogen and of androgen injection on serum phosphatases in metastatic carcinoma of the prostate. Cancer Res 1:293, 1943

54. Newmann F, Graf KJ, Hasan SH, et al: Central action of antiandrogens. In L Martini, M Motts (eds): Androgens and Antiandrogens. New York, Raven Press, 1977
55. Collip PJ, Kaplan SA, Boyle DC, et al: Constitutional isosexual prococious puberty: Effects of medroxyprogesterone acetate therapy. Amer J of Dis Child 108:359, 1964
56. Kaplan SA, Ling SM, Irani NG: Idiopathic sexual precocity: Therapy with medroxyprogesterone. Am J of Dis Child 116:591–598, 1968
57. Altman K, Gordon G, Southern AL, et al: On the mechanism of the antiandrogenic effect of medroxyprogesterone acetate. Endorcinol 90:1252–1260, 1972
58. Albin J, Vittek J, Gordon G, et al: On the mechanism of the antiandrogenic effect of medroxyprogesterone acetate. Endocrinology 93:417–422, 1973
59. Camacho AM, Williams LD, Montalvo JM: Alterations of testicular histology and chromosomes in patients with constitutional sexual precocity treated with medroxyprogesterone acetate. J Clin Endocrinol Metab 34:279–286, 1972
60. Meyer W, Walker P, Wiedeking C, et al: Pituitary function in adult males receiving medroxyprogesterone acetate. Fertil Steril 28:10:1072–1076, 1977
61. Moore R: Neuroendocrine regulation of reproduction. In S Yen, R Jaffe (eds): Reproductive Endocrinology. Philadephial, WB Saunders, 1978
62. Pelletier G, Dusan GL, Belanger A, et al: Further studies on the inhibitory effect of D-ala^6-des-gly-Na$_2$^{10}-LHRH ethylamide on spermatogenesis and steroidogenesis in the rat: Reversibility and effect of androgen administration. J Androl 1:171–181, 1980
63. Lemay A: Fertility. Fertil Steril 32:646, 1979
64. Lemay A, Aaure N: Sensitivity of gonadotropin and corpus luteum responses to single intranasal administration of [D-Ser(TBU)6-des-gly-NH$_2$^{10}] LHRH ethylamide (Buserelin) in normal women. Presented at the 63rd Annual Meeting of the Endocrine Society. Cincinnati, OH, June 17–19, 1981
65. Rivier C, Rivier J, Vale W: Antireproductive effects of a potent gonadotropin-releasing hormone antagonist in the male rat. Science 210:93–95, 1980

Future Directions

CHAPTER 15

The Endorphins

STEVEN R. GAMBERT

Perhaps no hormone or group of hormones has received such notoriety in such a short amount of time as have the endorphins. These neurotransmitters, sometimes referred to as endogenous opioid peptides, were first discovered in 1964 when C. H. Li at the Hormone Research Laboratory of the University of California in San Francisco isolated a 91-amino-acid molecule with recognized morphine-like effects from the pituitary gland [1]. Readers are referred to a more detailed review of the structure and physiologic actions of this group of peptides which has recently been published [2]. In brief, beta-endorphin is one fragment of the larger peptide, beta-lipotropin (endorphin: beta-lipotropin 61-91; enkephalin: beta-lipotropin 61-65). The entire beta-liporropin is a polypeptide hormone contained within a 31,000-dalton glycoprotein molecule known as pro-opiocortin, also containing ACTH within its structure [3-5].

Beta-endorphin is found not only in the pons intermedia and adenohypophysis portions of the pituitary gland, but also in the hypothalamus, corpus striatum, midbrain, and to a lesser degree, cerebrum [6-8]. Enkephalin has been found throughout the body in areas including brain, spinal cord, gastrointestinal tract, pancreas, sympathetic ganglia, and adrenal medulla [9,10,11-15].

Several forms of the endorphins have been noted as well as several opioid receptor subtypes. Three types of receptors have been clearly described using standard pharmacologic methodology; μ, k, and σ.

The μ receptor mediates the well-known effects of morphine, i.e., analgesia, euphoria, respiratory depression, miosis, and a specific abstinence syndrome after habituation.

Handbook of Psychiatric Diagnostic Procedures, vol. 2, edited by R. C. W. Hall and T. P. Beresford. Copyright © 1985 by Spectrum Publications, Inc.

Ketocyclazocine is the principal agonist for the k receptor, producing analgesia, motor incoordination, but sedation more than euphoria. K receptor agonists also lead to an abstinence syndrome after chronic administration.

The third receptor subtype, σ, is stimulated by the pharmacologic agent SKF (10047 (N-allylnormetazocine). Stimulation results in midriasis, euphoria, delusions, and hallucinations. A more detailed discussion concerning these receptors can be found in the literature [16–19].

Nallorphine is credited as being the first clinically available opiate antagonist. *In vivo* this agent has mixed agonist/antagonist activity, completely antagonizing μ receptors while partially activating other receptors [20]. Naloxone and naltrexone are considered to be pure opioid antagonists, with specific action at the μ receptor. Due to the fact that a higher dose of naloxone is required to block the effects mediated by the σ and k receptor, large doses (up to 50 times that required to antagonize morphine) have been generally employed in clinical studies. In low dosage, naloxone and naltrexone are considered safe and without appreciable side-effects in persons not on other medications. At high dosages, however, naltrexone has produced a distinct dysphoria [21].

It is of great interest that certain psychotomimetic agents appear to stimulate σ receptors. Phencyclidine (PCP, angel dust), a known hallucinogenic, is one such agent. In addition, both SKF 10047 and cyclazocine have psychotomimetic properties in man at certain doses.

It appears that certain pharmacologic agents may modify behavior mediated through specific opioid receptors.

Most of the literature to date exploring the role of the endorphins in mental illness have unfortunately only evaluated μ receptor agonists and antagonists. Clinical manifestations resulting from endorphin administration likewise have not been clearly linked to any receptor subtype.

Numerous studies have been conducted linking psychiatric illnesses and the endorphins with varied results.

ENDORPHINS AND MENTAL HEALTH–SCHIZOPHRENIA

Many investigators have attempted to prove a causal relationship between schizophrenia and either an excess or deficiency of endorphins. Some have even argued that the presence of an abnormal endorphin may alter mental health, though conclusive evidence is still lacking.

Although some argue that circulating basal levels of plasma beta-endorphin are too low to measure reliably, Ross and co-workers [22] did report no difference in plasma beta-endorphin immunoreactivity when comparing 98 schizophrenics to 41 normal controls.

In 1977, Wagenmaher and Cade [23] excited the psychiatric world by reporting resolution of psychotic symptoms in five of six schizophrenics during long term hemodialysis therapy. Palmour and Ervin [24] in analyzing the dialysate described Leu^5-beta-endorphin as present. Unfortunately, other attempts since have failed to confirm these observations [25,26].

Although cerebrospinal fluid (CSF) is the body fluid most closely associated with the brain, access is difficult. Despite this, several studies have evaluated the CSF for endorphins in mental illness with mixed results [27-29]. It is imperative that investigators control for the stress associated with blood drawing and lumbar puncture, as stress of any type has clearly been shown to be a major cause of increased beta-endorphin [30].

Beta-endorphin has been given to schizophrenics with limited success to date, perhaps in part due to small sample size, brevity of trials, and difficulty in documenting improvement in mental function [31-34]. Other studies have attempted to explore the possible relationship of opioid excess and schizophrenia. Davis et al [35] gave naloxone (0.4 mg IV) to 12 chronic schizophrenics while monitoring several parameters of psychosis. They reported a significant decrease in unusual thought content following the use of this opioid antagonist. Using higher doses of naloxone (10 mg), and a longer observation period, some improvement was noted in a majority of 11 patients studied. Although other studies have reported positive results, most have concluded negatively [36-39].

To date, the role of the endorphins in schizophrenia still remains in question. Discrepant results have arisen largely due to differing experimental design, data analysis, and assay procedures. In addition, work has focused almost exclusively on agonists and antagonists of the μ receptor. Until agonists and antagonists of other receptor types, especially σ, are studied in humans, no definitive statement can be made.

ENDORPHINS AND AFFECTIVE DISORDERS

Although several reports have linked the endorphins to affective illness, data remains speculative at this time. In 1970, Fink and co-workers [40] reported an antidepressant effect for cyclazocine, predominantly a σ receptor agonist. This finding arose during ongoing research on narcotic antagonists. Ten chronically depressed hospitalized patients who were refractory to conventional medications were given increasing doses from 0.2 mg to 3 mg per day orally. This dose was then decreased to 2 mg daily after three weeks. Eight of the ten subjects were reported to have either a complete or partial resolution of their depressive symptoms. Although predictable side effects were initially seen (e.g., drowsiness, dizziness, blurred vision, nausea, constipation and sleep disturbance), tolerance to these developed by the third week of the trial. In the same paper, the authors reported results from a drug trial on 19 subjects with acute depression. Ten reported moderate to marked improvement. Eight of the nine who had little or no response had dose limiting side effects. Cyclazocine has potent narcotic antagonistic effects at the μ receptor in man, but only modest analgesic potential. In addition, it can cause hallucinations and delusions making its clinical use limited at present.

In an interesting report, Davis et al [41] noted that affectively ill patients had a greater tolerance to painful stimuli from electrical shocks than normal volunteers. This lead to speculation that affective illness and an excess of endorphins may be causally related. Davis and co-workers then gave large doses of naloxone, 20 mg IV, to ten hospitalized patients suffering from mania [42]. Although this was done in a double-blind fashion using placebo and there was frequent and prolonged (up to 8 hours) evaluation, no effect was noted. This was in contrast to the small transient effect observed by Janowsky and co-workers [43], who administered lower doses of naloxone to 12 manic or hypomanic patients who were continued on their lithium and/or other psychotropic agents.

Pickar et al [34] administered beta-endorphin to four depressed patients without an observed effect. Catlin and co-workers [44] also reported minimal effects from an infusion of beta-endorphin to eight chronically depressed subjects. Two studies have reported a transient improvement in mood [31,33] following an infusion of beta-endorphin.

In an attempt to block morphine-like activity, methadone was administered intravenously to ten hospitalized depressives [45]. Although no change was noted in mental function following the infusion, previously elevated basal levels of cortisol returned to normal. This was of particular interest in light of the report of Carroll et al showing elevated plasma cortisol levels in patients with endogenous depression [46].

Although a few reports have appeared [47], no conclusive data is yet available regarding the relationship between levels of endorphins in the CSF and affective illness. In general, no definitive conclusion can be reached regarding any possible relatinship between the endorphins and affective illness.

CONCLUSIONS

Despite the wealth of data which has been accumulated on the endorphins and mental illness, no final conclusions have been reached. Once again, problems have arisen due to differences in study design and assay methodology. Unfortunately, most studies have almost exclusively examined agonist and antagonist agents acting at the μ receptor with little attention to other receptor types.

Much work still needs to be done to better define a possible relationship between endorphins and mental health. At present, the assay is too cumbersome to be widely utilized by the practicing clinician. Although "kits" are available to measure beta-endorphin, one must keep in mind that these are not very precise in terms of actual measurements. Any hope of giving endorphin analogs or antagonists on a large scale must await the development of agents with less potential risks and side effects.

Another major barrier to research on the endorphins stems from their possible role in so many physiologic functions. Subjects selected, whether with mental illness or not, must be carefully screened. It now appears that the opioids may be affected by age [48–49], stress [50-54], altered feeding behavior [55-69], body temperature [70,71], shock [72-74], and sexual activity [75-79].

Whatever barriers may presently exist, the future holds many promises. Ongoing and anticipated research will hopefully provide the answer as to whether there is truly a link between the endorphins and mental health. However, until a definitive link is established and methods developed for easy clinical use, the clinician has little practical use for any of the opioid agonists or antagonists in either diagnosing or treating mental illness.

LABORATORY DETERMINATION OF THE ENDORPHINS

Investigations to date have determined levels of the endogenous opioids in a variety of tissue using varied methodology. To date, no one method appears to be the only acceptable one. Problems have arisen due to differences in antibody specificity and in general low levels of the respective peptides in body fluids.

To accurately determine the exact amount of beta-endorphin, either an antibody must be used that will recognize this peptide exclusively or samples must first be chromatographically analyzed to eliminate competing peptides. There has not been much success in obtaining an antibody which recognizes only beta-endorphin, although a few report success. In several reports, cross-reactivity to beta-lipotropin has been reported as low as 10%; however, most antibodies available either commercially or from research laboratories throughout the country report cross-reactivity somewhere between 50 and 100%. This necessitates measurements of beta-endorphin being qualified with a statement that levels actually obtained more reflect "beta-endorphin immunoreactivity" and not true levels of beta-endorphin. This methodologic problem has led to a lot of confusion in the literature and may be the single most important barrier to better defining the role of the endorphins in clinical practice.

Not only is a chromatographic isolation of beta-endorphin time consuming, but it necessitates laboratory expertise and time often not readily available. In addition, a large amount of blood is required for this process further making it clinically undesirable.

A standardized protocol for accurately determining beta-endorphin in plasma is listed below.

Plasma Extraction Procedure

1. Blood is collected using a heparinized plastic syringe. At all times blood should be kept on ice.
2. 15-20 ml of plasma is mixed with silicic acid (60 mg/ml).
3. The mixture is then shaken for 20 minutes at $10°C$, after which it is centrifuged for 10 minutes at ~ 3000 rpm at $5°C$.
4. Precipitates are washed with 4 ml. of buffer (0.01 PB, 0.15 M NaCl, 0.1% human serum albumin). Misture is centrifuged (3000 rpm at $5°C$) and the supernatant discarded.
5. The precipitate is again washed, this time using 4 ml of cold distilled water and the supernatant is again discarded.
6. 4 ml of 40% acetone/60% 0.1 N HCl is added to the precipitate. This mixture is then vortexed for one minute at $5°C$, centrifuged at 3000 rpm at $5°C$, and the supernatant saved. Process is repeated.
7. Supernatants (extracts) are combined and lyophilized or evaporated under N_2 at $45°C$.

Chromatographic Separation of Beta-Endorphin*

8. Above extracts are reconstituted in 0.1 N acetic acid with 0.1% bovine serum albumin (BSA) (500 μl).
9. Samples are placed onto a 0.9 $\times$ 30 cm column packed with Sephadex G-50 (fine) mesh using 0.1 N acetic acid with 0.1% BSA (300 μl).
10. Fractions are collected (30, 1.0 ml fractions) and then lyophilized.
11. Using known beta-endorphin as a marker, appropriate fractions are saved for determination of beta-endorphin using standard radioimmunoassay techniques. Each laboratory must establish their own standards as many variables may influence where beta-endorphin actually elutes.

REFERENCES

1. Li, CH: Lipotropin, a new active peptide from pituitary glands. Nature 201: 924–927, 1964
2. Cheung AL, Goldstein A: Failure of hypophysectomy to alter brain content of opioid peptides (endorphins). Life Sci 25:1005–1008, 1976

---

*Necessary if antibody to be used in radioimmunoassay is not very specific.

3. Mains RE, Eipper BA, Ling M: Common precursor to corticotropins and endorphins. Proc Natl Acad Sci 74:3014–3018, 1977
4. Roberts JL, Herbert G: Characterization of a common precursor to corticotropin and β-lipotropin: Cell-free synthesis of the precursor and identification of corticotropin peptides in the molecule. Proc Natl Acad Sci 74:4826–4830, 1977
5. Rubinstein M, Stein S, Udenfriend S: Characterization of proopiocortin, a precursor to opioid peptides and corticotropin. Proc Natl Acad Sci 75:669–671, 1978
6. Bugnon C, Block B, Lenys D, et al: Infundibular neurons of the human hypothalamus simultaneously reactive with antisera against endorphins, ACTH, MSH and beta-LPH. Cell Tissue Res 199:177–1796, 1979
7. Rossier J, Veago TM, Minick S, et al: Regional distribution of β-endorphin and enkephalin content in rat brain and pituitary. Proc Natl Acad Sci 74:5162–5165, 1977
8. Gambert SR, Garthwaite TL, Pontzer CH: Age-related changes in central nervous system beta-endorphin and ACTH. Neuroendocrinol 31:252–255, 1980
9. Watson SJ, Akil H, Richard III, CW, et al: Evidence for two separate opiate peptide neuronal systems. Nature 275:226–228, 1978
10. Bloom RE, Battenberg E, Rossier J, et al: Endorphins are located in the intermediate and anterior lobes of the pituitary gland, not in the neurohypophysis. Life Sci 20:43–47, 1977
11. Schultzberg M, Hokfelt T, Lundbert JM, et al: Enkephalin-like immunoreactivity in nerve terminals in sympathetic ganglia and adrenal medulla and in adrenal medullary gland cells. Acta Physiol Scand 103:475–477, 1978
12. Schultzberg M, Lundbert JM, Hokfelt T: Enkephalin-like immunoreactivity in gland cells and nerve terminals of the adrenal medulla. Neuroscience 3:1169–1186, 1978
13. Lundberg JM, Hamberger B, Schultzberg M, et al: Enkephalin- and somatostalin-like immunoreactivities in human adrenal medulla and pheochromocytoma. Proc Natl Acad Sci 76:4079–4083, 1979
14. Lewis RV, Stern AS, Rossier J, et al: Putative enkephalin precursor in bovine adrenal medulla. Biochem Biophys Res Commun 89:822
15. Di Guilio AM, Yang HYT, Lutold BE, et al: Pharmacologist 20:167–170, 1978
16. Adler MW: The *in vivo* differentiation of opiate receptors. Life Sci 28:1543–1545, 1981
17. Martin WR: Multiple opioid receptors. Life Sci 28:1547–1554, 1981
18. Cowan A: Simple in vivo tests that differentiate prototype agonists of opiate receptors. Life Sci 28:1559–1570, 1981
19. Herling S, Woods JH: Discriminative stimulus effects of narcotics: Evidence for multiple receptor-mediated actions. Life Sci 28:1571–1584, 1981
20. Jaffe JH, Martin WR: Narcotic analgesics and antagonists. In LS Goodman, A Gilman (eds): The Pharmacological Basis of Therapeutics. 5th ed. New York, Macmillan Publishing Co, 1975
21. Mendelson JH, Ellingboe J, Keukule JC, et al: Effects of naltrexone on mood and neuroendocrine function in normal adult males. Psychoneuroendocrinol 3:231–236, 1979
22. Ross M, Berger PA, Goldstein A: Plasma β-endorphin immunoreactivity in schizophrenia. Science 205:1163–1164, 1979
23. Wagemaker H, Cade R: Use of hemodialysis in chronic schizophrenia. Am J Psych 134:684–685, 1977

24. Palmour RM, Ervin FR: Biochemical and physiological characteristics of a peptide from the hemodialysate of psychotic patients. Psychopharmacol Bull 15: 21-24, 1979
25. Lewis RV, Gerber CD, Stein S, et al: On β_h-Leu^5-endorphin and schizophrenia. Arch Gen Psych 36:237-239, 1979
26. Cohen IM, Schreiber SC, Yamamura H: Why should dialysis benefit schizophrenia? J Nerv Ment Dis 167:475-477, 1979
27. Lindstrom LH, Gunne LM, Wahlstrom A, et al: Endorphins in human CSF: Clinical correlations to some psychotic states. Acta Psychiatr Scand 57:153-164, 1978
28. Rimon R, Terenius L, Kampman R: Cerebrospinal fluid endorphin in schizophrenia. Acta Psych Scand 61:395-403, 1980
29. Domschke W, Dickschas, Mitznegg P: Cerebrospinal fluid β-endorphin in schizophrenia. Lancet 1:1024, 1979
30. Nakao K, Oki S, Tanaka I, et al: Immunoreactive β-endorphin and adrenocorticotropin in human cerebrospinal fluid. J Clin Invest 66:1383-1380, 1980
31. Guillemin R, Vargo T, Rossier J, et al: β-endorphin and adrenocorticotropin are secreted concomitantly by the pituitary gland. Science 197:1367-1369, 1977
32. Kline NS, Li CH, Lehmann HE, et al: β-endorphin induced changes in schizophrenia and depressed patients. Arch Gen Psych 34:1111-1113, 1977
33. Gerner RH, Catlin DH, Gorelick DA, et al: β-endorphins: Intravenous infusion causes behavioral changes in psychiatric inpatients. Arch Gen Psych 37:642-647, 1980
34. Pickar D, Davis GC, Schulz I, et al: Behavioral and biological effects of acute β-endorphin injection in schizophrenic and depressed patients. Am J Psych 138:160-166, 1981
35. Davis GC, Bunney WE, DeFraites EG, et al: Intravenous naloxone administration in schizophrenia and affective illness. Science 197:75-77, 1977
36. Volavka J, Mallya A, Baig S: Naloxone in chronic schizophrenia. Science 196: 1227-1228, 1977
37. Janowsky DS, Segal DS, Bloom F, et al: Lack of effects of naloxone on schizophrenic symptoms. Am J Psych 134:926-927, 1977
38. Kurland AA, McCabe OL, Hanlon TE, et al: The treatment of perceptual disturbances in schizophrenia with naloxone hydrochloride Am J Psych 134: 1408-1410, 1977
39. Lipinski J, Meyer R, Kornetsky C, et al: Naloxone in schizophrenia: Negative results. Lancet 1:1292-1293, 1979
40. Fink M, Simeon J, Itil T, et al: Clinical antidepressant activity of cyclazocine, a narcotic antatonist. Clin Pharm Ther 2:41-48, 1970
41. Davis GC, Buschsbaum M, Bunney Jr, WE: Analgesia to painful stimuli in affective illness. Am J Psych 136:1148-1152, 1979
42. Davis GC, Extein I, Reus V, et al: Failure of naloxone to reduce manic symptoms. Am J Psych 137:1583-1585, 1980
43. Janowsky D, Judd L, Huey L, et al: Naloxone effects on manic symptoms and growth hormone levels. Lancet 2:320-321, 1978
44. Catlin DH, Gorelich D, Gerner R, et al: Clinical effects of β-endorphin infusions. Adv Biochem Pharmacol 22:465-472, 1980
45. Extein I, Pickar D, Gold M, et al: Methadone and morphine in depression. Psychopharm Bull 17:29-33, 1981

46. Carroll BJ, Curtis GC, Mendels J: Neuroendocrine regulation in depression II. Discrimination of depressed from nondepressed patients. Arch Gen Psych 33:1051–1058, 1976
47. Terenius L, Wahlstrom A, Agren H: Naloxone treatment in depression: Clinical observations and effects on cerebrospinal fluid endorphins and monoamine metabolites. Psychopharmacol 54:31–33, 1977
48. Bayon A, Shoemaker WJ, Bloom FE: Perinatal development of the endorphin- and enkephalin-containing systems in the rat brain. Brain Res 179:93–95, 1979
49. Gambert SR: Interaction of age and thyroid hormone status on beta-endorphin content in rat corpus striatum and hypothalamus. Neuroendocrinol 32:114–117, 1981
50. Akil H, Madden J, Patrick RL: In HW Kosterlitz (ed): Opiates and Endogenous Opioid Peptides, Amsterdam, Elsevier, 1976
51. Hayes RL, Bennett GJ, Newlon P, et al: Neuroscience Abst 2:939–942, 1976
52. Chance WT, White AC, Krynock GM, et al: Conditional fear-induced antinociception and decreased binding of [^{3}H]-leu-enkephalin to rat brain. Brain Res 141:371–374, 1978
53. Chesher GB, Chan B: Footshock induced analgesia in mice: Its reversal by naloxone and cross-tolerance with morphine. Life Sci 21:1569–1574, 1977
54. Madeen JH, Akil RL, Barchas JD, et al: Stress-induced parallel changes in central opioid levels and pain responsiveness in the rat. Nature 265:358–360, 1977
55. Morley JE: The neuroendocrine control of appetite: The role of the endogenous opiates, cholecystokinin, TRH, gamma-aminobutyric acid and the diazepam receptor. Life Sci 27:355–368, 1980
56. Baile CA, Keim DA, Della-Fera MA: Opiate antagonists and agonists and feeding in sheep. Physiol Behav 26:1019–1023, 1981
57. King BM, Castellanos FX, Kastin AJ, et al: Naloxone-induced suppression of food intake in normal and hypothalamic obese rats. Pharmacol Biochem Behav 11:729–732, 1979
58. Brown DR, Holtzman SR: Suppression of deprivation-induced food and water intake in rats and mice by naloxone. Pharmacol Biochem Behav 11:567–573, 1979
59. Brands B, Thornhill JA, Hirst M, et al: Suppression of food intake and body weight gain by naloxone in rats. Life Sci 24:1773–1779, 1979
60. Sanger DJ, McCarthy PS, Metcalf G: The effects of opiate antagonists on food intake are stereospecific. Neuropharmacol 20:45–47, 1981
61. Holtzman SG: Suppression of appetitive behavior in the rat by naloxone: Lack of effect of prior morphine dependence. Life Sci 24:219–226, 1979
62. Morley JE, Levine AS: Stress-induced eating is mediated through endogenous opiates. Science 209:1259–1261, 1980
63. Schulz R, Wuster M, Herz A: Interaction of amphetamine and naloxone in feeding behavior in guinea pigs. Eur J Pharmacol 53:313–319, 1980
64. Margules DL, Moisset B, Lewis MJ, et al: β-endorphin is associated with overeating in genetically obese (ob/ob) and rats (fa/fa). Science 202:988–991, 1978
65. McGivern RF, Bernston GG: Mediation of diurnal fluctuations in pain sensitivity in the rat by food intake patterns: Reversal by naloxone. Science 210:210–211, 1980

66. Garthwaite, TL, Martinson DR, Tseng LF, et al: A longitudinal hormonal profile for the genetically obese mouse. Endocrinol 107:671–676, 1980
67. Rossier J, Rogers J, Shibasaki T, et al: Opioid peptides and a-melanocyte-stimulating hormone in genetically obest (ob/ob) mice during development. Proc Natl Acad Sci 76:2077–2080, 1979
68. Gambert SR, Garthwaite TL, Pontzer CH, et al: Fasting associated with decrease in hypothalamic β-endorphin. Science 210:1271–1272, 1980
69. McGivern R, Berka C, Bernston GG, et al: Effect of naloxone on analgesia induced by food deprivation. Life Sci 25:885–888, 1979
70. Wallace M, Fraser CD, Clements JA, et al: Naloxone, adrenalectomy, and steroid replacement: Evidence against a role for circulating β-endorphin in food intake. Endocrinol 108:189–192, 1981
71. Bloom A, Tseng LF: The effects of beta-endorphin and body temperature in the mouse. Soc Neurosci 5:524–530, 1979
72. Faden AI, Holaday JW: Experimental endotoxin shock: The pathophysiologic function of endorphins and treatment with opiate antagonists. J Infect Dis 142:229–238, 1980
73. Holaday JW, Faden AI: Naloxone reversal of endotoxin hypotension suggests a role of endorphins in shock. Nature 275:450–451, 1978
74. Reynolds DG, Gurll NJ, Vargish T, et al: Blockade of opiate receptors with naloxone improves survival and cardiac performance in endotoxic shock. Circulation 7:39–48, 1980
75. McDoubal JN, Marques PR, Burks TF: Thermic responses to morphine in cold and young rats. Proc West Pharmacol Soc 23:235–238, 1980
76. McIntosh TK, Vallano ML, Barfield RJ: Effects of morphine, β-endorphin, and naloxone on catecholamine levels and sexual behavior in the male rat. Pharmacol Biochem Behav 13:435–441, 1980
77. Ostrowski NL, Stapleton JM, Noble RG, et al: Morphine and naloxone's effects on sexual behavior of the female golden hamster. Pharmacol Biochem Behav 11:673–681, 1979
78. Pellegrini Quarantotti B, Corda MGl Paglietti E, et al: Inhibition of copulatory behavior in male rats by d-ala^2-met-enkephalin amide. Life Sci 23:673–678, 1978
79. Hetta J: Effects of morphine and naltrexone on sexual behavior of the male rat. Acta Pharmacol Toxicol 4(Suppl):53–58, 1977

CHAPTER 16

Computerized Psychiatric Practice

THOMAS P. BERESFORD and RICHARD C. W. HALL

INTRODUCTION

Each new technical advance in the understanding of health and disease has served to heighten the fear that man would one day come to view himself as a machine. So it was in the 17th century when William Harvey undertook his investigations of the human circulatory system. He published the results of his research many years after they had been completed in order to lessen their effect in placing human beings more in the proximity of the animal kingdom and further from the cherished view of ourselves as children of God.

In our age, one that is perhaps more akin to the Renaissance than to the Restoration, technical advances cause us to fear for the loss of our humanity. Much of this fear can be attributed to the technologic breakthroughs which resulted in the advent of atomic weapons. The destructive power of technology demonstrated at Hiroshima and Nagasaki cast a necessary doubt upon the optimistic view of human life occasioned by our increased understanding.

The greater part of our fear, however, is due to a more traditional cause: human ignorance and misunderstanding. As our knowledge of the world increases, so does the apparent complexity of that world. As complexity increases, as we realize how much we do not know, we want to hold tightly to our previous concepts and

Handbook of Psychiatric Diagnostic Procedures, vol. 2, edited by R. C. W. Hall and T. P. Beresford. Copyright © 1985 by Spectrum Publications, Inc.

modes of behavior. Most of us probably prefer to think romatically of ourselves as humanistic diagnosticians and therapists rather than as performing the more realistic and usually more tedious work of examining our own clinical assumptions and methods.

"Diagnosis," says R. D. Couch, "is the most hallowed and richly historic element of medicine. It is an activity in which every physician considers himself an expert. It is the heart that pumps the life and blood through medicine. To inquire of its' objectivity, to dissect its components, to improve on its efficiency or to relegate it to machines are all equally unthinkable and necessary.

"There is a diagnostic process, whether or not we agree exactly upon what it is or how it works. It can be described in explicit terms. It includes what is called 'clinical judgement' and what is in fact wisdom. Intuition in diagnosis is a myth and in reality is probably a 'pruned decision tree.' " [1]

The advent of widely available computer technology in the last few years has brought with it the fear Dr. Couch articulates. To make use of these new machines, to "talk" to computers, we must ourselves learn a new language. That language is necessarily terse, objective, and exceedingly simple. It is so because the machine itself can make use of information only on these terms. To the man using the machine, the language often appears complex because it is strange and often dull, because it is written to make use of a machine rather than for the poetic expression of human existence.

When using this language, one quickly realizes that the computer is no more than an adjunct to human observation and thought. Further, the demands of the highly specific language of computers necessitates our looking at our own methods of human observation and thought in minute detail in order to communicate them simply to the computer. As Sir William Harvey performed a step-wise examination of the anatomy and physiology of the circulatory system to make that knowledge useful in understanding health and disease, we have the opportunity in our age to examine our methods of observation and integration to the same purpose. Much work has already begun in this area of human understanding. The purpose of this chapter is to review some of it as it relates to the nature of psychiatric practice. Most of the knowledge in computer applications to health care lies ahead of us. As this understanding and its subsequent applications develop, it will undoubtedly appear as one more significant advance in that tradition of medical knowledge begun in the time of William Harvey and pursued, in Sir Francis Bacon's phrase, "to the accomplishment of all things possible." [2]

INFORMATION SYSTEMS

McDonald points out that over 50 hospitals in this country currently have large computer systems that allow them to establish banks of information on specific patients [3]. His own system at the University of Indiana currently has data on some 50,000 medicine patients. Typically, such large systems begin in hospitals in order to increase the effectiveness of fiscal management.

Nonetheless, software programs capable of managing clinical data on large numbers of patients have been developed in several centers. These include the PROMIS system at the University of Vermont, the MUMPS system at the Massachusetts General Hospital and the CARE and HELP systems at the University of Indiana. Large systems such as these usually include demographic data, the results of diagnostic studies including imaging studies, endoscopies, and tests of cardiovascular function, as well as records of diagnoses and medical treatments provided at the specific institution. Common to large systems also are items such as electronic display of medical records, record retrieval for purposes of research, patient appointment scheduling, and management statistics on hospital administrative functions.

The implications of a readily accessible data base involving large numbers of patients is immediate. Descriptive data on methods of clinical practice are far more accessible than ever before. One would expect from this a surge both in maintenance medical care as well as in clinical research.

The Indiana group, for example, has done significant research over the past several years in using their information system to construct a series of "physician reminders" that have added significantly to the provision of medical care [4]. Their hospital computer nightly scans the patient appointments list for the next day's ambulatory medical clinic. It combs the data base on each patient with regard to over 1400 statements of medical care "rules." These "rules" include recommendations for preventive care, such as immunization, testing for cervical cancer, completion of diagnostic work-ups and management, or initial follow up therapy. It then provides the patient's physician with a list of "reminders" such as the patient's need for a current immunization or diagnostic screening tests. Clinical trials of this method demonstrated that patients were more likely to receive preventive care procedures when their physicians were "reminded" in this way [5,6].

This type of data surveillance should serve to greatly increase the quality of medical care available to psychiatric patients. Many studies have demonstrated the high incidence of physical illness among psychiatric patients [7]. Properly designed and applied computer technology can serve to identify patients in need of preventive medical care as well as to surveil the ongoing medical diagnosis and therapy of patients already receiving care. To our knowledge, no such system is in effect for large numbers of psychiatric patients.

Another area of computer application has been that of the automated questionnaire. This does not refer to the program of open-ended questions constructed at the Massachusetts Institute of Technology in which a computer seemed to be conducting psychotherapy. We refer more to those specific questionnaires involving subjective, historical, and present symptoms which patients may "fill out" either by talking with a professional operating a computer terminal or by interacting with the terminal itself. Such questionnaires have been in use for many years. Analogous to these questionnaires are the automated mental status examination programs which are filled out by a professional administering the instrument.

The use of these automated devices has proved to be limited by the complex factors that go into any clinical examination. For example, specific terms such as mood or affect, often carry different connotations in different areas of the world [8]. Similarly, the meaning of terms commonly found in the mental status examination may vary among practitioners depending on their therapeutic orientation and extent of training or experience in clinical practice. Another compounding variable is the patient's ability to cooperate with an automated questionnaire. No matter how sophisticated the questionnaire or mental status examination program may be, a patient who is seriously ill may not have the capacity to perform the tasks of the automated interview.

Several studies have nonetheless demonstrated the usefulness of the automated interview, not because the machine can replace the man, but because the necessary rigor of the machine language insists on detail. As the large surveillance systems "remind" the physician of the health care "rules," so the automated interview or examination "reminds" the clinician of the "rules" involved in clinical practice. This does not mean that the clinician must give up his years of hard won diagnostic acumen only to laboriously punch in data at a terminal. The "reminders" work best when they are more specific.

For example, on one neurologic intensive care unit, a computer-guided neurologic assessment increased physician-nurse collaboration and sharpened clinical skills [9]. In another setting, computer-assisted interviews in a headache clinic furnished data which led the staff physicians to question their previous symptom assessment methods [10].

A third study found that alcoholic patients were more likely to give an accurate report of the amount of alcohol imbibed to the computer terminal than to the clinician [11]. In a fourth study, computer-assisted protocol provided physician assistants with a standard decision system that was easily audited by their physician supervisors [12]. Studies like these demonstrate the assistance computer technology can provide when properly used as a tool in providing medical care.

DIAGNOSTIC SYSTEMS

The difficulty in replacing man with machine is highlighted by studies of computerized psychiatric diagnostic efforts. These have resulted in widely varying degrees of diagnostic accuracy, from as low as 25% to as high as 85% accuracy depending on the syndrome examined and the method of investigation used [13]. These rates of validity are much less than those seen in other areas of clinical medicine and probably reflect the subtlety of psychiatric symptoms. The studies enjoying the highest rates of validity, comparing automated to clinical diagnosis, are those in which symptoms are most stridently clear, as, for example, in acute schizophrenia.

While the ability of the computer to diagnose psychiatric maladies is far from certain, it can provide invaluable diagnostic help. A diagnostic protocol has been devised on a pain service that assists in sorting psychologic and physical variables among chronic pain patients [14]. Another group of clinicians has designed an interactive program capable of demonstrating subtle memory losses seen in early dementia [15]. Applications such as these are feasible for the office clinician but will require further clinical research to assure our knowledge of their validity and reliability in the clinical setting. Their ultimate use will bring an added dimension to daily practice.

Screening evaluations on the basis of laboratory data have not been studied to nearly the same extent as diagnostic interviews. While psychiatric populations have been demonstrated to have a high yield of positive laboratory studies [16], little further research has been done in this area. The work of our own group [17] as well as of others [18] has demonstrated a potentially useful role for automated laboratory data evaluation in providing screening diagnoses for patients suffering from alcoholism. Other uses of this kind of technology, for example, in patients suffering from polysubstance abuse alone or in combination with other major psychiatric diagnoses, have yet to be examined. Such diagnostic methods, while not providing the validity or reliability of careful clinical diagnosis, are nonetheless able to provide the clinician with a sufficiently high index of suspicion to allow him to direct his efforts toward the areas of highest diagnostic yield.

THERAPEUTIC MONITORING

While diagnosis seems the most apparent application area for the computer and clinical psychiatry, therapeutic protocols probably offer the most applicable use of the computer in psychiatric practice. Once diagnosis is established, target symptoms are identified. Pharmacologic intervention, when indicated, is aimed specifically at the target symptoms. Therapy continues until these symptoms remit or unwanted side effects supervene. Efficacy may be improved with the introduction of other data such as blood levels of therapeutic agents discussed elsewhere in this volume. Target symptoms, drug intervention, and clinical assessment provide the ingredients of simple algorithms which may be easily translated into computer programs. These may then be put in place for large numbers of patients in a given institution. Similarly, algorithms already exist for the assessment of side effects of medications [19]. The technology of careful pharmacologic therapeutic surveillance exists and awaits only application to clinical practice.

CONSULTATION SYSTEMS

As these kinds of applications take place, diagnostic and therapeutic considerations may be analyzed not only within a practice or an institution but among practices and institutions.

As information networks grow, clinicians in turn will have much greater access to the medical information currently reposited in medical libraries throughout the country. With the advent of video discs, capable of as many as 50,000 entries per disc [3], vast quantities of medical information can be made available to the practicing physician within minutes. The American Medical Association and General Telephone and Electronics Corporation have announced plans for an electronic information system of this type [20]. Current library searches of such information take hours if not days.

As large computer information networks promise to improve our access to medical knowledge, small office microprocessors have already begun to improve doctor-to-doctor communication. One psychiatric consultation service, for example, has solved the problem of the illegible consultation report. Through an elegantly simple program, these clinicians have established a format that not only "reminds" the consultant or trainee of standard issues in the consultation but prints out a thorough consultation report as well [21]. Microprocessor systems will probably always have a role in clinical practice because of their ease of use and their ease of adaptation to day-to-day demands.

Greater access to information will lead to a revolution in the clinical practice of psychiatry. The term "standard practice" will take on a more specific meaning as information with regard to the norms of diagnosis and of therapeutic intervention become more widely shared and more widely scrutinized. This will in turn raise larger social issues, some of which have already begun to appear. The most obvious is that of confidentiality between patient and physician. A second issue will involve the legal definition of standard practice. Local standards will decrease in their meaning. More accurate judgements of treatment modality risks and benefits should become apparent as information access widens.

In short, improved information systems will have profound effects on the improvement of the quality of psychiatric care. While this change will be striking, it will nonetheless be limited by the skills and judgment of the practicing psychiatrist. The kind of information that goes into any automated data system is dependent upon the person who enters it. While information may be moved and analyzed in a myriad of ways, the worth of that information is solely dependent upon the physicians who provided it.

DECISION SYSTEMS

The newest and probably most jarring innovation on the horizon of computer application is that of artificial intelligence. This application uses the computer less as a purveyor of information and more as an integrator of information supplied to it. Based on that information the computer provides a specific action or states a specific plan. A simple-minded example is the home computer programmed to turn on the lights in a house when signaled to do so by a photoelectric cell. This signal process is made many more times complex in an artificial intelligence application such as that currently being developed at the University of Pittsburgh. The decision course, given a stated problem or set of observations, is programmed into the computer along with a prioritized series of responses. Contingent observations, decisions, and responses are likewise programmed into the computer. On the basis of these, the computer begins to plan not only diagnosis but therapeutic intervention as well.

This type of research is very early in its development, but several observers have predicted that it will make a major impact within the next ten years not only on medical practice but in other fields as well. Commercial interests see the promise of this area of technology as sufficiently strong to warrant large investments of economic resources [22].

CONCLUSION

This very brief survey of possible computer applications in psychiatric practice may call up the last fear of our technologic times: will the physician be supplanted by the machine? The likelihood of this is slim. Patients prefer to be treated by human beings rather than machines because of intangible attributes like hope and compassion. These have been responsible for the creation of medicine as a profession down through the ages. Automated data processing and even artificial intelligence will serve as physician-extenders rather than physician-replacers. Our task, like that of Sir William Harvey, is to understand the uses of our science and the technology of our day. With that understanding, we may one day give our children the kind of gift that Harvey's understanding has given us. Without the knowledge that comes of inquiry we will give them only the knowledge of the past.

"Physicians do not trust computers," writes R. D. Couch [1]. This distrust is largely based on misunderstanding or on experiences no longer relevant. Computer diagnosis, as a discipline, offers more for the physician to exploit than any other facet of automation. Fewer mistakes in planning and execution have occurred in computer diagnosis than in other machine applications. The physician stands to gain more, and lose less, in this discipline than in any other.

"The future of the computer in diagnosis is probably already set. There is much more to learn and discover. The physician's partnership with the computer will undoubtedly strengthen. That it may do so in a way that will benefit the important person in this system, the patient, is entirely up to us" [1].

REFERENCES

1. Couch RD: Computer diagnosis—review and comment. Pathol Annual 11: 141-151, 1976
2. Bacon Sir Francis: The New Atlantis
3. McDonald CJ: Computer technology and continuing medical education: A scenario for the future. Continuing Medical Education Newsletter of the American Medical Association 11:2-9, Sept 1982
4. McDonald CJ: Action Oriented Discussion in Ambulatory Medicine, Chicago, Yearbook Medical Publishers, 1981
5. McDonald CJ: Computer reminders, the quality of care and the nonperfectability of man. N Engl J Med 295:1351-1355, 1976
6. McDonald CJ, Wilson GA, McCabe GP: Physician response to computer reminders. JAMA 244:1579-1581, 1980
7. Hall RCW, Beresford TP, Gardner E, et al: The medical care of psychiatric patients. Hosp Community Psych 33:25-34, 1982
8. Overall JE, Woodward JA: Conceptual validity of a phenomenological classification of psychiatric patients. J Psych Res 12:215-230, 1975
9. Ropper AH, Griswold K, McKenna D, et al: Computer-guided neurologic assessment in the neurologic intensive care unit. Heart Lung 10:54-60, 1981
10. Bana DS, Leviton A, Slack WV, et al: Use of a computerized data base in a headache clinic. Headache 21:72-74, 1981
11. Lucas RW, Mullin PJ, Luna CBX, et al: Psychiatrists and a computer as interrogators of patients with alcohol-related illnesses: A comparison. Br J Psych 131:160-167, 1977
12. Cannon SR, Gardner R: Experience with a computerized interactive protocal system using HELP. Comput Biomed Res 13:399-409, 1980
13. Rogers W, Ryack B, Moeller G: Computer-aided medical diagnosis: Literature review. Int J Biomed Comput 10:267-289, 1979
14. Duncan GH, Gregg JM, Ghia J: The pain profile: A computerized system for assessment of chronic pain. Pain 5:275-284, 1978
15. Perez FI, Hruska N, Stell R, et al: Computerized assessment of memory performance in dementia. Can J Neurol Sci 5:307-312, 1978
16. Hall RCW, Popkin MK, DeVaul R, et al: Physical illness presenting as psychiatric disease. Arch Gen Psych 35:1315-1320, 1978
17. Beresford TP, Low D, Hall RCW, et al: A computerized diagnostic biochemical profile for the detection of alcoholism. Psychosomatics 23:713-720, 1982
18. Ryback RS, Eckardt MJ, Pautler CP: Biochemical and hematological correlates of alcoholism. Res Commun Chem Pathol Pharmacol 27:533-550, 1980
19. Kramer MS, Leventhol JM, Hutchinson MB, et al: An algorithm for the operational assessment of adverse drug reactions. JAMA 247:623-632, 1979
20. AMA Update. American Medical Association, 1983
21. Hale MS, DeLaune W: Microcomputer use on a consultation-liaison service. Psychosomatic 24:1003-1015, 1983
22. Business Week, March 6, 1982

CHAPTER 17

Positron Emission Transaxial Tomography

MONTE S. BUCHSBAUM and HENRY H. HOLCOMB

INTRODUCTION

The dramatic response of psychiatric patients to psychoactive medication and the subtle but pervasive genetic transmission of liability continue to inspire biologic approaches to the puzzles of psychopathology. In schizophrenia, clinical alleviation of symptoms appears related to the effects of neuroleptics on the action of dopamine as chemical messenger [1,2]. Similarly, drugs used to alleviate depression, modulate activity in the norepinephrine, serotonin and dopamine systems [3,4]. From this we might expect that a neurochemical dysfunction is involved in these illnesses and that a neurochemical test could diagnose the illness, predict treatment outcome, and assess longitudinal course. Unfortunately, despite the logical scientific basis of this approach, there has been great difficulty in discovering a reliable chemical indicator for schizophrenia and affective disorders. This difficulty may be due partly to biological heterogeneity of the disorders, i.e., the presence of several or even many biologic deficits responsible for the symptom clusters associated with schizophrenia or affective disorder [5].

No less severe may be the problems inherent in the indirect approach of the clinical neuroscientist to the brain; he relies on peripheral fluids to assess central and regional neurochemical processes. Blood, urine, and cerebrospinal fluid, although valuable reflectors of the neurochemical and neuropharmacologic activity

Handbook of Psychiatric Diagnostic Procedures, vol. 2, edited by R. C. W. Hall and T. P. Beresford. Copyright © 1985 by Spectrum Publications, Inc.

of the brain, are removed in time and place from disordered thought processes and diluted by the products of both functional and dysfunctional brain systems. Biopsy studies, which have aided the study of functional disorders of organs such as the liver, are destructive to the brain and less useful because, unlike these organs, the brain has a complex and varied structure. The experimental insights gained from experiments in animals which examine the pharmacology of individual cell groups in striatum or locus coeruleus, for example, cannot easily or unambiguously be applied in clinical populations. Positron emission topography (PET) is a versatile approach utilizing the mathematics of x-ray transmission scanning (CAT scans) to produce slice images of radioisotope distribution [6]. This opens an unlimited vista of metabolic studies. Positron emitters such as carbon-11 or fluorine-18 can be used to label glucose, amino acids, drugs, neurotransmitter precursors and many other molecules and examine their distribution and fate in discrete cell groups.

BLOOD FLOW, BRAIN WORK AND REGIONAL FUNCTION

The major energy source for the brain is glucose and its use is closely related to local functional activity, oxygen consumption and blood flow [7]. This coupling is not merely a generalized brain effect characterizing states such as coma or excitement, but is a localized mechanism affecting small brain areas. Before the development of PET techniques, cerebral blood flow was, together with the electroencephalogram, the major means of approaching regional brain function in clinical studies. In the earliest efforts, Kety et al [8] studied the cerebral blood flow correlates of schizophrenia with their nitrous oxide technique for the whole brain. No differences between their 22 patients and normal controls were found but they noted that "there remains the possibility that local disturbances confined to small but important regions may still occur since the method used yields only mean values for the entire brain."

Ingvar and Franzen [9] measured cerebral blood flow in 31 patients with schizophrenia and ten neurologically normal male alcoholics. They used the intraarterial xenon injection technique with 32 detectors to evaluate cortical flow. Subjects were tested resting, usually with their eyes closed. Control subjects had relatively higher frontal than posterior blood flow. Patients with schizophrenia had low frontal regions; low frontal flow was especially found in patients with symptoms of indifference, inactivity and autism. Flow increases in postcentral, temporal–occipital, and parietal regions were associated with symptoms of disturbed cognition. Chronic schizophrenics also showed smaller increases in frontal blood flow with simple tasks. In highly disturbed patients, the task of naming objects in pictures produced slight and nonsignificant frontal flow increases [10]. Controls showed large increases although a somewhat more difficult task (Raven's matrices) was used, which might increase blood flow more. However, postcentral flows increased about equally in both groups, tending to support the concept of hypofrontal function in schizophrenia.

The blood flow in the frontal lobes was further explored in studies of "motor ideation" [11]. Regional blood flow maps were obtained at rest, while subjects imagined a slow rhythmic clenching of the right hand, and during actual hand movements. Again, at rest, the subjects had higher flows in frontal than postcentral regions. When they imagined hand movements, flow increases appeared in premotor frontal regions especially in superior frontal, inferior frontal and temporal pole regions.

Subsequent reports on cerebral blood flow using inhalation of xenon-133 in schizophrenia [12] and depression [13] showed decreases in blood flow in the whole right hemisphere in schizophrenia and whole left hemisphere in depression. Higher right frontal than occipital values were found in controls (frontal/occipital ratio 1.05) than in schizophrenics (1.00) but this difference did not reach statistical significance. Ariel et al [14] did confirm statistically significant differences in anteroposterior blood flow between normals and schizophrenics. It is important to note that high individual differences in regional blood flow make within subject regional comparisons such as ratios a critical test of the hypotheses.

POSITRON EMISSION TOMOGRAPHY (PET) METHODS

The method of xenon-133 washout blood flow measurement, like rheoencephalography and electroencephalography, is basically a two-dimensional technique. Flow values in the gray matter of the cortex or underlying white are assessed and plotted on a two-dimensional projection of the cortical surface. PET is a three dimensional technique, developing consecutive slice images and assessing each cubic cm of brain tissue. The historical development of PET scanning technology is well reviewed by Phelps et al [15]. Based on the mathematics of computed tomography images of the distribution of an extensive variety of positron-emitting radiopharmaceuticals can be produced.

What molecules should be imaged in psychiatry? The therapeutic success of neuroleptics suggests examining their binding site distribution. The results of Ingvar [16] suggest the dynamic imaging of blood flow or local metabolism. These two types of PET imaging are only the beginning of the potential approaches to the varied problems in psychiatry and human behavior.

RECEPTOR IMAGING

Neuroleptics have a higher binding affinity for the dopaminergic receptors in the brain than for other receptors. Thus, a positron-emitting labeled drug, such as chlorpromazine, might reveal the location and density of dopamine receptors. The PET scan values could reflect the number of receptors/unit volume, receptor affinity for the labeled compound and the concentrations of natural receptor agonists available. Thus, it is a dynamic experiment reflecting the neurochemical status of the dopamine system at the time of the scan. Unfortunately, other factors would also affect labeling. Neuroleptic ligands bind to receptors other than the dopamine receptor. Multiple dopamine receptors with different affinities complicate the direct interpretation of the quantitative image. Metabolic products of neuroleptics which retained the positron-emitting isotope would appear, although perhaps with a time course slower than the half-life of the isotope (see Comar et al [17]). In addition, these drugs are lipid soluble and enter myelin and fatty material. The resultant image reflects all of these influences on radiolabel distribution.

The first clinical PET study with neuroleptics used ^{11}C-chlorpromazine in 22 schizophrenic patients who had not been treated with neuroleptics for several months before the study [17]. Their images are not entirely dissimilar to those obtained with glucose where gray matter labeled more strongly than white matter. The cerebellum, where dopaminergic receptors are not thought to occur, appeared clearly, indicating relatively high nonspecific binding. Because of these findings, radioligands with more specific binding, two-scan subtraction procedures using displacement or pretreatment with nonradioactive agonists, and other dynamic maneuvers will be necessary to exploit this approach.

BLOOD FLOW

Blood flow can be measured with a number of tracers including krypton-77, oxygen-15 labeled water, ^{13}NH$_3$, and molecules labeled with ^{18}F (see Phelps et al [15]). The short half-life of ^{15}O and ^{13}N$_3$ (2 min and 10 min) make them suitable for behavioral studies where a series of scan studies can be done to compare different psychological tasks within a space of 30 minutes to 2 hours. The studies of Ingvar and co-workers emphasize not only the large changes in blood flow with mental activity, with many brain areas changing flow more than 50% (e.g., Ingvar and Philipson [11]), but also the possibility of schizophrenia/normal differences in these dynamic shifts. The rigorous testing of any of the major psychological theories of schizophrenia, such as a selective attentional deficit, requires at least two scans on a patient, one while the patient is doing the attentional task and a contrasting control. Since most tasks used in schizophrenia research involve motor, perceptual, and cognitive phases, many scan studies comparing isolated components of the task in normal controls will be necessary to characterize the nature of the deficit. One possible disadvantage of the very short-life flow studies with ^{15}O and ^{13}N is that the entire isotope administration and scan process takes place in less than 10 minutes; the psychological task must take place in the scanner room and the subject must do the task, be positioned, and scanned. With some kinetic models, scanning must actually be done during the task (see discussion in Phelps et al [15]), making complete sensory control and stimulus administration difficult. These short-lived isotopes also require an on-site cyclotron for their production.

METABOLIC RATE OF GLUCOSE

PET imaging of glucose metabolic rate rather than blood flow has both advantages and disadvantages for psychiatric studies. The Sokoloff technique [18] uses an ^{18}-Fluorine labeled analogue of glucose, 2-deoxy glucose (FDG).

FDG is taken up by the brain much as glucose itself. But glucose is rapidly metabolized to CO_2 and H_2O. Since CO_2 is a gas, it diffuses rapidly across tissues and prevents us from obtaining high resolution images and precise quantification of metabolic rates. The unusual structure of 2DG allows its metabolism to the first step in the glycolytic pathway (to 2-deoxy-glucose-6-phosphate), but no further. Since metabolism stops at this point, the cells are labeled in proportion to their glucose uptake. After injection, FDG is almost entirely taken up over the next 30-40 minutes, the majority consumed in the first 10. This step can be done in a separate and psychologically controlled environment. The scan, started at 50 minutes, thus reflects glucose use during the initial controlled period after injection, not the scan operation. Thus, psychological tasks, directed interviews about emotional subjects, or even REM sleep could be studied. The need to sustain the activity for 30 minutes limits the time resolution, however, and the habituated response to sensory stimulation could predominate in the glucose use image. Nevertheless, FDG has been the tracer predominantly used in psychiatric studies to date.

INTERPRETING THE GLUCOSE IMAGE

Local cerebral glucose use (CGU) reflects cellular work [19]. The energy for this work comes from the oxidation of glucose to carbon dioxide and water. This process provides for the production of high energy phosphate bonds in adenosine triphosphate (ATP). The action potential of a nerve cell does not require glucose. Instead it is the recovery work to return the cell to an excitable state which requires ATP's energy. Action potentials are propagated by membrane depolarization along the entire cell. Propagation is associated with cellular potassium loss and sodium gain across this membrane. Only by actively pumping these two ions against their respective gradient can the cell regain its transmembrane potential and its excitable state following discharge. The recovery work or ion transport is accomplished by Na^+-K^+-ATPase, which consumes a large share of the ATP generated by glucose oxidation, perhaps 30-50% of neuronal metabolism. It is through this enzyme's action and the concomitant use of ATP that nerve cell firing serves to pace the rate of glucose metabolism. Membrane-bound ATPase uses energy obtained from the hydrolysis of ATP to adenosine diphosphate (ADP) to achieve coupled transport of sodium out and potassium into the cell. The enzyme is apparently stimulated by sodium moving into the cell during depolarization. Products of ATP hydrolysis and associated ion transport, adenosine diphosphate (ADP) and phosphate, subsequently promote increased glucose use by stimulating regulatory enzymes in the glycolytic pathway (phosphofructokinase in particular). Glucose movement or flux through glycolysis and the tricarboxylic acid cycle is modulated by a number of inhibitory and facilitatory intermediates and byproducts; ADP is particularly important in this role.

Initially, glucose is phosphorylated to glucose-6-phosphate, isomerized to fructose-6-phosphate and then a second phosphorylation by phosphofructokinase yields fructose diphosphate. It is at this second phosphorylation step that multiple regulatory factors, including ADP, ATP, phosphocreatine citrate, cyclic AMP, phosphate, and fructose, are importance. Additionally, glucose-6-phosphate is inhibitory to the phosphorylation of glucose. The net result of these interlocking regulatory forces is to reduce glucose flux when cellular ATP is high and to increase flux when ADP and phosphate are high. Generally, this is equivalent to elevated LCGU when neurons are actively engaged in ionic transport and using large amounts of Na^+-K^+-ATPase. Conversely, low firing rates are accompanied by relatively higher levels of ATP and reduced phosphofructokinase activity levels. The work of maintaining the nerve cell ionic gradient occurs over its entire surface. Due to the high surface area/volume ratio characteristic of dendrites, presynaptic terminals are the major contributor to cerebral glucose metabolism. The presynaptic input to a brain area uses glucose regardless of whether the input is inhibitory or stimulatory to the postsynaptic cell. The pathways with cell bodies in the substantia nigra and terminals in the globus pallidus provide an example. Either chemical ablation (with 6-hydroxydopamine [20], or stimulation (electrical) of these nigra cell bodies [21,22]) result in increased glucose use in the globus pallidus. The selective depletion of dopamine in the substantia nigra by 6-hydroxydopamine may increase pallidal glucose use directly or indirectly. Reduced inhibitory input to the pallidus may disinhibit interneurons within the globus pallidus. Indirectly, reduced inhibitory nigral dopaminergic input to the caudate nucleus may enhance its input to the globus pallidus. In contrast, nigral stimulation directly increases presynaptic activity in the globus pallidus.

This example illustrates the importance of considering circuitry in understanding metabolic topography. Different circuits often use different neurotransmitters. A change in glucose use thus reflects total neurotransmitter release (TNR) in the region. When metabolic mapping is combined with chemical measurements of activated areas, demonstrated by autoradiographic and PET studies, neurotransmitter identity and the regional contribution to behavior will be determined.

TOMOGRAPHIC MAPPING OF GLUCOSE USE
AND SENSORY STIMULATION

As was observed in studies of blood flow and psychological tasks, local glucose use is highly sensitive to sensory stimulation. Visual stimulation in one hemifield is associated with increases in glucose use in the contralateral visual cortex [23] and more glucose is used when two eyes are stimulated than when one eye is stimulated [24]. As visual stimulation increased from eyes closed to simple white light, checkerboard pattern reversal, and viewing a park outside the laboratory, visual cortex glucose use, increased twofold [24,25]. Somatosensory and auditory stimulation also increased glucose use in the primary sensory areas [23]. Electrical stimulation of the right forearm was associated with greater left than right glucose use in the region of the postcentral but not precentral gyrus [26]. Whole brain use was little changed by visual stimulation [25]. Thus control of sensory stimulation and mental activity (recall Ingvar's experiments with imagining the hand clenching) is critical to reliable and interpretable results in the psychiatric patient.

GLUCOSE USE IN PATIENTS WITH SCHIZOPHRENIA

The earliest report was by Farkas et al [27] who studied a 45-year-old patient with a history of schizophrenia since the age of 16. This patient had taken no neuroleptic medication before the scan. The patient showed a 40% depression in frontal glucose use in comparison to an unspecified control population. A second scan obtained when the patient was on phenothiazines showed an apparent return toward normal. They also noted a relative left hemisphere diminution in glucose use, especially in temporal and motor cortex.

The hypofrontal pattern of glucose use seen by Farkas et al parallels the blood flow findings of Ingvar and co-workers. This case report of hypofrontality was consistent with a subsequent larger series of patients in a preliminary report [28]. Details of drug dosage, ages, sex distribution and statistical analysis are not available at this writing.

In our recent report [29] local cerebral uptake of ^{18}F labeled 2-fluoro-2-deoxy-D-glucose (2^{18}FDG) use was measured in eight patients with schizophrenia who were off-medication and six age-matched normal volunteers by positron emission tomography. Subjects sat resting in an acoustically treated, darkened room with eyes closed following injection of 3-5 mCi FDG. Following uptake, we obtained 7-8 horizontal brain scans parallel to the canthomeatal line (a line connecting the outer canthus of the eye with the external auditory meatus). Scans were treated digitally, with a 2 cm strip peeled off each slice and ratios to whole slice activity computed. Patients with schizophrenia showed lower ratios in frontal cortex, indicating relatively lower glucose use than normal controls; this was consistent with previously reported studies of regional cerebral blood flow. No clear evidence of left-right difference was found in the cortex. Patients also showed diminished ratios for a 2 cm square positioned over central gray matter areas on the left, but not right side (a region including the anterior thalamus, caudate, globus pallidus, internal capsule, and part of the ventricles).

In this initial exploration of glucose metabolism, we chose the resting eyes closed condition for direct comparison with blood flow data [9,16]. These authors found lower frontal blood flow in schizophrenic patients, and did not compare both hemispheres. Thus, the absence of cortical asymmetries, especially in normals, is not altogether unexpected with this condition. Subjects were merely instructed to rest with their eyes closed for 30 minutes, an entirely unstructured task with no clear hemispheric assignment.

In our second series of patients, we chose somatosensory stimulation of the right forearm as the condition. This was done because Ingvar [16] noted that frontal blood flow increased in subjects who inserted their hands in a bucket of ice water and observed a smaller increase in schizophrenics. This was consistent with the observations by ourselves and others (see Davis et al [30]; also Davis and Buchsbaum [31]) of diminished pain sensitivity in schizophrenia (see Buchsbaum et al [32]; also Davis et al [33]). Animal studies of bradykinin perfusion of the right lower extremity of cats also showed increases of left frontal but not occipital cerebral blood flow [34]. We anticipated that in addition to a possibly enhanced hypofrontality in schizophrenia, we might observe some lateralized indication of the affective response to pain.

In this second series we studied 16 patients with schizophrenia and 11 patients with affective disorder as a control comparison (Figures 1-3). Patients were off all medication a minimum of 14 days and an average of 39.8 days. The subjects were administered the FDG just before receiving a 34 minute 1/sec series of unpleasant electrical stimuli to their right forearm while resting with their eyes closed in a darkened, acoustically attenuated psychophysiologic testing chamber. Following monitored stimulation in the controlled environment, subjects were scanned and images converted to values of glucose use in $\mu m/100$ g/min according to Sokoloff's model. Data were analyzed with a 4-way ANOVA with independent groups (normals, schizophrenics, and affectives) and repeated measures for slice level (supra-, mid-, and infraventricular), hemisphere (right, left), and anteroposterior position (4 sectors). Normals and patients both showed a significant anteroposterior gradient in glucose use with highest values in the frontmost sector. Patients with both schizophrenia and affective illness showed less of an anteroposterior gradient, especially at superior levels, which was statistically confirmed by ANOVA. Absolute glucose levels in patients, which were actually higher in posterior regions rather than lower in frontal regions, were the largest contributors to the effect. No significant correlation was observed between A/P ratios and length of time off neuroleptics, body weight, or sex. PET studies in the well-known Genain quadruplets [35]

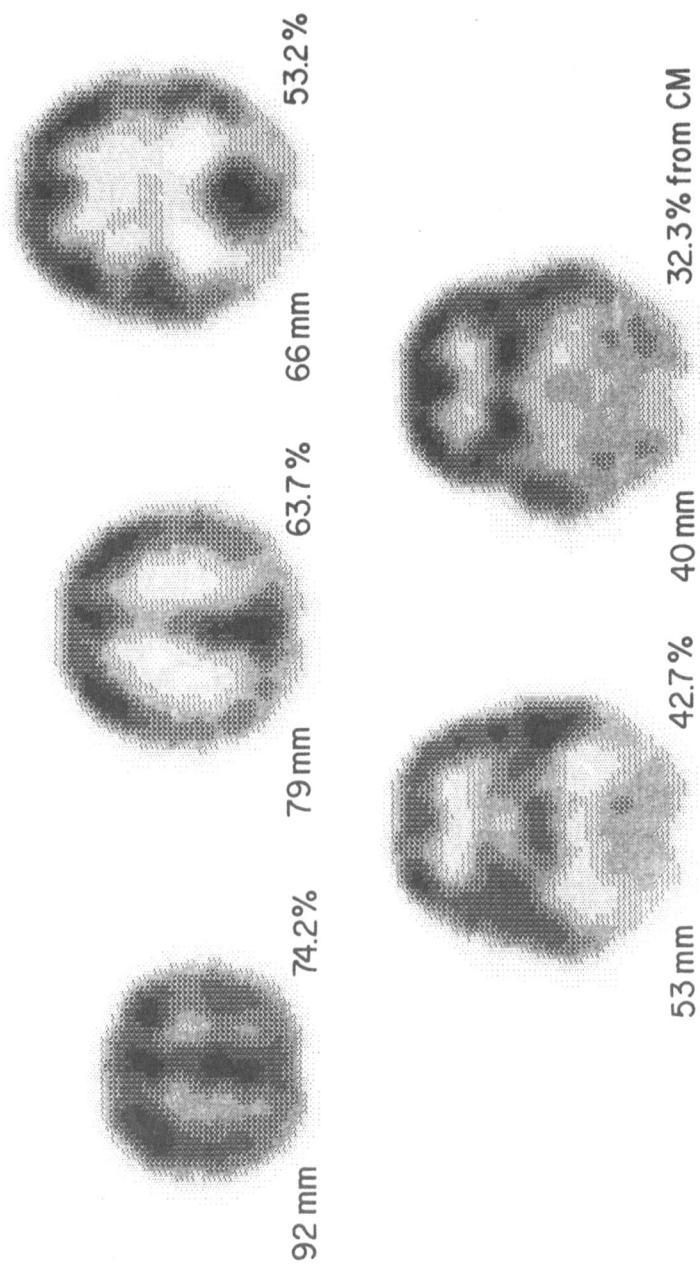

Figure 1. Typical PET scans for one normal individual displayed as 9-level dot density gray scale. Slice heights given as mm above the line joining the canthus of the eye and the external auditory meatus (CM line) and as percentage of CM-top head distance. Note pattern of greater frontal than posterior glucose use extends from 92 to 40 mm.

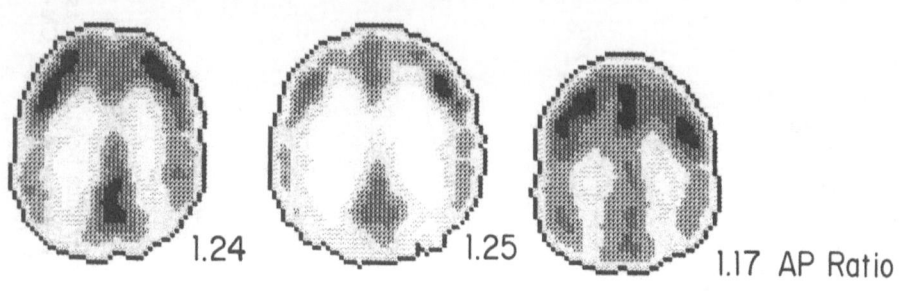

Schizophrenia

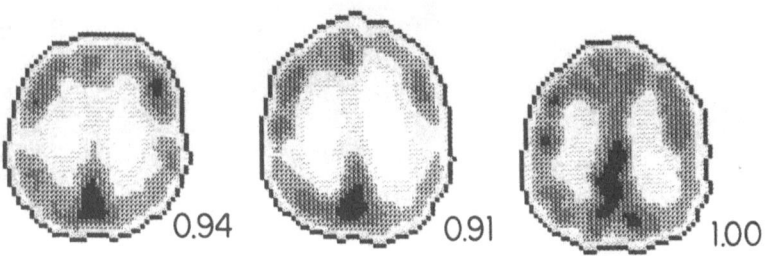

Affective Disorder

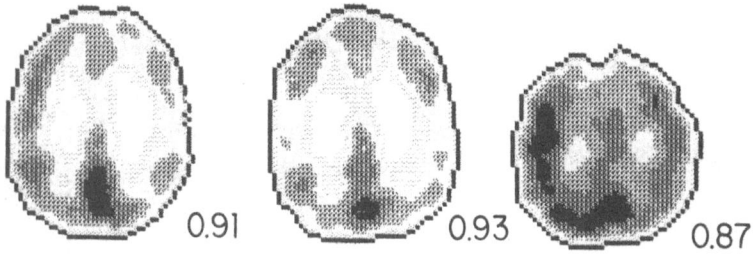

Figure 2. PET images in horizontal plane (parallel to and about 8 cm above the canthomeatal line) at supraventricular level. Three scans typical of normal controls, patients with affective disorder and patients with schizophrenia are shown. A ratio of anterior to posterior cortex glucose use was calculated as in Buchsbaum et al [29] and is shown to the lower right of each slice.

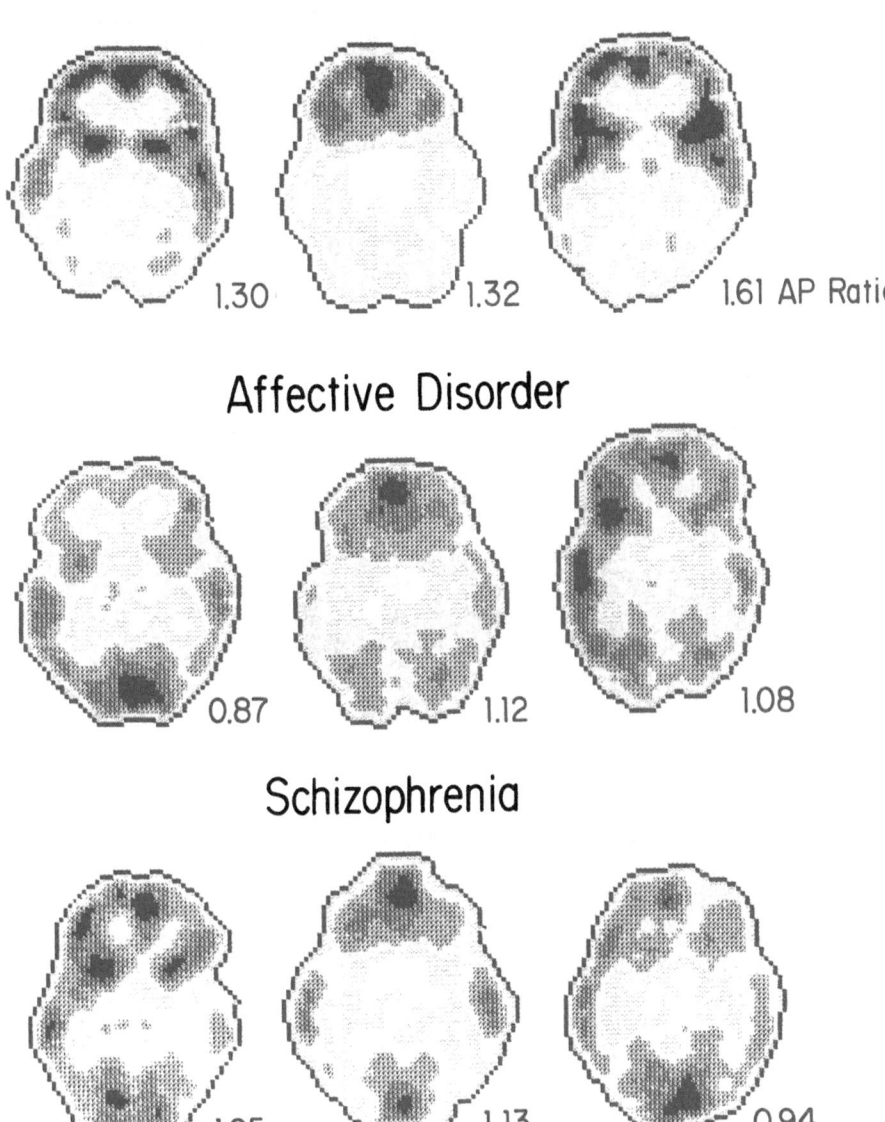

Figure 3. PET images at intraventricular level, as shown in Figure 2.

produced rather similar relative hypofrontality (Figure 4). Neither group differences in whole brain glucose use nor left-right asymmetries reached statistical significance. These results are consistent with our earlier reports of a relative hypofrontal function in schizophrenia compared with controls, with the blood flow studies of Ingvar and coworkers [9] and Arie et al [14] as well as with the original Kety et al [8] finding of no total brain metabolic differences.

Artifacts of the effects of drugs on PET scans are another increasingly important question as patients who have never been treated with a neuroleptic are increasingly difficult to find. Neuroleptics seem to decrease glucose use throughout the brain in autoradiographic studies of rats [36]. Blood flow stuaies in patients also seem to indicate neuroleptics lowering blood flow [37], perhaps in frontal regions especially, but specific statistical confirmation of this regional effect is lacking. However, it should be noted that the first patient of Farkas et al [27] had never been treated with neuroleptics and showed similar results to ours [29] who are off medication an average of 37.6 days.

Patients with schizophrenia and affective illness did not differ in anteroposterior ratios. The possibility of missing a true group difference was increased by the relatively small sample size, diagnostic heterogeneity within the affective disorder sample, mood heterogeneity, and the limited number of brain areas so far assessed. This lack of diagnostic specificity may well indicate that relative hypofrontality is a general feature of illness and/or hospitalization, familiarity with hospital procedures, differential anxiety in patients and controls, or other factors. However, other more extensively studied biological markers, including smooth pursuit eye movements, platelet monoamine oxidase, and attentional deficits also show affective/schizophrenia overlap. All of these biologic markers may well indicate some important commonality between these two functional psychoses.

BRAIN IMAGING AND THE FUTURE OF PSYCHIATRY

Two new imaging techniques have appeared which complement and extend positron emission tomography: nuclear magnetic resonance and electroencephalographic topography. Neither use radioactivity so they are well suited to combine with PET studies.

NMR Imaging

Nuclear magnetic resonance (NMR) imaging is based on reception of radiofrequencies emitted by nuclei of different elements in the brain following application of a magnetic field [6,38]. Using principles similar to x-ray CT scan reconstruction, a slice image can be obtained. The first clinical use has been to image the hydrogen nucleus; mostly in H_2O, it provides a water distribution picture. Since

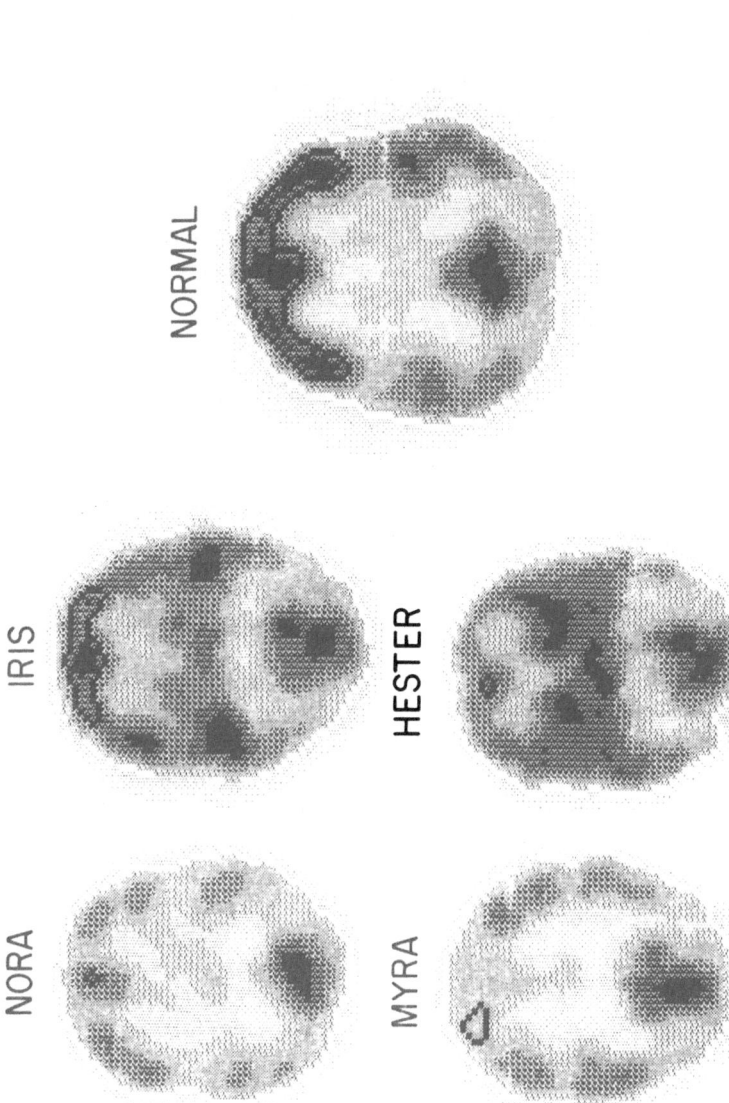

Figure 4. PET scans of four 51-year-old monozygotic quadruplets concordant for schizophrenia and one normal control, all resting with their eyes closed. Gray scale indicates glucose use with darker areas being higher use. Each slice is scaled to its own range of glucose values. Next, the topographic contour is positioned at 75% of the highest mean level observed in an approximately 1-sq cm block of cortex. The quadruplets have a "hypofrontal" pattern with relatively lesser frontal than occipital glucose use in contrast with "hyperfrontal" pattern seen in normal subject (see Buchsbaum et al [29]). Note also that contour forms a complete mushroom-shaped cap around frontal lobes in the normal—a pattern not seen in the quadruplets.

gray and white matter differ significantly in water content, gray matter structures may be more easily separated than with CT scanning which images x-ray transmission (little difference between gray and white). No psychiatric studies have been done, but measurements of the size and shape of the basal ganglia and limbic structures are obvious targets of interest for studies in schizophrenia and affective illness.

NMR will make possible a detailed anatomic horizontal image to match the functional PET images. It must be noted that FDG does not provide an anatomic image, only a functional one. This can lead to ambiguous interpretataions; a hot spot in the region of the basal ganglia could be caudate in one group and putamen in another. NMR can provide a detailed gray/white atlas for each subject for transfer to metabolic images.

The NMR technique has a potential for going beyond anatomic studies and measuring other nuclei, such as ^{31}P cell energy metabolism and NMR, sensitive labeled pharmaceuticals. But the low concentrations of these nuclei make the production of high resolution slice images currently unattainable.

Electroencephalographic Imaging

Brain wave recording has been used for years to detect tumors, epilepsy, and other brain diseases, as well as to study psychological functioning. EEG patterns are exquisitely sensitive to drug effects and can be used to predict action or dosage of new drugs. EEG can also be an imaging technique when signals from electrodes placed all over the scalp are collected and analyzed by spectral analysis to yield amplitude measures for each of the major EEG frequency patterns—delta, alpha, and beta. A map of the electrical activity on the surface of the brain can be constructed by interpolating values between each observed point [39]. In initial studies, this method has shown frontal increases in delta activity [40,41] (Figure 5) in schizophrenics which may match the relative hypofrontality seen with blood flow and PET.

Using briefly presented words or tones and a computer technique known as averaging, an "evoked potential"—the specific brain response to the stimulus—can be recorded. Evoked potentials from scalp EEG leads spaced 1 cm apart can reveal the sensory stations on the cortex of parts of the body as close together as wrist and finger. The possibilities for exploring the entire cortex of the brain with mapping techniques and better defining neurophysiological and pharmacological effects are great. Preliminary data reveal decreases in EP amplitude, especially in parietal areas. With leads attached to a flexible helmet and rapid computer sampling, arrays of 64 to 128 leads can be handled as a clinical procedure.

This entirely hazard-free technology will be significantly enhanced by combination with PET and NMR imaging to provide a strengthened functional basis for interpretation.

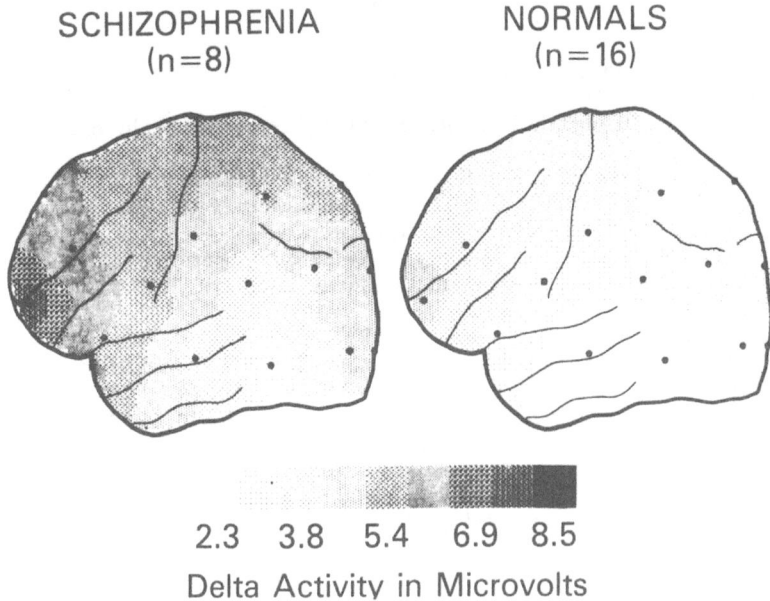

SCHIZOPHRENIA   NORMALS
    (n=8)   (n=16)

2.3   3.8   5.4   6.9   8.5
Delta Activity in Microvolts

Figure 5. Delta activity in 16 normals and eight off-medication schizophrenics. Note frontal distribution in patients with schizophrenia, consistent with their diminished glucose use as assessed by PET scan. Differences were statistically confirmed by ANOVA.

CONCLUSION

A review of PET studies in psychiatry may be criticized as premature today. As of this writing, only a single article on psychiatric patients has appeared as a regular article in a scientific journal [29]. It is the promise of the technique for investigation of specific brain structures in the future which makes it noteworthy at this time. In combination with new clinical anatomical imaging techniques such as electroencephalographic topography, nuclear magnetic resonance [6], and insights from animal data obtained with autoradiography, a level of scientific approach previously unattainable will be realized.

ACKNOWLEDGMENT

The authors wish to thank Ms. Erin Hazlett for her assistance with illustrations and manuscript preparation.

342   BUCHSBAUM AND HOLCOMB

REFERENCES

1. Meltzer HY, Stahl SM: The dopamine hypothesis of schizophrenia: A review. Schizophr Bull 2:19–76, 1976
2. Meltzer HY: Biochemical studies in schizophrenia. Schizophr Bull 2:10–18, 1976
3. Randrup A, Munkvad I, Fog R, et al: Mania, depression, and brain dopamine. In WB Essman, L Valzelli (eds): Current Development in Psychopharmacology Vol II. New York, Spectrum Publications, Inc., 1975
4. Charney DS, Menkes DB, Heninger GR: Receptor sensitivity and the mechanism of action of antidepressant treatment. Arch Gen Psychiatry 38:1160–1180, 1981
5. Buchsbaum MS, Haier RJ: Biological homogeneity, symptom heterogeneity, and the diagnosis of schizophrenia. Schizophr Bull 4:473–475, 1978
6. Brownell GL, Budinger TF, Lauterbur PC, et al: Positron tomography and nuclear magnetic resonance imaging. Science 215:619–626, 1982
7. Sokoloff L: Relationships among local functional activity, energy metabolism, and blood flow in the central nervous system. Fed Proc 40:2311–2316, 1981
8. Kety SS, Woodford RB, Harmel MH, et al: Cerebral blood flow and metabolism in schizophrenia. Am J Psych 104:765–770, 1948
9. Ingvar DH, Franzen G: Distribution of cerebral activity in chronic schizophrenia. Lancet 2:1484–1486, 1974
10. Franzen G, Ingvar DH: Absence of activation in frontal structures during psychological testing of chronic schizophrenics. J Neurol Neurosurg Psych 38:1027–1032, 1975
11. Ingvar DH, Philipson L: Distribution of cerebral blood flow in the dominant hemisphere during motor ideation and motor performance. Ann Neurol 2:230–237, 1977
12. Mathew R, Meyer JS, Frances DJ, et al: Regional cerebral blood flow in schizophrenia: A preliminary report. Am J Psych 138:112–113, 1981
13. Mathew RJ, Meyer JS, Francis DJ, et al: Cerebral blood flow in depression. Am J Psych 137:1449–1450, 1980
14. Ariel RN, Golden CJ, Berg RA, et al: Regional cerebral blood flow in schizophrenics. Arch Gen Psych 40:258–263, 1983
15. Phelps ME, Mazziotta JC, Huang SC: Study of cerebral function with positron computed tomography. J Cerebral Blood Flow and Metabolism 2:113–162, 1982
16. Ingvar DH: Abnormal distribution of cerebral activity in chronic schizophrenia; A neurophysiological interpretation. In CF Baxter, T Melnechuck (eds): Perspectives in Schizophrenia Research. New York, Raven Press, 107–125, 1980
17. Comar D, Zarifian E, Verhas M, et al: Brain distribution and kinetics of ^{11}C-chloropromazine in schizophrenics. Psych Res 1:23–29, 1979
18. Sokoloff L: The radioactive deoxyglucose method. In BW Agranoff, MH Aprison (eds): Advances in Neurochemistry 4:1–81. Plenum Publishing Corp, 1982
19. Siesjo BK: In Wiley (ed): Brain Energy Metabolism. New York, Interscience Publication, 1978
20. Wooten GF, Collins RC: Metabolic effects of unilateral lesion of the substantia nigra. J Neurosci 13:285–291, 1981
21. Pert A, Eurist HD, Holcomb HH, et al: Metabolic mapping of nigral connections with the 2-[^{14}C] deoxyglucose method. Neurosci Abstracts, 1982 (In Press)

22. Savaki NE, Desban M, Glowinski J, et al: Local cerebral glucose consumption in the rat Part II: Effects of unilateral substantia nigra stimulation in conscious and in halothane-anesthetized animals. Neurosci Abstracts, 1982 (In Press)

23. Greenberg JH, Reivich M, Alavi A, et al: Metabolic mapping of functional activity in human subjects with the [18F] fluoro-deoxyglucose technique. Science 212:678-680, 1981

24. Phelps ME, Kuhl DE, Mazziotta JC: Metabolic mapping of the brain's response to visual stimulation: Studies in humans. Science 211:1445-1448, 1981

25. Phelps ME, Mazziotta JC, Kuhl DE, et al: Tomographic mapping of human cerebral metabolism: Visual stimulation and deprivation. Neurology 31:517-529, 1981

26. Buchsbaum MS, Holcomb HH, Johnson J, King AC, Kessler R: Cerebral metabolic consequences of electrical stimulation in normal individuals. Human Neurobiology 2:35-38, 1983

27. Farkas T, Reivich M, Alavi A, et al: The application of 18F 2-deoxy-2-fluoro-D-glucose and positron emission tomography in the study of psychiatric conditions. In JV Passonneau, RA Hawkins, WD Lust, FA Welsh (eds): Cerebral Metabolism and Neural Function. Baltimore, Williams and Wilkins, 1980

28. Farkas T, Wolf AP, Jaeger J, et al: Regional cerebral glucose utilization in chronic schizophrenia. III World Congress of Biological Psychiatry. Symposium on Cerebral Circulation and Metabolism Related to Psychopathology. Stockholm, June 28-July 3, 1981

29. Buchsbaum MS, Ingvar DH, Kessler R, et al: Cerebral glucography with positron tomography. Arch Gen Psych 39:251-259, 1982

30. Davis GC, Buchsbaum MS, van Kammen DP, et al: Analgesia to pain stimuli in schizophrenics reversed by naltrexone. Psych Res 1:61-69, 1979

31. Davis GC, Buchsbaum MS: Pain sensitivity and endorphins in functional psychoses. In TA Ban et al (eds): Modern Problems of Pharmacopsychiatry. Basel, Switzerland, S. Karger, 1981

32. Buchsbaum MS, Davis GC, van Kammen DP: Diagnostic classification and the endorphin hypothesis of schizophrenia: Individual differences and Psychopharmacological strategies. In C Baxter, T Meinechuk (eds): Perspectives in Schizophrenia Research, New York, Raven Press, 1980

33. Davis GC, Buchsbaum MS, Bunney WE Jr: Research in endorphins and schizophrenia. Schizophr Bull 5:244-250, 1979

34. Tsubokawa T, Katayama Y, Ueno Y, et al: Evidence for involvement of the frontal cortex in pain-related cerebral events in cats: Increase in local cerebral blood flow by noxious stimuli. Brain Res 217:179-185, 1981

35. Rosenthal D: The Genain Quadruplets, New York, Basic Books, 1963

36. McCulloch J, Savaki HE, Sokoloff L: Distribution of effects of haloperidol on energy metabolism in the brain. Brain Res 243:81-90, 1982

37. Risberg J: Regional cerebral blood flow measurements by 133Xe-inhalation: Methodology and applications in neuropsychology and psychiatry. Brain Lang 9:9-34, 1980

38. James AE Jr, Price RR, Rollo FD, et al: Nuclear magnetic resonance imaging: A promising technique. JAMA 247:1331-1334, 1982

39. Buchsbaum MS, Rigal F, Coppola R, Cappelletti J, King AC, Johnson J: A new system for gray-level surface distribution maps of electrical activity. Electroenceph Clin Neurophysiol 53:237-742, 1982

40. Morihisa JM, et al: Topographic analysis of computer processed electroenceph-

alography in schizophrenia. In E Usdin, I Hanin (eds): Biological Markers in Psychiatry and Neurology. New York, Pergamon Press, 1982

41. Buchsbaum MS, Cappelletti J, Coppola R, et al: New methods to determine the CNS effects of antigeriatric compounds: EEG topography and glucose use. Drug Dev Res 2:489–496, 1982.

Index

Sensory function, 156
Septic arthritis, 218–219
Severe acquired immune deficiency
   syndrome (AIDS), 221
Sex offenders, 274
Sexual
   acting out, 188
   disorders, assessment, 241–243
   dysfunction, neurologic assessment
      in, 243
   phobias, 238
   response cycle, 238
Sexuality, 23
Shared electrophysiologic activity, 145
Sickle cell disease, 192
Side effects, 323
Sigmoidoscopic examination, 190
Signal averaging equipment, 114
Silastic rods, 254
Silent areas, in EEG, 20
Sjögren's syndrome, 249
Skin temperature, 186
Skull x-rays, 175, 193
Sleep, 52–54
   apnea, 49, 61, 62
   architecture, 54
   deprivation, 36
   deprivation, EEG, 36
   in the diagnosis of sexual disorders,
      67
   diaries, 51
   disorders of excessive sleepiness,
      62–64
   disorders of initiating and maintain-
      ing sleep, 59–61
   drunkenness, 66
   EEG, 76
   EEG variables, definition, 79
   evaluation outside the sleep clinic,
      51–52
   initiation, 54
   maintenance, 54
   paralysis, 63
   parasomnias, 65
   quantity, 54
   recording, EEG, 32, 37

[Sleep]
   research, 2
   spindles, 63
   stages and their characteristics, 55–
      56
   states, 55
   talking, 66
   walking, 52, 65
Sleep-deprived EEGs, 37
Sleep induced
   autonomic behavior, 37
   behavior, 49
   penile tumescence, 66
Slow-wave sleep, 55
Snoring, 52
Sodium, 189
Somatosensory-evoked potential, 97
Somnambulism, 65
Somnolence, 2
Space occupying lesions, 125, 161
Spatial shifts, 155
Specificity, 172, 178
Spectral coherence analysis, 145
Spectral density, 138
Spectral window, 146, 148
Speech pause time, 88
Sphenoidal electrodes, in EEG, 36
Spike discharges, 5
Spike-wave complexes, 22
Spinal cord, 97
   lesions, 241
Spindles, 60
Spongiform leukencophalopathy, 219
Standard practice, 324
Starvation, 181, 183
State of consciousness, 176
Statistical modeling, EEG, 142
Status epilepticus, 174, 217
Steroid administration, 161
Steroid medication, 248
Stimulants, 60
Stool fat, 192
Stroke, 128
Structural brain disease, 153, 166
Subacute bacterial endocarditis, 192,
   194